ELSEVIER

1600 John F. Kennedy Boulevard • Suite 1800 • Philadelphia, Pennsylvania, 19103-2899

http://www.theclinics.com

RADIOLOGIC CLINICS OF NORTH AMERICA Volume 57, Number 5
September 2019 ISSN 0033-8389, ISBN 13: 978-0-323-68248-0

Editor: John Vassallo (j.vassallo@elsevier.com)
Developmental Editor: Donald Mumford

Radiologic Clinics of North America (ISSN 0033-8389) is published bimonthly by Elsevier Inc., 360 Park Avenue South, New York, NY 10010-1710. Months of issue are January, March, May, July, September, and November. Periodicals postage paid at New York, NY and additional mailing offices. Subscription prices are USD 508 per year for US individuals, USD 933 per year for US institutions, USD 100 per year for US students and residents, USD 594 per year for Canadian individuals, USD 1193 per year for Canadian institutions, USD 683 per year for international individuals, USD 1193 per year for international institutions, and USD 315 per year for Canadian and international students/residents. To receive student and resident rate, orders must be accompanied by name of affiliated institution, date of term and the signature of program/residency coordinatior on institution letterhead. Orders will be billed at individual rate until proof of status is received. Foreign air speed delivery is included in all *Clinics* subscription prices. All prices are subject to change without notice. **POSTMASTER:** Send address changes to *Radiologic Clinics of North America*, Elsevier Health Sciences Division, Subscription Customer Service, 3251 Riverport Lane, Maryland Heights, MO63043. **Customer Service: Telephone: 1-800-654-2452** (U.S. and Canada); **1-314-447-8871** (outside U.S. and Canada). **Fax: 1-314-447-8029. E-mail: journalscustomerservice-usa@ elsevier.com (for print support); journalsonlinesupport-usa@elsevier.com (for online support)**.

Reprints. For copies of 100 or more of articles in this publication, please contact the Commercial Reprints Department, Elsevier Inc., 360 Park Avenue South, New York, New York 10010-1710. Tel.: +1-212-633-3874; Fax: +1-212-633-3820; E-mail: reprints@elsevier.com.

Radiologic Clinics of North America also published in Greek Paschalidis Medical Publications, Athens, Greece.

Radiologic Clinics of North America is covered in *MEDLINE/PubMed (Index Medicus)*, *EMBASE/Excerpta Medica, Current Contents/Life Sciences, Current Contents/Clinical Medicine, RSNA Index to Imaging Literature, BIOSIS, Science Citation Index,* and *ISI/BIOMED*.

Printed in the United States of America.

Contributors

CONSULTING EDITOR

FRANK H. MILLER, MD, FACR
Lee F. Rogers MD Professor of Medical
Education, Chief, Body Imaging Section and
Fellowship Program, Medical Director, MRI,
Department of Radiology, Northwestern
Memorial Hospital, Northwestern University
Feinberg School of Medicine, Chicago, Illinois,
USA

EDITORS

GIUSEPPE GUGLIELMI, MD
Professor, Department of Radiology, University
of Foggia, Foggia, Italy

ALBERTO BAZZOCCHI, MD, PhD
Diagnostic and Interventional Radiology,
IRCCS Istituto Ortopedico Rizzoli, Bologna,
Italy

AUTHORS

DOMENICO ALBANO, MD
Università degli Studi di Palermo, Dipartimento
di Biomedicina, Neuroscienze e Diagnostica
Avanzata, Palermo, Italy

HAILEY ALLEN, MD
Assistant Professor, Department of Radiology
and Imaging Sciences, University of Utah
School of Medicine, Salt Lake City, Utah,
USA

FRANCISCO APARISI, MD, PhD
Department of Radiology, Hospital Nisa Nueve
de Octubre, Valencia, Spain

**MARIA PILAR APARISI GÓMEZ, MBChB,
FRANZCR**
Departments of Radiology and Ultrasound,
National Women's Hospital, Auckland City
Hospital, Greenlane Clinical Center, Auckland
District Health Board, Grafton, Auckland,
New Zealand; Department of Radiology,
Hospital Nisa Nueve de Octubre, Valencia,
Spain

FRANCESCO ARRIGONI, MD
Department of Biotechnological and Applied
Clinical Sciences, University of L'Aquila,
Coppito, L'Aquila (AQ), Italy

LAURA W. BANCROFT, MD, FACR
Department of Radiology, AdventHealth
Orlando, Orlando, Florida, USA

ANTONIO BARILE, MD
Department of Biotechnological and Applied
Clinical Sciences, University of L'Aquila,
Coppito, L'Aquila (AQ), Italy

GIUSEPPE BATTISTA, MD
Department of Experimental, Diagnostic
and Specialty Medicine, University of Bologna,
Sant'Orsola-Malpighi Hospital, Bologna,
Italy

ALBERTO BAZZOCCHI, MD, PhD
Diagnostic and Interventional Radiology,
IRCCS Istituto Ortopedico Rizzoli, Bologna,
Italy

DONNA G. BLANKENBAKER, MD
Professor, Department of Radiology, University of Wisconsin-Madison School of Medicine and Public Health, Madison, Wisconsin, USA

MIKAEL BOESEN, MD, PhD
Professor, Department of Radiology, Parker Institute, Bispebjerg and Frederiksberg Hospital, Copenhagen University, Department of Clinical Medicine, University of Copenhagen, Copenhagen, Denmark

AGNIESZKA BORON, BS
University of Central Florida College of Medicine, Orlando, Florida, USA

MIRIAM A. BREDELLA, MD
Professor of Radiology, Harvard Medical School, Division of Musculoskeletal Imaging and Intervention, Vice Chair, Department of Radiology, Massachusetts General Hospital, Boston, Massachusetts, USA

LUCA BRUNESE, MD
Department Life and Health "V. Tiberio," University of Molise, Campobasso, Italy

FEDERICO BRUNO, MD
Department of Biotechnological and Applied Clinical Sciences, University of L'Aquila, Coppito, L'Aquila (AQ), Italy

VICTOR CASSAR-PULLICINO, LRCP, MRCS, DMRD, FRCR, MD
Department of Radiology, Robert Jones and Agnes Hunt Orthopaedic Hospital NHS Foundation Trust, Oswestry, United Kingdom

CARLO CATALANO, MD
Department of Radiologic, Oncologic and Pathologic Sciences, La Sapienza University of Rome, Rome, Italy

LUIS CEREZAL, PhD
Department of Radiology, Diagnostico Médico Cantabria, Santander, Spain

BRIAN Y. CHAN, MD
Assistant Professor, Department of Radiology and Imaging Sciences, University of Utah School of Medicine, Salt Lake City, Utah, USA

VITO CHIANCA, MD
IRCCS Istituto Ortopedico Galeazzi, Milano, Italy

TECK YEW CHIN, MBChB, MSc, FRCR
Consultant Radiologist, Department of Diagnostic Radiology, Khoo Teck Puat Hospital, Singapore, Republic of Singapore

HONG CHOU, MBBS, FRCR
Consultant Radiologist, Department of Diagnostic Radiology, Khoo Teck Puat Hospital, Singapore, Republic of Singapore

ANDREW CIBULAS, MD, MSME
Department of Radiology, AdventHealth Orlando, Orlando, Florida, USA

GEORGE CIBULAS II, MD, PharmD
Department of Orthopaedic Surgery, University of Michigan, Ann Arbor, Michigan, USA

KIRKLAND W. DAVIS, MD, FACR
Professor, Department of Radiology, University of Wisconsin-Madison School of Medicine and Public Health, Madison, Wisconsin, USA

BERT DEGRIECK, MD
Department of Radiology, Ghent University UZ-Gent, Gent, Belgium

JOHN DENNISON, MD
Department of Radiology, AdventHealth Orlando, Orlando, Florida, USA

ERNESTO DI CESARE, MD
Department of Biotechnological and Applied Clinical Sciences, University of L'Aquila, Coppito, L'Aquila (AQ), Italy

DAVIDE MARIA DONATI, MD
Department of Orthopaedic Oncology, IRCCS Istituto Ortopedico Rizzoli, Department of Biomedical and Neuromotor Sciences, University of Bologna, Bologna, Italy

CESARE FALDINI, MD
1st Orthopaedic and Traumatologic Clinic, IRCCS Istituto Ortopedico Rizzoli, Department of Biomedical and Neuromotor Sciences, University of Bologna, Bologna, Italy

MICHAEL FOSS, BS
Lake Erie College of Osteopathic Medicine – Bradenton, Bradenton, Florida, USA

ANDREA GIOVAGNONI, MD
Department of Radiology, Ospedali Riuniti, Università Politecnica delle Marche, Ancona, Italy

ALI GUERMAZI, MD, PhD
Professor, Department of Radiology, Boston
University School of Medicine, Boston,
Massachusetts, USA

GIUSEPPE GUGLIELMI, MD
Professor, Department of Radiology, University
of Foggia, Foggia, Italy

BRETT GUTTERMAN, MD
Department of Radiology, AdventHealth
Orlando, Orlando, Florida, USA

JON A. JACOBSON, MD
Professor, Department of Radiology,
Division of Musculoskeletal Radiology,
University of Michigan Hospital,
Main Campus, Ann Arbor, Michigan,
USA

VIVEK KALIA, MD, MPH, MS
Assistant Professor, Department of Radiology,
Division of Musculoskeletal Radiology,
University of Michigan Hospital, Main
Campus, Ann Arbor, Michigan,
USA

KIMIA KANI, MD
University of Maryland, Baltimore, Maryland,
USA

ARA KASSARJIAN, MD
Founder, Elite Sports Imaging, SL, Pozuelo de
Alarcón, Madrid, Spain

ARVIN B. KHETERPAL, MD
Division of Musculoskeletal Imaging and
Intervention, Department of Radiology,
Massachusetts General Hospital, Harvard
Medical School, Boston, Massachusetts,
USA

RADHESH LALAM, MBBS, MRCS, FRCR
Department of Radiology, Robert Jones
and Agnes Hunt Orthopaedic Hospital
NHS Foundation Trust, Oswestry, United
Kingdom

ALEXANDER LEYVA, MD
Department of Radiology, AdventHealth
Orlando, Orlando, Florida, USA

EVA LLOPIS, MD
Department of Radiology, Hospital de la
Ribera, Valencia, Spain

MARIO MAAS, MD, PhD
Professor, Department of Radiology, AMC
Hospital, Amsterdam, the Netherlands

NICOLA MAGGIALETTI, MD
Department Life and Health "V. Tiberio,"
University of Molise, Campobasso, Italy

ALESSANDRO MARINELLI, MD
Shoulder and Elbow Surgery, IRCCS Istituto
Ortopedico Rizzoli, Bologna, Italy

CARLO MASCIOCCHI, MD
Department of Biotechnological and Applied
Clinical Sciences, University of L'Aquila,
Coppito, L'Aquila (AQ), Italy

CARMELO MESSINA, MD
IRCCS Istituto Ortopedico Galeazzi,
Dipartimento di Scienze Biomediche per la
Salute, Università degli Studi di Milano, Milano,
Italy

VITTORIO MIELE, MD
Department of Radiology, Careggi University
Hospital, Florence, Italy

ALESSANDRO NAPOLI, MD, PhD
Department of Radiologic, Oncologic and
Pathologic Sciences, La Sapienza University of
Rome, Rome, Italy

RAFFAELE NATELLA, MD
Department of Precision Medicine,
University of Campania "Luigi Vanvitelli,"
Napoli, Italy

MIKKEL ØSTERGAARD, MD, PhD, DMSc
Professor, Department of Clinical Medicine,
University of Copenhagen, Copenhagen,
Denmark; Department of Rheumatology,
Rigshospitalet Glostrup, Copenhagen
University, Glostrup, Denmark

PIERPAOLO PALUMBO, MD
Department of Biotechnological and Applied
Clinical Sciences, University of L'Aquila,
Coppito, L'Aquila (AQ), Italy

**WILFRED C.G. PEH, MBBS, MD, FRCP
(Glasg), FRCP (Edin), FRCR**
Professor, Senior Consultant, Department
of Diagnostic Radiology, Khoo Teck
Puat Hospital, Singapore, Republic of
Singapore

JACK PORRINO, MD
University of Washington Medicine, Seattle, Washington, USA; Yale School of Medicine, New Haven, Connecticut, USA

GRAZIA POZZI, MD
IRCCS Istituto Ortopedico Galeazzi, Milano, Italy

SILVIA PRADELLA, MD
Department of Radiology, Careggi University Hospital, Florence, Italy

ALFONSO REGINELLI, MD
Department of Precision Medicine, University of Campania "Luigi Vanvitelli," Napoli, Italy

RODRIGO RESTREPO, MD
Cedimed, Medellin, Colombia

FRANK W. ROEMER, MD, PhD
Professor, Department of Radiology, Boston University School of Medicine, Boston, Massachusetts, USA; Department of Radiology, Friedrich-Alexander University Erlangen-Nürnberg (FAU) and Universitätsklinikum Erlangen, Erlangen, Germany

ROBERTO ROTINI, MD
Shoulder and Elbow Surgery, IRCCS Istituto Ortopedico Rizzoli, Bologna, Italy

KURT SCHERER, MD
Department of Radiology, AdventHealth Orlando, Orlando, Florida, USA

LUCA MARIA SCONFIENZA, MD, PhD
IRCCS Istituto Ortopedico Galeazzi, Dipartimento di Scienze Biomediche per la Salute, Università degli Studi di Milano, Milano, Italy

PAOLO SPINNATO, MD
Diagnostic and Interventional Radiology, IRCCS Istituto Ortopedico Rizzoli, Bologna, Italy

ALESSANDRA SPLENDIANI, MD
Department of Biotechnological and Applied Clinical Sciences, University of L'Aquila, Coppito, L'Aquila (AQ), Italy

LENE TERSLEV, MD, PhD
Associate Professor, Department of Rheumatology, Rigshospitalet Glostrup, Copenhagen University, Glostrup, Denmark

DANIEL VANEL, MD
Department of Pathology, IRCCS Istituto Ortopedico Rizzoli, Bologna, Italy

KOENRAAD VERSTRAETE, MD
Department of Radiology, Ghent University UZ-Gent, Gent, Belgium

TIMOTHY WOO, MBChB, MA, FRCR
Department of Radiology, Robert Jones and Agnes Hunt Orthopaedic Hospital NHS Foundation Trust, Oswestry, United Kingdom

MARCELLO ZAPPIA, MD
Department Life and Health "V. Tiberio," University of Molise, Campobasso, Italy

Contents

The anatomy of the upper limb is complex and allows for exceptional functionality. The movements of the joints of the shoulder, elbow, and wrist represent a complex dynamic interaction of muscles, ligaments, and bony articulations. A solid understanding and of the characteristics and reciprocal actions of the anatomic elements of the joints of the upper limb helps explain the mechanisms and patterns of injury. This article focuses on the anatomy and functionality of the shoulder, elbow, and wrist, with emphasis on the stabilizing mechanisms, to set the foundation for understanding the occurrence of pathologic conditions.

Acute shoulder injury is commonly encountered by clinicians, surgeons, and radiologists. A comprehensive evaluation of the shoulder by the radiologist is essential to accurately relay findings that have a direct impact on acute and long-term management. In this review, imaging features of acute injuries involving the proximal humerus, glenohumeral joint, rotator cuff, tendon of the long head of the biceps brachii, and acromioclavicular joint are discussed. Modalities include ultrasound examination, conventional radiography, computed tomography scans, and MR imaging. Emphasis is placed on radiographic features that have an impact on patient management.

This article discusses the most common and important overuse injuries of the shoulder with attention to MR imaging and ultrasound findings. Pathologic conditions occurring in athletes and nonathletes are included, with review of relevant anatomy, predisposing factors, and treatment considerations. Specific overuse injuries involving the rotator cuff, long head of the biceps tendon, and subacromial-subdeltoid bursa are reviewed. Impingement syndromes of the shoulder, Little Leaguer's shoulder, and stress-induced distal clavicular osteolysis are also discussed.

The acutely injured elbow can present as a diagnostic challenge, encompassing a spectrum of conditions that involve the various osseous and soft tissue structures of this complex joint. Imaging plays a vital role in the management of these patients by providing an accurate interpretation of the underlying trauma sustained, which can have important implications on the preservation of joint function and stability. This article examines the mechanisms, patterns, classifications, and imaging findings of acute elbow injuries, providing key concepts for the radiologist in the interpretation of these injuries.

Repetitive microtrauma in the elbow from chronic overuse occurs in athletes and nonathletes. Although the diagnosis is often made clinically, imaging is helpful to confirm the diagnosis, grade the injury, and guide treatment. MR imaging is particularly helpful in evaluating overuse injuries in the elbow, as tendons, ligaments, and bones/cartilage can be assessed. Tendinopathy can be distinguished from partial- or full-thickness tears, and reactive changes in the bone marrow can be easily identified. This article focuses on the MR imaging appearance of overuse injuries of the elbow involving tendons, ligaments, and bones.

Wrist traumas are a frequent clinical emergency for which instrumental imaging assessment is required. The purpose of this article is to review the role of imaging assessment of traumatic wrist injuries, with particular reference to fractures and associated lesions.

Overuse is defined as repetitive microtrauma that overwhelms the tissues' ability to adapt. Microtrauma represents damage at molecular level and can be produced by either a tension or shear load. The wrist and hand are vulnerable to upper extremity overuse injuries related to work or sports activities that require repetitive movements, often coupled with weight bearing. These injuries create challenges for orthopedic surgeons and radiologists because of the demands on athletes and employees. A thorough understanding of the mechanism of injury, activities, and magnetic resonance imaging findings is necessary for accurate diagnosis, providing key information to perform adequate therapeutic planning.

Imaging has a paramount role in postsurgical assessment. Radiologists need to be familiar with the different surgical procedures to be able to identify expected postsurgical appearances and also detect potential complications. This article reviews the indications, normal expected postsurgical appearances, and complications of the most frequently used surgical procedures in the shoulder, elbow, and wrist. The emphasis is on points that should not be overlooked in the surgical planning.

Imaging of Common Rheumatic Joint Diseases Affecting the Upper Limbs   1001

Mikael Boesen, Frank W. Roemer, Mikkel Østergaard, Mario Maas, Lene Terslev, and Ali Guermazi

Imaging plays an important role in diagnosis and monitoring of rheumatic diseases of the upper limb. Many rheumatic diseases present with similar clinical pictures, especially in the early stages. Imaging findings in inflammatory and degenerative joint diseases often are nonspecific, especially in the early stages. Imaging findings should be interpreted in light of the clinical context—clinical and paraclinical findings. Good referrals with short clinical history, main clinical findings, disease-involved joint(s), pain distribution, and relevant blood tests increase the likelihood of a correct diagnosis.

Imaging of Upper Limb Tumors and Tumorlike Pathology   1035

Timothy Woo, Radhesh Lalam, Victor Cassar-Pullicino, Bert Degrieck, Koenraad Verstraete, Davide Maria Donati, Giuseppe Guglielmi, Daniel Vanel, and Alberto Bazzocchi

Bone and soft tissue sarcomas are uncommon tumors that can occur within the upper extremity as well as elsewhere within the body. However, certain histopathological subtypes have increased affinity for the upper limb and even certain sites within the arm and hand. Other benign masses and tumor mimics, such as infection and traumatic lesions, are more common and imaging appearances can sometimes overlap with malignant lesions making diagnosis difficult. In this article, we explore the current options for imaging of these lesions as well as typical imaging appearances of the more common upper limb tumors.

MR Imaging of the Upper Limb: Pitfalls, Tricks, and Tips   1051

Federico Bruno, Francesco Arrigoni, Raffaele Natella, Nicola Maggialetti, Silvia Pradella, Marcello Zappia, Alfonso Reginelli, Alessandra Splendiani, Ernesto Di Cesare, Giuseppe Guglielmi, Vittorio Miele, Andrea Giovagnoni, Luca Brunese, Carlo Masciocchi, and Antonio Barile

MR imaging is the modality of choice to evaluate musculoskeletal pathologies of the upper limb in most settings. However, due to the complexity in anatomy, MR imaging can give a false pathologic appearance and lead to several errors in the interpretation of MR imaging findings. Also, several artifacts can be confused with pathologic entities. This article reviews the most frequently encountered conditions in shoulder, elbow, and wrist MR imaging that can represent diagnostic pitfalls mimicking true pathology, together with some possible tips and tricks that can be useful to solve these equivocal cases and achieve a correct diagnosis.

Imaging of Peripheral Nerves of the Upper Extremity   1063

Vivek Kalia and Jon A. Jacobson

Peripheral neuropathy (often defined as weakness of sensory loss in one limb) of the upper extremity is a common clinical musculoskeletal scenario. The most common include carpal tunnel syndrome, cubital tunnel syndrome, and cervical radiculopathy. A combination of clinical examination, electrodiagnostic testing, and imaging studies, chiefly MR imaging and ultrasonography, is often needed to identify a specific diagnosis for an individual patient. In many cases, ultrasonography is preferred because of ease of access, the possibility of quick contralateral extremity imaging for comparison, and lower cost profile. MR imaging is preferred for deeper nerve structures and large-field-of-view evaluation.

Luca Maria Sconfienza, Vito Chianca, Carmelo Messina, Domenico Albano, Grazia Pozzi, and Alberto Bazzocchi

Ultrasound has been reported to be a quick, cheap, and effective imaging modality to guide the interventional procedures in the musculoskeletal system. The use of ultrasound results in increased accuracy of needle placement associated with a reduction of complications. In the upper limb, ultrasound-guided procedures are applied to joints and soft tissues around the shoulder, elbow, wrist, and hand. This article reviews the clinical and technical aspects of the most common procedures performed in this anatomic area.

PROGRAM OBJECTIVE
The objective of the *Radiologic Clinics of North America* is to keep practicing radiologists and radiology residents up to date with current clinical practice in radiology by providing timely articles reviewing the state of the art in patient care.

TARGET AUDIENCE
Practicing radiologists, radiology residents, and other healthcare professionals who provide patient care utilizing radiologic findings.

LEARNING OBJECTIVES
Upon completion of this activity, participants will be able to:
1. Review common US-guided procedures performed in the musculoskeletal system of the upper limb.
2. Discuss imaging techniques used in the diagnosis and monitoring of rheumatic diseases affecting the upper limb.
3. Recognize the role of imaging in the diagnosis of and treatment considerations for shoulder and elbow overuse injuries.

ACCREDITATION
The Elsevier Office of Continuing Medical Education (EOCME) is accredited by the Accreditation Council for Continuing Medical Education (ACCME) to provide continuing medical education for physicians.

The EOCME designates this journal-based CME activity for a maximum of 14 *AMA PRA Category 1 Credit*(s)™. Physicians should claim only the credit commensurate with the extent of their participation in the activity.

All other healthcare professionals requesting continuing education credit for this enduring material will be issued a certificate of participation.

DISCLOSURE OF CONFLICTS OF INTEREST
The EOCME assesses conflict of interest with its instructors, faculty, planners, and other individuals who are in a position to control the content of CME activities. All relevant conflicts of interest that are identified are thoroughly vetted by EOCME for fair balance, scientific objectivity, and patient care recommendations. EOCME is committed to providing its learners with CME activities that promote improvements or quality in healthcare and not a specific proprietary business or a commercial interest.

The planning committee, staff, authors and editors listed below have identified no financial relationships or relationships to products or devices they or their spouse/life partner have with commercial interest related to the content of this CME activity:
Domenico Albano, MD; Hailey Allen, MD; Francisco Aparisi, MD, PhD; Maria Pilar Aparisi Gómez, MBChB, FRANZCR; Francesco Arrigoni, MD; Antonio Barile, MD; Giuseppe Battista, MD; Alberto Bazzocchi, MD, PhD; Agnieszka Boron, BS; Miriam A. Bredella, MD; Luca Brunese, MD; Federico Bruno, MD; Victor Cassar-Pullicino, LRCP, MRCS, DMRD, FRCR, MD; Carlo Catalano, MD; Luis Cerezal, PhD; Brian Y. Chan, MD; Vito Chianca, MD; Teck Yew Chin, MBChB, MSc, FRCR; Hong Chou, MBBS, FRCR; Andrew Cibulas, MD, MSME; George Cibulas II, MD, PharmD; Bert Degrieck, MD; John Dennison, MD; Ernesto Di Cesare, MD; Davide Maria Donati, MD; Cesare Faldini, MD; Michael Foss, BS; Andrea Giovagnoni, MD; Giuseppe Guglielmi, MD; Brett Gutterman, MD; Jon A. Jacobson, MD; Vivek Kalia, MD, MPH, MS; Kimia Kani, MD; Ara Kassarjian, MD; Alison Kemp; Arvin B. Kheterpal, MD; Pradeep Kuttysankaran; Radhesh Lalam, MBBS, MRCS, FRCR; Alexander Leyva, MD; Eva Llopis, MD; Mario Maas, MD, PhD; Nicola Maggialetti, MD; Alessandro Marinelli, MD; Carlo Masciocchi, MD; Carmelo Messina, MD; Vittorio Miele, MD; Frank H. Miller, MD, FACR; Alessandro Napoli, MD, PhD; Raffaele Natella, MD; Pierpaolo Palumbo, MD; Wilfred C.G. Peh, MBBS, MD, FRCP (Glasg), FRCP (Edin), FRCR; Jack Porrino, MD; Grazia Pozzi, MD; Silvia Pradella, MD; Alfonso Reginelli, MD; Rodrigo Restrepo, MD; Roberto Rotini, MD; Kurt Scherer, MD; Luca Maria Sconfienza, MD, PhD; Paolo Spinnato, MD; Alessandra Splendiani, MD; Daniel Vanel, MD; John Vassallo; Koenraad Verstraete, MD; Timothy Woo, MBChB, MA, FRCR; Marcello Zappia, MD.

The planning committee, staff, authors and editors listed below have identified financial relationships or relationships to products or devices they or their spouse/life partner have with commercial interest related to the content of this CME activity:
Laura W. Bancroft, MD, FACR: receives royalties from Thiele Medical Publishers, Inc. and Lippincot and Wolters Kluwer.
Donna G. Blankenbaker, MD: receives royalties from Elsevier.
Mikael Boesen, MD, PhD: owns stock, participates in speakers bureau, and is a consultant/advisor for IAG and participates in speakers bureau and is a consultant/advisor for Eli and Lilly Company, Esaote Spa, Celgene, Pfizer Inc., AbbVie Inc., Canon Medical Systems, Siemens Medical Solutions USA, and AstraZeneca.
Kirkland W. Davis, MD, FACR: receives royalties from Elsevier.
Ali Guermazi, MD, PhD: owns stock in BICL and is a consultant/advisor for Pfizer Inc., Kolon TissueGene, Inc., Merck Sharp & Dohme Corp., a subsidiary of Merck & Co., Inc., EMD Serono, Inc., AstraZeneca, Galapagos NV, and F. Hoffmann-La Roche Ltd.
Mikkel Østergaard, MD, PhD, DMSc: participates in speakers bureau and is a consultant/advisor for Bristol-Myers Squibb Company, Boehringer Ingelheim International GmbH, Eli Lilly and Company, Pfizer Inc, Janssen Pharmaceuticals, Inc., Novo Nordisk A/S, Orion Corporation, Pfizer Inc., Regeneron, F. Hoffmann-La Roche Ltd, and UCB, Inc.; participates in speakers

bureau, is a consultant/advisor for, and receives research support from AbbVie, Inc., Celgene Corporation, Merck Sharp & Dohme Corp., a subsidiary of Merck & Co., Inc, and Novartis AG; receives research support from Johnson & Johnson Services, Inc.

Frank W. Roemer, *MD, PhD*: *owns stock in BICL.*

Lene Terslev, *MD, PhD*: *participates in speakers bureau for F. Hoffmann-La Roche Ltd, Pfizer Inc., Medical Specialties Distributors, Bristol-Myers Squibb Company, Novartis AG, Celgene Corporation, and General Electric Company.*

UNAPPROVED/OFF-LABEL USE DISCLOSURE

The EOCME requires CME faculty to disclose to the participants:

1. When products or procedures being discussed are off-label, unlabelled, experimental, and/or investigational (not US Food and Drug Administration [FDA] approved); and
2. Any limitations on the information presented, such as data that are preliminary or that represent ongoing research, interim analyses, and/or unsupported opinions. Faculty may discuss information about pharmaceutical agents that is outside of FDA-approved labelling. This information is intended solely for CME and is not intended to promote off-label use of these medications. If you have any questions, contact the medical affairs department of the manufacturer for the most recent prescribing information.

TO ENROLL

To enroll in the *Radiologic Clinics of North America* Continuing Medical Education program, call customer service at 1-800-654-2452 or sign up online at http://www.theclinics.com/home/cme. The CME program is available to subscribers for an additional annual fee of USD $327.60.

METHOD OF PARTICIPATION

In order to claim credit, participants must complete the following:

1. Complete enrolment as indicated above.
2. Read the activity.
3. Complete the CME Test and Evaluation. Participants must achieve a score of 70% on the test. All CME Tests and Evaluations must be completed online.

CME INQUIRIES/SPECIAL NEEDS

For all CME inquiries or special needs, please contact elsevierCME@elsevier.com.

RADIOLOGIC CLINICS OF NORTH AMERICA

RELATED SERIES

Magnetic Resonance Imaging Clinics
Neuroimaging Clinics
PET Clinics

Preface
Imaging of the Upper Limb

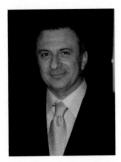 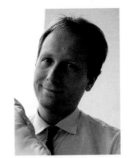

Giuseppe Guglielmi, MD   Alberto Bazzocchi, MD, PhD
Editors

Whether working in a private or a public setting, whether in an emergency department or a specialized orthopedic hospital, not a single day will go by without admitting a patient complaining of pain or other symptoms of the upper limb. Imaging examination comes right thereafter, and radiologists should be confident with the clinical background too.

The relationship between Radiology, Orthopedics, Physiatry, and other musculoskeletal-related health care professions should be close and open, and radiologists should be familiar with the conservative and surgical options of treatment. Clearly, radiologists are fully involved in the management of patients and are responsible for finding the cause and the solution of upper-limb disorders.

The aim of this issue of *Radiologic Clinics of North America* is to provide the reader with a comprehensive and up-to-date imaging interpretation of disorders and hot topics related to the upper limb. This issue includes 13 review articles covering different aspects of imaging of the upper limb, with the invaluable contribution of several internationally acclaimed and credited authors.

The upper limb is constantly stressed by daily activities, from domestic tasks to work and sports. It is directly or indirectly involved when traumas happen. It comprises different joints with completely different anatomy, therefore with significant differences in functions at different levels but still in a complex interaction. That is why it is so important to approach imaging diagnosis after reviewing the anatomy from a functional and surgical point of view. Several articles cover the different aspects of traumatic injuries and overuse pathology, joint by joint. The correct approach to evaluation of the postsurgical patient is discussed in 1 article. What is that lump? The incidence and features of specific rheumatic diseases and tumors, including the difficulties in differential diagnosis, are discussed in 2 different articles. Two special focus articles address tricks in MR imaging, and peripheral nerve imaging of the upper limb, respectively. At the end of the issue, a review of several interventional imaging-guided procedures on the upper limb is also included.

Giuseppe Guglielmi, MD
Department of Radiology
University of Foggia
Viale Luigi Pinto 1
71100 Foggia, Italy

Alberto Bazzocchi, MD, PhD
Diagnostic and Interventional Radiology
IRCCS Istituto Ortopedico Rizzoli
Via G. C. Pupilli 1
40136 Bologna, Italy

E-mail addresses:
giuseppe.guglielmi@unifg.it (G. Guglielmi)
abazzo@inwind.it (A. Bazzocchi)

Radiol Clin N Am 57 (2019) xv
https://doi.org/10.1016/j.rcl.2019.06.001
0033-8389/19/© 2019 Published by Elsevier Inc.

Functional and Surgical Anatomy of the Upper Limb
What the Radiologist Needs to Know

Maria Pilar Aparisi Gómez, MBChB, FRANZCR[a,b,*],
Francisco Aparisi, MD, PhD[b], Giuseppe Battista, MD[c],
Giuseppe Guglielmi, MD[d], Cesare Faldini, MD[e,f],
Alberto Bazzocchi, MD, PhD[g]

KEYWORDS

• Shoulder • Elbow • Wrist • Anatomy • Joints • Stability

KEY POINTS

- The anatomy of the upper limb allows for exceptional functionality but this comes at the price of a wide range of potential lesions.
- The upper limb joints have different stabilizing structures, grossly divided into static (bones, ligaments) and dynamic (tendons, muscles).
- A good understanding of the anatomy and biomechanics of the upper limb joints provides a useful tool for accurate diagnosis and, therefore, has a positive impact on selection of treatment and prognosis.

INTRODUCTION

The anatomy of the upper limb is complex, allowing for exceptional functionality. The movements of the joints of the shoulder, elbow, and wrist represent a complex dynamic synergy of muscles, ligaments, and bony articulations. A solid knowledge and of the characteristics and interactions of the anatomic elements of the joints of the upper limb will help in understanding the mechanisms and patterns of injury.

Musculoskeletal pathologic conditions of the upper limb are extremely frequent and have a very high impact on the quality of life.

SHOULDER

The shoulder has a greater range of motion than any other joint in the human body.

The authors have no conflicts of interest or funding information to disclose.

[a] Department of Radiology, National Women's Hospital, Auckland City Hospital, Greenlane Clinical Center, Auckland District Health Board, 2 Park Road, Grafton, Auckland 1023, New Zealand; [b] Department of Radiology, Hospital Nisa Nueve de Octubre, Calle Valle de la Ballestera, 59, Valencia 46015, Spain; [c] Department of Experimental, Diagnostic and Specialty Medicine, University of Bologna, Sant'Orsola-Malpighi Hospital, Via Massarenti 9, 40138 Bologna, Italy; [d] Department of Radiology, University of Foggia, Viale Luigi Pinto 1, Foggia 71100, Italy; [e] 1st Orthopaedic and Traumatologic Clinic, IRCCS Istituto Ortopedico Rizzoli, Via G. C. Pupilli 1, Bologna 40136, Italy; [f] Department of Biomedical and Neuromotor Sciences, University of Bologna, Via U. Foscolo 7, Bologna 40123, Italy; [g] Diagnostic and Interventional Radiology, IRCCS Istituto Ortopedico Rizzoli, Via G. C. Pupilli 1, Bologna 40136, Italy
* Corresponding author. Department of Radiology/Department of Ultrasound, National Women's Hospital, Auckland City Hospital, Greenlane Clinical Center, Auckland District Health Board, 2 Park Road, Grafton, Auckland 1023, New Zealand.
E-mail addresses: pilucaparisi@yahoo.es; pilara@adhb.govt.nz

Radiol Clin N Am 57 (2019) 857–881
https://doi.org/10.1016/j.rcl.2019.03.002
0033-8389/19/

Bony Anatomy

Bony architecture, with the relatively large humeral head and small glenoid, relies on stabilizers such as ligaments and muscles.

Proximal humerus

In the proximal humerus, the head is inclined with respect to the shaft, approximately 130° to 150°, and retroverted with respect to the plane of the epicondyles (26°–31°).[1]

The greater tuberosity has 3 facets for the insertion of the supraspinatus, infraspinatus, and teres minor. The subscapularis inserts in the lesser tuberosity.

Fractures generally involve the tuberosities. Displacement of fragments is modulated by muscular attachments.

The surgical neck corresponds to the metaphyseal region. It is a common fracture site in the elderly, in the context of insufficiency fractures.[2]

Scapula

The scapula has a flat configuration. Fractures normally involve the processes.

The spine forms the base of the acromion and is part of the insertion of the trapezius and the origin of the deltoid.

The acromion is the lever arm for function of the deltoid. It articulates with the distal end of the clavicle. Variations in the shape of the acromion can result in impingement (type III)[3] (**Fig. 1**). The acromion may also demonstrate lateral downsloping, which is a predisposing factor for impingement (**Fig. 2**). Banas and colleagues[4] described a strong association of an angle of less than 70° with rotator cuff tears. An os acromiale is an anatomic variation resulting from failure of fusion of the acromial accessory ossification center, occurring with a frequency of 1.3% to 15%. It can be a cause for impingement.[5] A summary of anatomic variations with the potential to lead to misdiagnosis or be clinically significant is listed in **Table 1**.

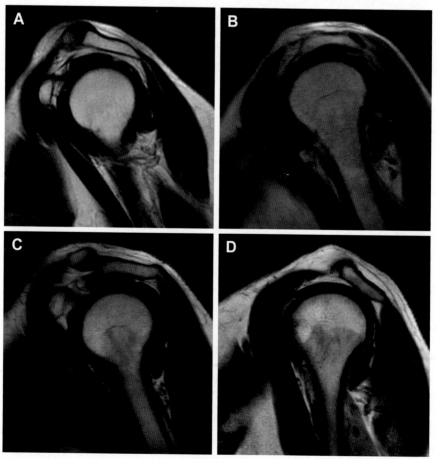

Fig. 1. Oblique sagittal T1-weighted images of the different types of acromial undersurface shape. (*A*) Type I, flat. (*B*) Type 2, curved. (*C*) Type 3, hooked. (*D*) Type 4, convex.

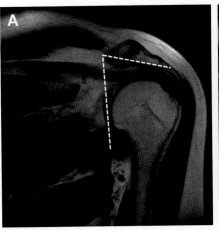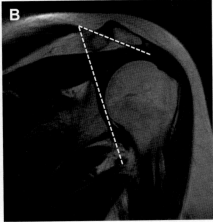

Fig. 2. Measurement of lateral downsloping of the acromion. This represents the angle between the glenoid surface and the orientation of the undersurface of the acromion (*dotted lines*). (*A*) Normally the acromion is almost parallel to the longitudinal axis of the clavicle. (*B*) An angle of less than 70° has been linked to rotator cuff pathologic conditions.

The coracoid is the origin of coracoclavicular, coracoacromial, and coracohumeral ligaments; and the coracobrachialis muscle, the short head of the biceps, and the pectoralis minor muscle.

The glenoid fossa is the articulating surface for the humerus. Its surface is only one-third to one-fourth of that of the surface of the humeral head and provides negligible contribution to stability.

Table 1
Anatomic variants around the shoulder: description and significance

Variant	Description	Significance
Shape of the undersurface of the acromion	Type I: flat Type II: curved Type III: hooked Type IV: convex	Association with pathologic rotator cuff type III
Lateral downsloping acromion	Narrow angles between clavicle and acromion	Rotator cuff and impingement symptoms
Os acromiale	Accessory ossification center tip acromion	Rotator cuff and impingement symptoms
Labral attachment variations	Sublabral recess Sublabral foramen	Possible pitfall when diagnosing labral tears
Variations glenohumeral ligaments	Common origin MGHL + SGHL Common origin of the SGHL + biceps tendon Common origin of MGHL + IGHL Bifid MGHL Cordlike thickening of the MGHL absence of the anterosuperior portion of the labrum (Buford complex)	Possible pitfall interpretation labral and ligamentous lesions
Capsular insertion	Type I, type II, type III (less to more distance from glenoid)	Decreased stability in type III
Insertion of the LHB	Broad-based or thin-based Predominantly anterior-posterior	Association with posterior extension of tears in predominantly posterior insertions

Abbreviations: IGHL, inferior glenohumeral ligament; LHB, long head biceps; MGHL, medial glenohumeral ligament; SGHL, superior glenohumeral ligament.

The articular surface is retroverted, on average 4° to 12°, with respect to the scapular plane. The scapular plane lies 30° to 45° anterior with respect to the coronal plane of the body.[6]

Moor and colleagues[7] were the first to suggest the association between the individual anatomy of the scapula and the development of osteoarthritis of the glenohumeral joint through the concept of the critical shoulder angle (a combination of the measurement of the inclination of the glenoid and the lateral extension of the acromion) (**Fig. 3**). This concept has been validated by other groups for the development of osteoarthritis with small angles (less than 30°, odds ratio 2.25)[8] and extended to the pathogenesis of rotator cuff tears, with inconsistent results.[8,9]

The acromion, along with the coracoacromial ligament and coracoid form the acromial arch, which contains the supraspinatus and infraspinatus muscles and tendons. If the humeral head and rotator cuff impinge against these structures, tendinitis and bursitis develop.[3]

Clavicle
The clavicle represents a bony strut, connecting the trunk to the shoulder. It has a double curve and is subcutaneous in its whole extent. The flat outer third is an attachment point for muscles and ligaments. The remainder of it is tubular and accepts axial loading.

The clavicle is a site for muscle attachments, a barrier to protect structures, and a stabilizing strut for the shoulder.[10]

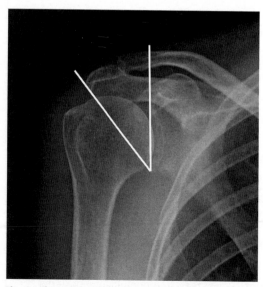

Fig. 3. The critical shoulder angle is the angle resulting from the inclination of the glenoid surface and a line from the inferior margin of the glenoid to the lateral aspect of the acromion (*solid lines*).

Joints

Glenohumeral joint
The glenohumeral join has extreme mobility, provided by the large humeral head in comparison with a small glenoid articular surface. Only 25% to 30% of the humeral head is in contact with the glenoid fossa at any given time. Even though there is lack of coverage, a normally working shoulder precisely constrains the humeral head to within 1 to 2 mm of the center of the glenoid cavity, through most of the arc of motion, owing to the static and dynamic stabilizers.[11]

This is important because injury to these stabilizers through a single traumatic event or repetitive microtrauma will result in instability. The direction of the instability will depend on the injured structure or it will be a combination.

Surgical treatment aims toward restoration of structural integrity of the components and rehabilitation is important to strengthen the dynamic stabilizers.

Static stabilizers
Articular surfaces The radius of curvature of the glenoid is larger (flatter) than the radius of the humeral head. This discrepancy is in part bridged by a physiologic thickening of the articular cartilage toward the periphery of the glenoid.[12]

This additional conformity is the basis for the concavity compression effect provided by the dynamic stabilizers.[12]

Labrum The labrum is a dense fibrous structure that is triangular in cross-section. Anatomic variation in its shape is possible and frequent (**Fig. 4**).

The labrum has the role of extending the conforming articular surfaces, which increases the contact surface area and, therefore, stability. Simultaneously, the concavity of the socket is enhanced by the labrum (an average of 9 mm in the superoinferior plane, and 5 mm in the anteroposterior plane[12]) and, therefore, if injury to the labrum occurs, the resistance to translation decreases by 20%.[11]

Also, the labrum is the anchor point for capsuloligamentous structures. Bankart[13] was the first to describe injury to the labrum as the culprit in recurrent anterior dislocation, through loss of an anchor for the inferior and medial glenohumeral ligaments, and loss of the enhancement in depth that the labrum provides in the anterior-anteroinferior regions. It has been proved that if there is a lesion of the superior labrum or biceps anchor anteroposterior and superoinferior translations increase in the lower and middle ranges of elevation.[14]

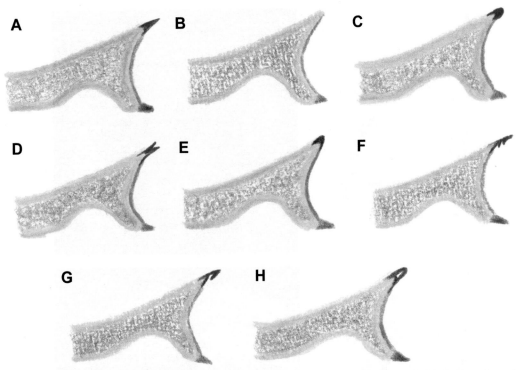

A **B** **C** **D** **E** **F** **G** **H**

Fig. 4. Labral shape variants. (*A*) Triangular. (*B*) Absent. (*C*) Rounded. (*D*) Cleaved. (*E*) Comma-shaped. (*F*) Notched. (*G*) Lineal hyperintensity. (*H*) Central hyperintensity.

Variations in the configuration of the anterosuperior labrum are frequent (approximately 35%).[15] The anterosuperior labrum is frequently partially detached, creating a space between the glenoid and the labrum, called sublabral foramen. A second potential space, known as sublabral recess, can exist between the superior labrum and the glenoid (**Fig. 5**). The presence of variation in the anterosuperior labrum has been linked to development of pathologic conditions,[16] especially type II superior labrum anterior-posterior lesions (SLAP).[17] The variations themselves do not seem to contribute to instability.[15]

Ligaments The ligaments are summarized in **Table 2**.

The coracohumeral ligament and the superior glenohumeral ligament (SGHL) run parallel and have similar functions. They constitute the rotator interval region together with the anterior margin of the supraspinatus and the superior margin of the subscapularis.[18]

The middle glenohumeral ligament (MGHL) is the most variable and can be absent in 8% to 30% of shoulders but also varies in configuration[19] and is associated with labral variation.

The inferior glenohumeral ligament (IGHL) is the thickest and most consistent ligament. It is complex, containing an anterior band, axillary pouch, and posterior band. Injury results in recurrent instability.[19]

Anatomic variants in the origin of the ligaments are common (**Fig. 6**): common origin of MGHL and SGHL, common origin of the SGHL and biceps tendon, common origin of MGHL and IGHL, bifid MGHL and cordlike thickening of the MGHL with or without absence of the anterosuperior portion of the labrum (Buford complex).

Joint capsule The joint capsule is truncated in shape and the axillary pouch (inferior aspect) is redundant (**Fig. 7**). The capsule and ligaments are intimately related anatomically. The capsuloligamentous structures harmonically tighten or loosen in the midrange spectrum of movement. In this range, stability is mainly provided by the rotator cuff and biceps. They become truly important in the extremes of motion, when these mechanisms may fail.[11]

The anterior capsular insertion can be divided in 3 types (**Fig. 8**). In general, the further the anterior capsular insertion is from the glenoid margin, the more unstable the glenohumeral joint is. This needs to be assessed in neutral position because it obviously demonstrates a slight variation with external-internal rotation.[20]

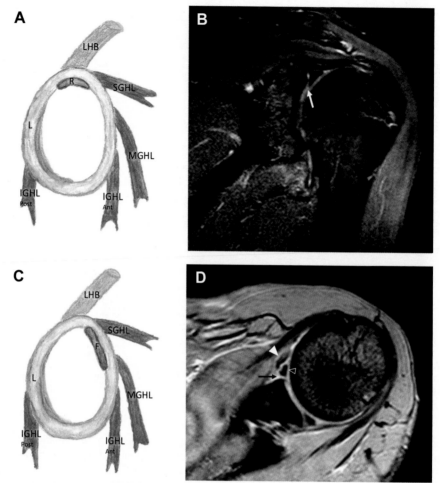

Fig. 5. Labral attachment variants. (*A*) Schematic of the potential space between the superior labrum and the glenoid, known as sublabral recess (R). (*B*) Coronal T2-weighted fat-saturated image demonstrates a hyperintense linear cleft at the base of the superior labrum, in keeping with a sublabral recess (*black arrow*). (*C*) Schematic of the potential space between the glenoid and the anterosuperior labrum, called sublabral foramen (F). (*D*) Axial gradient-recalled echo T2*-weighted image demonstrates a space (*white arrow*) between the glenoid and ante-rosuperior labrum (*open arrowhead*). The MGHL is seen separately from the labrum (*white arrowhead*). Ant, anterior band; IGHL, inferior glenohumeral ligament; L, labrum; LHB, long head biceps; MGHL, medial glenohum-eral ligament; Post, posterior band; SGHL, superior glenohumeral ligament.

Dynamic stabilizers

Rotator cuff muscles The rotator cuff muscles are summarized in **Table 3**.

As a group, they act as a mechanism to dynam-ically steer the humeral head (see **Fig. 7**). The movements of the humeral head ultimately result from the interplay between these and the static stabilizers. They are strategically located close to the center of rotation on which they act, with a short lever arm but also a small generated force.[21]

The supraspinatus tendon blends into the supe-rior joint capsule, and the subscapularis is inti-mately associated with the anterior capsule.

The long head of the biceps must be considered in association with the rotator cuff tendons because the functions are closely related. This acts as a depressor of the humeral head (similar to supraspinatus, infraspinatus, and teres minor) and as a stabilizer.[14]

Bursae

The subacromial-subdeltoid bursa is located between the rotator cuff and the acromion or the deltoid. It does not communicate with the joint in normal circumstances. On MR imaging, it is not visible unless there is fluid within.

The subcoracoid bursa is located between the subscapularis and the coracoid, and it does not

Table 2
Glenohumeral ligaments: anatomy and function

	Origin	Insertion	Function	Characteristics
Coracohumeral	Base of lateral coracoid	Greater and lesser tuberosities	Stabilize humeral head from inferior translation in adduction and from posterior translation in forward flexion, adduction, and internal rotation Constrains humeral head on glenoid	Extracapsular
Superior glenohumeral	Anterior base of the glenoid	Top of lesser tuberosity	Stabilize humeral head from inferior translation in adduction and from posterior translation in forward flexion, adduction, and internal rotation	Capsular reinforcement
Middle glenohumeral	Supraglenoid tubercle superior labrum scapular neck	Medial aspect of the lesser tuberosity	Limit anterior translation of the humerus in lower ranges of abduction and inferior translation in the adducted position	Capsular reinforcement
Inferior glenohumeral	Anteroinferior labrum and glenoid lip	Lesser tuberosity	Primary stabilizer against anterior translation in throwing position (abduction and external rotation)	Capsular reinforcement

communicate with the joint. It can communicate with the subacromial-subdeltoid bursa in 20% of cases.[22] On MR imaging, it is not visible unless there is fluid within. The subscapularis recess is located between the anterior surface of the scapula and the subscapularis muscle, and it communicates with the joint.

Neurovascular Structures

- The suprascapular nerve and vessels run under the suprascapular ligament in the suprascapular notch (**Fig. 9**). The nerve gives branches for the supraspinatus and the infraspinatus. The branches for the infraspinatus run under the spinoglenoid ligament in the posterior aspect glenoid margin. Labral cysts in the suprascapular or spinoglenoid notch can cause compressive neuropathies and denervation.

- The axillary nerve and vessels pass through the quadrilateral space between the humeral shaft, triceps muscle, and teres major and minor. The nerve gives branches for the teres minor and deltoid. Repetitive trauma or compression of the quadrilateral space (eg, use of crutches or backpacks), or acute trauma in anterior dislocation, can damage the axillary nerve.

Acromioclavicular joint

The acromioclavicular joint is a diarthroidal joint. It has a small surface area that transfers high axial loads, which can potentially result in early failure (osteolysis, osteoarthritis)

The primary stabilizers are the capsule, the intraarticular disc, and the ligaments (superior, inferior anterior, and posterior) (**Fig. 10**).

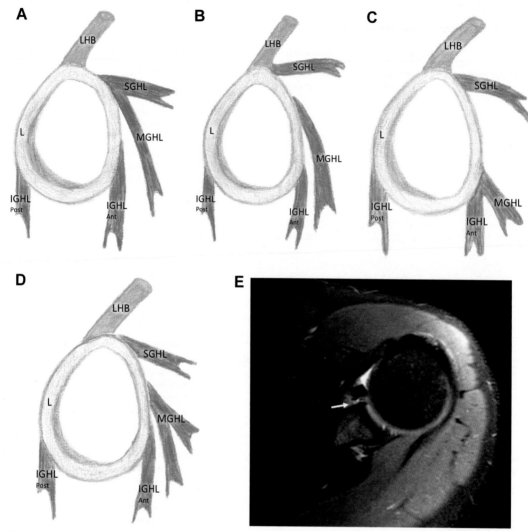

Fig. 6. Variations on configuration of the glenohumeral ligaments. (*A*) Common origin of MGHL and SGHL. (*B*) Common origin of the SGHL and biceps tendon. (*C*) Common origin of MGHL and IGHL. (*D*) Bifid MGHL. (*E*) Buford complex. Axial T1-weighted fat-saturated image with intraarticular gadolinium demonstrates a space between the glenoid and a thickened MGHL (*white arrow*). The labrum is absent.

The capsule is thicker in the superior and anterior aspects. The strongest ligament is the superior. The intraarticular disc degenerates very rapidly and is not present in most people in their fourth decade.

Secondary stability is provided by the coracoclavicular ligaments: trapezoid and conoid. These are the primary suspensory ligaments of the upper extremity. Both originate from the superior aspect of the coracoid and insert into the trapezoid ridge and conoid tuberosity of the clavicle, respectively (average distance 13 mm).[23]

Sternoclavicular joint

The sternoclavicular joint is the only true articulation between the upper extremity and the axial skeleton. It is a sellar joint between the medial aspect of the clavicle and the upper portion of the sternum. There is an important discrepancy in the size of the components. The clavicular end is large and bulbous, and the sternal end is small and not deep. Stability is provided by a strong ligamentous complex, which extends to the first ribs, and an intraarticular disc.[21]

Scapulothoracic joint

The scapulothoracic joint consists of a space that lodges in the neurovascular, muscular, and bursal structures that cushion the movement between the scapula and thorax. This articulation allows increased shoulder movement, beyond the 120° that would be achieved by the glenohumeral joint

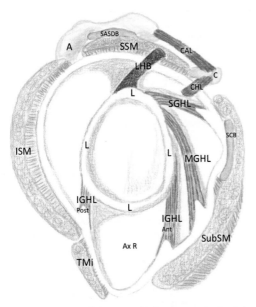

Fig. 7. Schematic of the capsule, ligaments, and rotator cuff muscles. A, acromion; Ax R, axillary recess; C, coracoid; CAL, coracoacromial ligament; CHL, coracohumeral ligament; ISM, infraspinatus; SASDB, subacromial-subdeltoid bursa; SCB, subcoracoid bursa; SSM, supraspinatus; SubSM, subscapularis; TMi, teres minor.

only. Many muscles (14) attach or originate in the scapula.

Scapulothoracic muscles

The scapulothoracic muscles stabilize the scapula and facilitate scapulothoracic motion, which adds to the range of mobility of the shoulder. These can be used in reconstructive surgery.[24] These muscles are summarized in **Table 4**.

ELBOW

The primary function of the elbow is to position the hand in space, to constitute a fulcrum for the forearm, and to allow for power grasping and fine motions of the hand and wrist. It is a stable joint and is highly congruous.

Bony Anatomy

Distal humerus

The medial epicondyle is the attachment of the ulnar collateral ligament and flexor-pronator group. The lateral epicondyle is the attachment for the lateral collateral ligament and the extensor-supinator group.[25] In the anterior aspect, the coronoid and radial fossae accommodate these structures in flexion; in the posterior aspect, the olecranon fossa accommodates this structure in extension.[26]

The trochlea is pulley-shaped and is larger medially than laterally. It articulates with the sigmoid notch of the ulna. In the lateral aspect, the capitellum articulates with the humeral head.

The capitellum and trochlea are covered in hyaline cartilage. These surfaces are oriented 30° anterior and are in 5° of internal rotation, and in 6° of valgus.[27]

Radius

The head of the radius has a cylindrical shape, with a slight central depression in the articular facet for the capitellum, and a slightly elevated rim. Approximately 240° of the circumference of the facet is covered by hyaline cartilage, and the anterior third is free of it. The head and shaft describe a medially oriented angle of

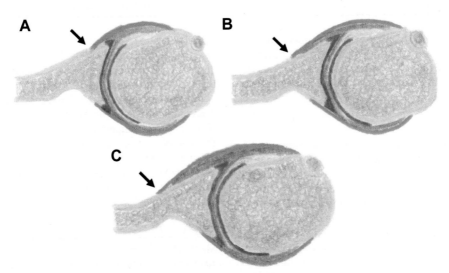

Fig. 8. Types of anterior capsular insertion. (*A*) Immediate vicinity to the glenoid rim and/or labral base. (*B*) More proximal but less than 1 cm from glenoid margin. (*C*) Beyond 1 cm from the glenoid margin.

Table 3
Rotator cuff muscles and long head biceps: anatomy and function

	Origin	Insertion	Function	Innervation
Supraspinatus	Supraspinous fossa	Superior aspect of the greater tuberosity	Stabilizer and elevator of arm with deltoid	Suprascapular
Infraspinatus	Infraspinatus fossa	Middle facet of the greater tuberosity	Primary external rotation force and stabilizes glenohumeral joint against the posterior subluxation	Suprascapular
Teres Minor	Mid to upper regions of axillary border of scapula	Most inferior facet of the greater tuberosity	External rotator and stabilizer	Axillary
Subscapularis	Subscapular fossa	Lesser tuberosity	Internal rotator, especially in maximum internal rotation	Upper and lower subscapular
LHB	Supraglenoid tuberosity and superior labrum (posterior and anterior)	Bicipital tuberosity of the radius	Contraction during the cocking phase of throwing reduces anterior translation and increases torsional rigidity resisting external rotation In lower elevated positions the long head tendon stabilizes the joint anteriorly when the arm is internally rotated and posteriorly when the arm is externally rotated	Musculo-cutaneous

approximately 15°. The medial aspect of the radial head articulates with the radial notch of the ulna. Distal to the radial neck is the radial tuberosity, which is the site of insertion of the distal biceps tendon.[27]

Ulna

The shape of the ulna provides a primary passive stabilizer of the elbow, through congruence of the ulnohumeral joint, especially in elbow extension. The proximal ulna consists of the coronoid process for insertion of the brachialis and the olecranon process, for insertion of the triceps. The sigmoid notch is the articular surface between these 2 processes. It is saddle-shaped, ellipsoid on itself, and articulates with the trochlea of the humerus. It is covered by hyaline cartilage, except for the mid portion where there is a small region covered by fatty tissue.[28] The arc of the greater sigmoid notch is approximately 190°.[28]

In the lateral coronoid, the semilunar notch articulates with the radial head.

In the proximal ulna, on the lateral aspect, the crista supinatoris is the attachment of the lateral ulnar collateral ligament. On the medial aspect, the anterior portion of the medial collateral ligament attaches to the coronoid.[25,29]

Anatomic variants that can represent a source of misdiagnosis or potential clinical significance are listed in **Table 5**.

Elbow Joint

Static stabilizers
Articular surfaces The elbow is a joint composed of 3 different articulations, all surrounded by the same synovial capsule (**Table 6**).

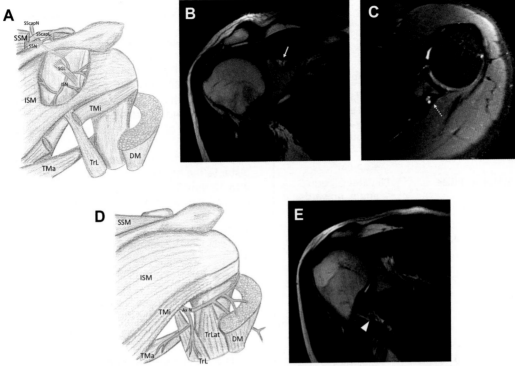

Fig. 9. Neurovascular structures around the shoulder. (*A*) Schematic of the course of the suprascapular nerve. (*B*) Coronal PD image demonstrating the suprascapular nerve in the suprascapular notch (*white arrow*). (*C*) Axial PD fat-saturated image demonstrating the infraspinatus nerve in the spinoglenoid notch (discontinuous *white arrow*). (*D*) Schematic of the course of the AxN. (*E*) Coronal PD image demonstrating the axillary nerve in the quadrilateral space (*white arrowhead*). AxN, axillary nerve; DM, deltoid muscle; ISN, infraspinatus nerve; SGL, supraglenoid ligament; SScapL, suprascapular ligament; SScapN, suprascapular nerve; SSN, supraspinatus nerve; TMa, teres major; TrL, long head triceps; TrLat, lateral head triceps.

The physiologic range of motion is 0° to 140° for flexion-extension movements and 0° to 180° for pronation-supination movements.[27]

The ulnotrochlear joint is the most important osseous stabilizer of the elbow; it provides primary stability at less than 20° or more than 120°of flexion.[30]

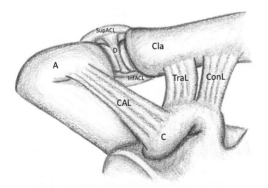

Fig. 10. Schematic of the acromioclavicular joint. Cla, clavicle; ConL, conoid ligament; D, disc; InfACL, inferior acromioclavicular ligament; SupACL, superior acromioclavicular ligament; TraL, trapezoid ligament.

The carrying angle of the elbow, formed by the longitudinal between humerus and ulna with elbow in full extension, has a slight valgus (11°–14° in men and 13°–16° in women). The orientation changes to varus in flexion.[27]

Capsule The joint capsule is thin anteriorly. It is taut in extension and lax in flexion. The joint has a maximal capacity of approximately 30 mL in intermediate flexion.[31]

Ligaments The ligaments are summarized in **Tables 7** and **8**.

Ligamentous of the elbow include the medial collateral ligament and the lateral collateral ligament[25,32,33] (**Fig. 11**).

Dynamic stabilizers

Muscles The muscles are summarized in **Table 9**.

These can be divided in 4 groups: posterior, anterior, lateral, and medial. The posterior groups are extensors, the anterior are flexors, the lateral comprise the wrist and finger extensors and supinator and the medial muscles are the flexor-pronator groups.

Table 4 Scapulothoracic other muscles: anatomy and function	
Scapulothoracic Muscles	**Function**
Trapezius	Scapular retractor and elevator of the lateral angle of the scapula
Rhomboids	Retract and elevate scapula
Levator scapulae	Elevates superior angle, upward and medial rotation of the scapular body
Serratus anterior	Scapular protraction and upward rotation
Pectoralis minor	Protracts and rotates scapula inferiorly
Deltoid	Anterior and middle elevate the scapular plane, assist in forward elevation
Other Muscles	**Function**
Latissimus dorsi	Adduct, extend, internally rotate humerus
Teres major	Internal rotator and adductor of the shoulder, extender of arm
Coracobrachialis	Flexes and adducts glenohumeral joint
Pectoralis major	Adduction and internal rotation of the humerus

The stabilizers of the elbow are summarized in **Table 10**.

Neurovascular Structures

The median nerve runs through the medial anterior aspect of the elbow, with the brachial artery. The radial nerve runs anterolateral and the ulnar nerve is posteromedial (**Fig. 12**).

WRIST

The wrist allows movement in 3 planes: flexion-extension, radial-ulnar deviation (abduction-adduction), and pronation-supination.

Bony Anatomy

Distal radius

The articular surface has 2 facets covered by hyaline cartilage: a lateral facet (triangular) for the scaphoid and a medial facet (quadrilateral) for the lunate. The medial surface of the distal radius articulates with the ulnar head. The lateral surface of the lateral radius extends into a styloid process, which is the attachment for the brachioradialis muscle.

Normally, the styloid process of the radius lies distal to the styloid of the ulna by approximately 9 to 12 mm. There is normally an average of 23° of volar angulation and 11° of lateral inclination.[34]

Distal ulna

The distal ulna comprises 2 eminences: the head and the styloid process. The head has an oval articular surface to articulate distally and a lateral surface to articulate with the distal radius.

The styloid process is separated from the head by a small depression that serves as an attachment for the fibrocartilage. The styloid is nonarticular.[35]

Ulnar variance reflects the relationship between the distal ends of the radius and the ulna (positive: the ulna projects more distally; negative: the ulna projects more proximally). This varies with wrist position in normal circumstances (in pronation becomes more positive, in supination becomes more negative) and also with a clenched fist. The variance is more accurately assessed on radiographs (MR imaging allows an estimate but does not quantify) with the shoulder abducted 90° and the elbow flexed 90°. In this position, a distance of +2.5 mm or −2.5 mm from the level of the radius will indicate a positive or negative variance. Positive variance has been associated with ulnar impaction syndrome; degenerative tear of the triangular fibrocartilage complex (TFCC); and chondromalacia of the lunate, triquetrum, and distal ulna.[36] Negative variance has been hypothesized to play a role in ulnar impingement and Kienböck disease[37]; however, the association with the latter remains controversial.[38]

Carpal bones

The carpal bones are organized in 2 rows that allow outlining of 3 arcs (Gilula arcs).[39] The first circumscribes the proximal joint surface of the first row; the second, the distal joint surface of the first row; and the third, the opposing joint formed by the convexity of the capitate and hamate (**Fig. 13**).

Metacarpal bases

The metacarpal bases have a cuboid configuration, broader in the dorsal aspect than the front.

Table 5
Anatomic variants around the elbow: description and significance

Variant		Description	Pitfall or Significance
Bones	Supracondylar spur	Spur in the anterior aspect (1% population)	Mistaken for exostosis Possible median nerve compression
	Bony flange lateral humerus	Bony flange lateral humerus	Mistaken for periosteal reaction
	Nonunited inferior olecranon	Small ossicle in the inferior olecranon	Mistaken for fracture
	Pseudodefect capitellum	Indentation between capitellum and the nonarticular surface of the lateral epicondyle	Mistaken for osteochondral defect
	Trochlear ridge	Mild elevation in the contour of the groove	Mistaken for osteophyte
	Pseudonotch	Indentation in articular surface at the junction of the coronoid and olecranon	Mistaken for osteochondral defect
Ligaments	Synovial invagination	Focal linear increased signal deep to the humeral attachment of the anterior bundle of the ulnar collateral ligament complex	Mistaken for a ligament tear
Tendons or muscles	Anconeus epitrochlearis	Accessory muscle arising from the medial epicondyle, and inserting on the olecranon, passing over the ulnar nerve	Compressive neuropathy

The dorsal and volar aspects are where the carpometacarpal ligaments attach.

Anatomic variants around the wrist that can represent a source of misdiagnosis are extremely numerous and beyond the scope of this review. Multiple accessory ossicles and variations in morphology of each of the bones have been described. Of note, lucencies with sclerotic margins and nutrient channels are very commonly seen and represent intraosseous ganglion cysts.

Table 6
Components of the elbow joint

Joint	Type	Movement
Ulnotrochlear	Hinge: ginglymus	Flexion or extension
Radiocapitellar	Hinge and pivot	Pronation or supination
Radioulnar	Pivot: throchoid	Pronation or supination

Joints

The wrist is not a single joint but, instead, a highly complex group of several joints that work in synergy. These are summarized in **Table 11**.

Distal radioulnar joint

The distal radioulnar joint (DRUJ) is formed by the distal radius, ulna, and interosseous membrane, and has the configuration of a uniaxial pivot joint. The DRUJ is 1 of 2 joints (together with the proximal radioulnar joint) that work simultaneously to allow pronation and supination of the forearm.

In this joint, the ulnar head is a fixed structure, around which the distal radius rotates.

This articulation also moves anteriorly and posteriorly with forearm pronation-supination (the radius moves proximally as it pronates and distally as it supinates).[34]

Radiocarpal joint

The radiocarpal joint occurs between the distal radius and proximal surfaces of the scaphoid and lunate.

Table 7
Lateral collateral ligament elbow: anatomy and function

	Components	Origin	Insertion	Function
Lateral collateral ligament	Annular ligament (encircles the radial head)	Anterior lesser sigmoid notch	Posterior lesser sigmoid notch	Primary stabilizer of the proximal radioulnar joint
	Radial collateral ligament	Anterior margin of the lateral epicondyle	Annular ligament fascia of the supinator muscles	Uniformly taut throughout flexion-extension
	Ulnar collateral ligament (lateral ulnar collateral ligament)	Lateral epicondyle	Supinator crest of the ulna	Major stabilizer of the elbow to varus forces (lateral stabilizer of the ulnohumeral) Prevents posterolateral rotatory instability
	Accessory radial collateral ligament	Fibers of the annular ligament	Tubercle of the supinator crest	Stabilizes the annular ligament during varus stress

This is a condyloid joint, which allows for flexion-extension, adduction and abduction, and circumduction. Stabilizing ligaments in the volar aspect include the radial collateral (to the styloid process), the radioscaphocapitate, the radiolunate, and the radioscapholunate. The dorsal aspect includes the radioscaphoid, the radiolunate, and the radiotriquetral (extrinsic ligaments) (**Fig. 14**).

Ulnocarpal joint

The ulnocarpal joint is in medial continuity with the radiocarpal joint. An articular disc extends from the medial aspect of the radius to form an elliptical

Table 8
Medial collateral ligament elbow: anatomy and function

	Components	Origin	Insertion	Function
Medial collateral ligament	Anterior Cordlike structure (4–5 mm wide)	Medial epicondyle	Anteromedial margin of the coronoid process (on the sublime tubercle)	Major passive stabilizer of the elbow to valgus forces
	Posterior Capsular thickening (5–6 cm wide)	Inferior aspect of the medial epicondyle	Posteromedial aspect of the trochlear notch of the ulna (the medial aspect of the olecranon)	Floor of the cubital tunnel Stabilizer of the elbow when the joint is flexed more than 90°
	Transverse Thickening of the joint capsule	Distal attachment of the posterior bundle of the medial collateral ligament (olecranon)	Distal attachment of the anterior bundle of the medial collateral ligament (coronoid process)	(No significant contribution to elbow stability)

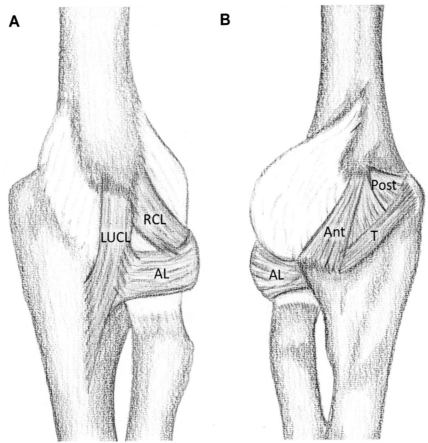

Fig. 11. Schematic of the elbow ligaments. (*A*) Lateral collateral ligament. AL, annular ligament; LUCL, lateral ulnar collateral; RCL, radial collateral. (*B*) Medial collateral ligament. T, transverse bundle.

concave surface to articulate with the proximal aspect of the first row of carpal bones.

The TFCC is a fibrocartilage (**Fig. 15**) ligament complex that acts as a strong condensation of stabilizing structures, attaching the distal ulna to the hand and to the radius.

This complex consists of the triangular fibrocartilage (proper disc), meniscus homologue, the ulnolunate and ulnotriquetral ligaments, the proximal ligamentous component, the volar and dorsal radioulnar ligaments, and the ulnar collateral ligament.[40,41] The extensor carpi ulnaris (ECU) subsheath is also considered a component.

Fibrocartilage disc The fibrocartilage disc attaches medially to the radius and laterally to the ulna. This has a biconcave or bowtie-shaped configuration, and is thinner in the central region and thicker in the periphery. The ulnar artery and palmar and dorsal branches of the anterior interosseous constitute the supply for the disc, which is peripheral. The central region and radial attachment are avascular. The periphery can, therefore,

be repaired but not the central area, which is weaker to injury and prone to degeneration.[42]

The ulnar attachment is formed by 2 ligaments (triangular ligaments). One attaches into the ulnar styloid tip (distal lamina) and the other into the fovea (proximal lamina). The tissue between these ligaments is richly vascularized and named the ligamentum subcruentum. It normally appears hyperintense on water-sensitive sequences.[43]

The morphology of the disc is strongly associated with ulnar variance. If this is neutral, the disc more or less follows the line of the articular surface of the radius, with a slight tilt. If the variance is positive, the disc is thin and stretched distally, forming an arc. If the variance is negative, the disc is more horizontal, thicker, and shorter.[44]

Radioulnar ligament The radioulnar ligaments are reinforcing fibers that travel from the radius to the base of the ulnar styloid in the dorsal and volar aspects.

Extensor carpi ulnaris tendon The ECU tendon changes position in supination-pronation. It

Table 9
Muscles around the elbow: anatomy and function

Posterior	Origin	Insertion	Function	Innervation
Triceps	Long: infraglenoid tuberosity; Lateral, medial: spiral groove humerus	Long and lateral heads into olecranon; Medial olecranon	Elbow extension	Radial nerve C7–C8
Anconeus	Posterolateral epicondyle	Dorsolateral proximal ulna	Elbow extension, abduction, stabilization	Motor branch of medial head of the triceps C7–C8
Extensor carpi ulnaris	Lateral epicondyle	5th metacarpal	Wrist extension ulnar deviation	PIN C6–C7
Extensor digitorum communis	Anterolateral epicondyle	Extensor mechanism fingers	Metacarpal phalangeal joint extension	PIN C7–C8
Anterior	**Origin**	**Insertion**	**Function**	**Innervation**
Biceps	Long: supraglenoid tubercle scapula; Short: coracoid	Bicipital tuberosity radius; Aponeurosis into forearm fascia and ulna	Elbow flexion, supination in flexion	Musculocutaneous C5–C6
Pronator teres (humeral head, ulnar head)	Humeral: medial epicondyle (anterosuperior); Ulnar: coronoid	Pronator tuberosity of the radius	Forearm pronation (elbow flexion)	Median nerve C6–C7
Flexor carpi radialis	Medial epicondyle (anteroinferior)	2nd and 3rd metacarpals	Wrist flexion (forearm pronation)	Median nerve C6–C7
Palmaris longus	Medial epicondyle	Palmar aponeurosis	Wrist flexion	Median nerve C7–C8–T1
Flexor carpi ulnaris (humeral head, ulnar head)	Humeral: medial epicondyle; Ulnar: medial olecranon, proximal ulna	Pisiform and 5th metacarpal	Wrist flexion; Ulnar deviation	Ulnar nerve C7–C8–T1

Medial	Origin	Insertion	Function	Innervation
Flexor digitorum superficialis	Medial epicondyle, Ulnar collateral ligament, Medial coronoid, Proximal radius	Middle phalanges	Flexion PIP	Median nerve C7–C8
Flexor digitorum profundus	Medial olecranon, Proximal ulna	Distal phalanges	Flexion DIP	2nd and 3rd median nerve; 4th and 5th ulnar nerve

Lateral	Origin	Insertion	Function	Innervation
Extensor carpi radialis brevis	Lateral epicondyle (inferior-lateral)	3rd metacarpal	Wrist extension	PIN C6–C7
Extensor carpi radialis longus	Lateral supracondylar ridge	2nd metacarpal	Wrist extension	Radial nerve C6–C7
Brachioradialis	Lateral supracondylar ridge	Radial styloid	Elbow flexion with forearm in neutral rotation	Radial nerve C5–C6
Supinator	Anterolateral lateral epicondyle, Lateral collateral ligament, Supinator crest ulna	Proximal and middle 3rd of radius	Forearm supination	PIN C5–C6

Abbreviations: DIP, distal interphalangeal joint; PIN, posterior interosseous nerve; PIP, proximal interphalangeal joint.

Table 10
Summary of stabilizers of the elbow

	Position		Stabilizer
Static	Valgus	Flexion	Medial collateral ligament
	—	Extension	Medial collateral ligament
			Anterior capsule ulnohumeral joint
	Varus	Flexion-extension	Ulnohumeral joint
			Lateral ulnar collateral ligament
	Distraction	Extension	Anterior capsule
	—	Flexion	Medial collateral ligament
Dynamic	Supination-pronation Flexion-extension	—	Muscles

constitutes an important stabilizer of the ulnar side of the TFCC.[45]

Meniscus homologue The meniscus homologue is a fibrous tissue on the ulnar aspect, extending from the tip of the ulnar styloid to the ulnar aspect of triquetrum and lunate.[41]

Ulnar collateral ligament Thin and fibrous, the ulnar collateral ligament lies superficial to the meniscus homologue. Many investigators do not consider it a ligament as such but, instead, as the ulnar aspect of the capsule. In most cases, it blends with the ECU and the meniscus homologue.[46]

Ulnolunate, ulnotriquetral, and ulnocapitate ligaments The ulnolunate, ulnotriquetral, and ulnocapitate ligaments represent the ulnocarpal ligamentous complex.[41] They merge with the volar radioulnar ligament and extend to insert into the volar aspect of the triquetrum, capitate and lunate.

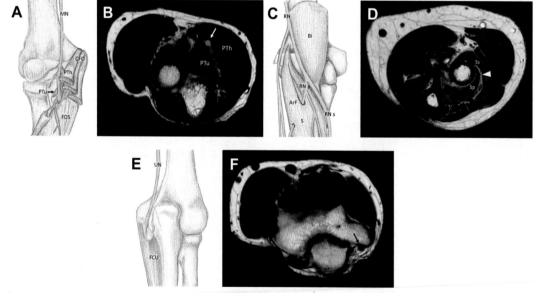

Fig. 12. Neurovascular structures around the elbow. (A) Schematic of the median nerve. CFO, common flexor origin; FDS, flexor digitorum superficialis; MN, median nerve; PTh, pronator teres humeral head; PTu, pronator teres ulnar head (the nerve courses between). (B) Axial T1-weighted image demonstrates the medial nerve between heads of the pronator teres (circled, white arrow). (C) Radial nerve. ArF, arcade of Frohse (deep branch courses between this fibrous arch; this is a location for entrapment); Bi, biceps; RN p, deep branch; RN s, superficial branch; RN, radial nerve; S, supinator muscle. (D) Axial T1-weighted image demonstrates the interosseous nerve between heads of the supinator, in the arcade of Frohse (white arrowhead). Sp, supinator profundus; Ss, supinator superficial. (E) Ulnar nerve. FCU, flexor carpi ulnaris; UN, ulnar nerve. (F) Axial T1-weighted image demonstrates the ulnar nerve in the cubital tunnel (black arrow).

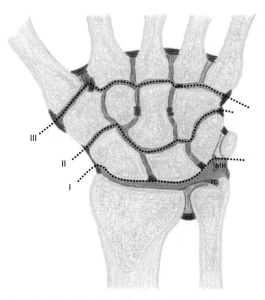

Fig. 13. Schematic of Gilula arches (I, II, III). The synovial compartments are represented in different colors: gray, pisotriquetral; green, intercarpal; light green, radiocarpal; orange, distal radioulnar; purple, first carpometacarpal; red, common carpometacarpal-midcarpal. FC, fibrocartilage; MH, meniscus homologue.

Proximal carpal joints

The proximal carpal joints are the joints between the scaphoid, the lunate, and the triquetrum. These bones are mainly connected and stabilized by the scapholunate and lunotriquetral ligaments, which are intrinsic ligaments.

The scapholunate ligament has 3 components: dorsal, longitudinal, and volar.

The longitudinal component is fibrocartilaginous and thin. The dorsal component is the strongest and is the main stabilizer of the scaphoid, restraining translation between the scaphoid and lunate. Injury results in dorsal intercalated segment instability deformity, which is the ultimate type of instability (static instability) and may result in scaphoid lunate advanced collapse. The scaphotrapezial ligaments, which are scaphocapitate (intrinsic across the mid carpal joint) and radioscaphocapitate (extrinsic), are secondary stabilizers of the scaphoid. If these are preserved, a tear of the scapholunate will result in lesser degrees of instability (dynamic instability).[47]

The lunotriquetral ligament also has 3 components: dorsal, longitudinal, and volar. The dorsal component restrains rotation but the volar is the strongest and thickest, and transmits extension momentum of the triquetrum. Injury is less common than injury to the scapholunate and may result in volar intercalated segment instability deformity. Secondary stabilizers for the joint are the radiotriquetral, the dorsal, and the volar radiolunate ligaments (extrinsic).[48]

The dorsal and volar portions of these ligaments are biomechanically more important than the longitudinal portion and, therefore, axial images on MR imaging may be more helpful to perform an accurate assessment than coronal images.

The pisiform articulates with the triquetrum. They form a synovial joint that is not communicated with the ulnocarpal joint in up to 25% of the cases.[49] The pisiform is the attachment for the flexor carpi ulnaris and abductor digiti minimi.

Midcarpal joints

The midcarpal joint is shaped as an S. This is the joint between the proximal and the distal rows of bones. There is some variability in the anatomy of this joint.

The lunate may simply articulate with the capitate or have a type II morphology, which confers it with a small articular facet for the hamate in its distal aspect. This configuration has been described as prevalent in half of the population,[50,51] and linked to the presence of chondromalacia.[50]

The triquetrum-hamate joint is a helical joint. This allows the triquetrum to rotate around the hamate.

Table 11 Joints composing the wrist joint	
Distal radioulnar joint	Distal radius, ulna, and interosseous membrane
Radiocarpal joint	Distal radius and proximal surfaces of the scaphoid and lunate
Ulnocarpal joint	Distal ulna and triangular fibroelastic cartilage, which connects ulna with lunate and triquetrum
Proximal carpal joints	Connect scaphoid, lunate, and triquetrum
Midcarpal joints	Capitate, hamate, trapezium, and trapezoid bones
Carpometacarpal and intermetacarpal joints	Connect trapezium, trapezoid, capitate, and hamate with metacarpals, and 2nd to 5th metacarpals among themselves

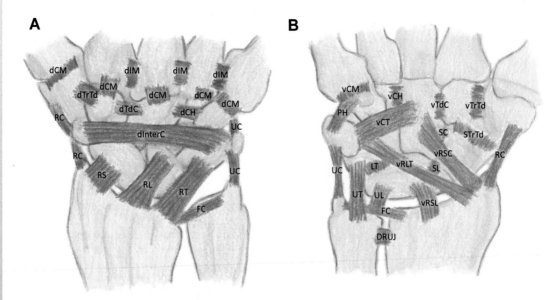

Fig. 14. Carpal ligaments. (*A*) Dorsal view. dCH, dorsal capitate hamate; dCM, dorsal carpometacarpal; dIM, dorsal intermetacarpal; dTdC, dorsal trapeziocapitate; dTrTd, dorsal trapeziotrapezoid; RL, radiolunate; RS, radioscaphoid; RT, radiotriquetral; UC, ulnar collateral. (*B*) Volar view. LT, lunotriquetral; PH, pisohamate; SC, scaphocapitate; SL, scapholunate; STrTd, scaphotrapezotrapezoidal; UL, ulnolunate; UT, ulnotriquetral; vCH, volar capitohamate; vCM, volar carpometacarpal; vCT, volar capitotriquetral; vRLT, volar radiolunotriquetral; vRSC, volar radioscaphocapitate; vRSL, volar radioscapholunate; vTdC, volar trapezoid capitate.

The intercarpal joints between the bones of each row are strongly stabilized by the radiate and pisohamate ligaments, and by the volar, interosseous, and dorsal intercarpal ligaments.

The second row of bones is tightly connected by the intercarpal ligaments and also has reinforcements from the pisometacarpal and carpometacarpal ligaments (volar and dorsal), resulting in very little mobility between the bones.

Carpometacarpal and intermetacarpal joints

The first carpometacarpal joint is a sellar joint between the base of the first metacarpal and the

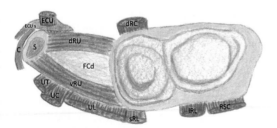

Fig. 15. Representation of the triangular fibrocartilage complex. C, capsule; dRC, dorsal radiocarpal; dRU, dorsal radioulnar ligament; ECU, extensor carpi ulnaris; ECU s, sheath; FCd, fibrocartilage disc; IRL, long radiolunate; RSC, radioscaphocapitate; S, styloid; sRL, short radiolunate; vRU, volar radioulnar ligament.

trapezium. Stability is maintained mainly by the anterior oblique ligament, the ulnar collateral ligament, the first intermetacarpal ligament, the posterior oblique ligament, and the dorsoradial ligament.[52]

Three other synovial articulations in vicinity are related to this joint (trapezium-scaphoid, trapezium-trapezoid, and base of the first metacarpal and radial side of base of the second metacarpal). These constitute the basal joint complex and allow for a very ample range of movement of the thumb.[53]

The second to fifth carpometacarpal joints are synovial ellipsoidal (condyloid) and only allow for flexion-extension. The bases of the second to fifth metacarpals also articulate in a row with the neighboring bases. These joints are stabilized by the strong dorsal and volar carpometacarpal ligaments and the dorsal, interosseous, and volar intermetacarpal ligaments.

Muscles

The muscles are summarized in **Table 12.**

Neurovascular Structures

The main nerves crossing the wrist are the median and ulnar.

The median nerve passes through the carpal tunnel, a fibroosseous tunnel formed laterally by

Table 12
Muscles around the wrist: anatomy and function

Volar Surface	Origin	Insertion	Function	Innervation
Flexor digitorum superficialis	Medial epicondyle Ulnar collateral ligament Medial coronoid Proximal radius	Middle phalanges	Flexion PIP	Median nerve C7–C8
Flexor digitorum profundus	Medial olecranon Proximal ulna	Distal phalanges	Flexion DIP	2nd and 3rd median nerve 4th and 5th ulnar nerve
Flexor carpi radialis	Medial epicondyle (anteroinferior)	2nd and 3rd metacarpals	Wrist flexion (forearm pronation)	Median nerve C6–C7
Flexor carpi ulnaris	Humeral: medial epicondyle Ulnar: medial olecranon, proximal ulna	Pisiform and 5th metacarpal	Wrist flexion Ulnar deviation	Ulnar nerve C7–C8–T1
Flexor pollicis longus	Anterior proximal radius Interosseous membrane Coronoid–medial epicondyle	Base distal phalanx thumb	Flexor phalanges thumb Flexor wrist (assist)	Median nerve C8–T1
Palmaris longus	Medial epicondyle	Palmar aponeurosis	Wrist flexion	Median nerve C7–C8–T1

(continued on next page)

Table 12
(continued)

Dorsal Surface	Origin	Insertion	Function	Innervation
Extensor carpi radialis longus	Lateral supracondylar ridge	2nd metacarpal	Wrist extension	Radial nerve C6–C7
Extensor carpi radialis brevis	Lateral epicondyle (inferolateral)	3rd metacarpal	Wrist extension	PIN C6–C7
Extensor pollicis longus	Posterior middle 3rd of ulna Interosseous membrane	Base distal phalanx thumb	Extends distal phalanx thumb Extends carpometacarpal Extends interphalangeal	PIN C7–C8
Extensor digitorum	Anterolateral epicondyle	Extensor mechanism fingers	Metacarpal phalangeal joint extension	PIN C7–C8
Extensor indices	Distal posterior ulna Interosseous membrane	Joins ulnar aspect of the common extensor for 2nd digit	Extends index finger Extends wrist Extends midcarpal joints	PIN C7–C8
Extensor digiti minimi	Lateral epicondyle humerus	Joins ulnar aspect of the common extensor for 5th digit	Extends 5th digit Extends metacarpophalangeal Extends interphalangeal	PIN C7–C8
Extensor carpi ulnaris	Lateral epicondyle	5th metacarpal	Wrist extension ulnar deviation	PIN C6–C7
Radial Surface	**Origin**	**Insertion**	**Function**	**Innervation**
Abductor pollicis longus	Posterior surface ulna, radius, interosseous membrane	Base 1st metacarpal	Abducts thumb and extends it at 1st metacarpophalangeal joint	PIN C7–C8
Extensor pollicis brevis	Posterior surface radius, interosseous membrane	Base proximal phalanx thumb	Extends proximal phalanx thumb at metacarpophalangeal joint	PIN C7–C8

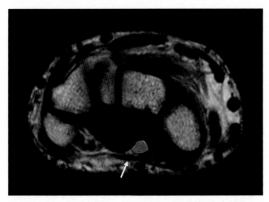

Fig. 16. Median nerve at the wrist. Axial T1-weighted image demonstrates the medial nerve in the carpal tunnel (*circled*), deep to the flexor retinaculum (*white arrow*).

the tubercles of the scaphoid and trapezium, medially by the pisiform and hook of the hamate, dorsally by the carpal bones, and volarly the flexor retinaculum (**Fig. 16**).

The ulnar nerve passes through Guyon canal, a fibroosseous tunnel formed medially by the pisiform and pisohamate, laterally by the hook of the hamate, dorsally the flexor retinaculum, and volarly the superficial transverse carpal ligament (**Fig. 17**).

SUMMARY

The anatomy of the upper limb is complex, allowing for a very wide range of movements and functionality. This article has briefly reviewed the structural components of the shoulder, elbow, and wrist, with emphasis on the stabilizing mechanisms, to set the foundations for the understanding of mechanisms and patterns of injury.

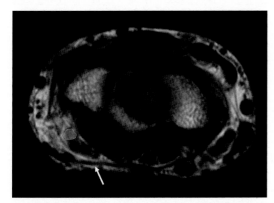

Fig. 17. Ulnar nerve at the wrist. Axial T1-weighted image demonstrates the ulnar nerve in the Guyon canal (*circled*), deep to the transverse ligament (*white arrow*).

ACKNOWLEDGMENTS

The authors would like to acknowledge the help of Arran Bird and Elena Uriel with the drawings for the artwork

REFERENCES

1. Kronberg M, Broström LA, Söderlund V. Retroversion of the humeral head in the normal shoulder and its relationship to the normal range of motion. Clin Orthop Relat Res 1990;(253):113–7.
2. Aparisi Gómez MP. Nonspinal fragility fractures. Semin Musculoskelet Radiol 2016;20(4):330–44.
3. Chang EY, Moses DA, Babb JS, et al. Shoulder impingement: objective 3D shape analysis of acromial morphologic features. Radiology 2006;239(2): 497–505.
4. Banas MP, Miller RJ, Totterman S. Relationship between the lateral acromion angle and rotator cuff disease. J Shoulder Elbow Surg 1995;4(6): 454–61.
5. Park JG, Lee JK, Phelps CT. Os acromiale associated with rotator cuff impingement: MR imaging of the shoulder. Radiology 1994;193(1):255–7.
6. Morrey BF, Itoi E, Kai-Nan A. Biomechanics of the shoulder. In: Rockwood CA Jr, Matsen FA III, editors. The shoulder, vol. I. Philadelphia: WB Saunders; 1998. p. 233–63.
7. Moor BK, Bouaicha S, Rothenfluh DA, et al. Is there an association between the individual anatomy of the scapula and the development of rotator cuff tears or osteoarthritis of the glenohumeral joint?: a radiological study of the critical shoulder angle. Bone Joint J 2013;95-B(7):935–41.
8. Bjarnison AO, Sørensen TJ, Kallemose T, et al. The critical shoulder angle is associated with osteoarthritis in the shoulder but not rotator cuff tears: a retrospective case-control study. J Shoulder Elbow Surg 2017;26(12):2097–102.
9. Beeler S, Hasler A, Götschi T, et al. The critical shoulder angle: acromial coverage is more relevant than glenoid inclination. J Orthop Res 2019;37(1): 205–10.
10. Craig EV. Fractures of the clavicle. In: Rockwood CA Jr, Matsen FA, editors. The shoulder, vol. I. Philadelphia: WB Saunders; 1998. p. 428–82.
11. Lippitt SB, Vanderhooft JE, Harris SL, et al. Glenohumeral stability from concavity-compression: a quantitative analysis. J Shoulder Elbow Surg 1993; 2:27–35.
12. Soslowsky U, Flatow EL, Bigliaoi LU, et al. Articular geometry of the glenohumeral joint. Clin Orthop 1992;285:181–90.
13. Bankart ASB. The pathology and treatment of recurrent dislocation of the shoulder joint. Br Med J 1923; 2:1132–3.

14. Pagnani M, Deng XD, Warren R, et al. Effect of lesions of the superior portion of the glenoid labrum on glenohumeral translation. J Bone Joint Surg Am 1995;77:1003–10.

15. Rao AG, Kim TK, Chronopoulos E, et al. Anatomical variants in the anterosuperior aspect of the glenoid labrum: a statistical analysis of seventy-three cases. J Bone Joint Surg Am 2003;85-A(4): 653–9.

16. Ilahi OA, Cosculluela PE, Ho DM. Classification of anterosuperior glenoid labrum variants and their association with shoulder pathology. Orthopedics 2008;31(3):226.

17. Kanatli U, Ozturk BY, Bolukbasi S. Anatomical variations of the anterosuperior labrum: prevalence and association with type II superior labrum anterior-posterior (SLAP) lesions. J Shoulder Elbow Surg 2010;19(8):1199–203.

18. Boardman ND III, Debski RE, Warner JJP, et al. Tensile properties of the superior glenohumeral ligament and coracohumeral ligaments. J Shoulder Elbow Surg 1996;5:249–54.

19. Turkel SJ, Panio MW, Marshall JL, et al. Stabilizing mechanisms preventing anterior dislocation of the glenohumeral joint. J Bone Joint Surg Am 1981;63: 1208–17.

20. Chen Q, Miller T, Padron M, et al. Normal shoulder. In: Pope TL, Bloem HL, Beltran J, et al, editors. Imaging of the musculoskeletal system. 2nd edition. Philadelphia: Saunders Elsevier; 2015. p. 70–86.

21. Terry GC, Chopp TM. Functional anatomy of the shoulder. J Athl Train 2000;35(3):248–55.

22. Grainger AJ, Tirman PF, Elliott JM, et al. MR anatomy of the subcoracoid bursa and the association of subcoracoid effusion with tears of the anterior rotator cuff and the rotator interval. AJR Am J Roentgenol 2000;174(5):1377–80.

23. McCluskey GM, Todd J. Acromioclavicular joint injuries. J South Orthop Assoc 1995;4:206–13.

24. Crowe MM, Elhassan BT. Scapular and shoulder girdle muscular anatomy: its role in periscapular tendon transfers. J Hand Surg Am 2016;41(2): 306–14.

25. Morrey BF, An KN. Functional anatomy of the elbow ligaments. Clin Orthop 1985;201:84–90.

26. Morrey BF, editor. The elbow and its disorders. Philadelphia: WB Saunders; 2000.

27. Bryce CD, Armstrong AD. Anatomy and biomechanics of the elbow. Orthop Clin North Am 2008; 39(2):141–54.

28. Sorbie C, Shiba R, Siu D, et al. The development of a surface arthroplasty for the elbow. Clin Orthop 1986; 208:100–3.

29. Aparisi F, Aparisi MP. The value of multislice computed tomography in the diagnosis of elbow fractures. Semin Musculoskelet Radiol 2013;17(5): 437–45.

30. Bazzocchi A, Aparisi Gómez MP, Bartoloni A, et al. Emergency and trauma of the elbow. Semin Musculoskelet Radiol 2017;21(3):257–81.

31. O'Driscoll SW, Morrey BF, An KN. Intraarticular pressure and capacity of the elbow. Arthroscopy 1990;6: 100–3.

32. Bucknor MD, Stevens KJ, Steinbach LS. Elbow imaging in sport: sports imaging series. Radiology 2016;279(1):12–28.

33. Binaghi D. MR imaging of the elbow. Magn Reson Imaging Clin N Am 2015;23(3):427–40.

34. Lees VC. Functional anatomy of the distal radioulnar joint in health and disease. Ann R Coll Surg Engl 2013;95(3):163–70.

35. Vezeridis PS, Yoshioka H, Han R, et al. Ulnar-sided wrist pain. Part I: anatomy and physical examination. Skeletal Radiol 2010;39(8):733–45.

36. Cerezal L, del Piñal F, Abascal F, et al. Imaging findings in ulnar-sided wrist impaction syndromes. Radiographics 2002;22(1):105–21.

37. Bonzar M, Firrell JC, Hainer M, et al. Kienbock disease and negative ulnar variance. J Bone Joint Surg Am 1998;80:1154–7.

38. D'Hoore K, De Smet L, Verellen K, et al. Negative ulnar variance is not a risk factor for Kienbock's disease. J Hand Surg Am 1994;19:229–31.

39. Metz VM, Wunderbaldinger P, Gilula LA. Update on imaging techniques of the wrist and hand. Clin Plast Surg 1996;23:369–84.

40. Palmer AK, Werner FW. The triangular fibrocartilage complex of the wrist–anatomy and function. J Hand Surg Am 1981;6(2):153–62.

41. Nakamura T, Yabe Y, Horiuchi Y. Functional anatomy of the triangular fibrocartilage complex. J Hand Surg Br 1996;21(5):581–6.

42. Thiru RG, Ferlic DC, Clayton ML, et al. Arterial anatomy of the triangular fibrocartilage of the wrist and its surgical significance. J Hand Surg Am 1986; 11(2):258–63.

43. Burns JE, Tanaka T, Ueno T, et al. Pitfalls that may mimic injuries of the triangular fibrocartilage and proximal intrinsic wrist ligaments at MR imaging. Radiographics 2011;31(1):63–78.

44. Yoshioka H, Tanaka T, Ueno T, et al. Study of ulnar variance with high-resolution MRI: correlation with triangular fibrocartilage complex and cartilage of ulnar side of wrist. J Magn Reson Imaging 2007;26(3): 714–9.

45. von Borstel D, Wang M, Small K, et al. High-resolution 3T MR imaging of the triangular fibrocartilage complex. Magn Reson Med Sci 2017;16(1): 3–15.

46. Skalski MR, White EA, Patel DB, et al. The traumatized TFCC: an illustrated review of the anatomy and injury patterns of the triangular fibrocartilage complex. Curr Probl Diagn Radiol 2016;45(1): 39–50.

47. Berger RA. The anatomy of the ligaments of the wrist and distal radioulnar joints. Clin Orthop Relat Res 2001;(383):32–40.

48. Watanabe A, Souza F, Vezeridis PS, et al. Ulnar-sided wrist pain. II. Clinical imaging and treatment. Skeletal Radiol 2010;39(9):837–57.

49. Pessis E, Drape JL, Bach F, et al. Direct arthrography of the pisotriquetral joint. AJR Am J Roentgenol 2006;186:800–4.

50. Malik AM, Schweitzer ME, Culp RW, et al. MR imaging of the type II lunate bone: frequency, extent, and associated findings. AJR Am J Roentgenol 1999; 173:335–8.

51. Pfirrmann CW, Theumann NH, Chung CB, et al. The hamatolunate facet: characterization and association with cartilage lesions-magnetic resonance arthrography and anatomic correlation in cadaveric wrists. Skeletal Radiol 2002;31(8): 451–6.

52. Imaeda T, An KN, Cooney WP III, et al. Anatomy of trapeziometacarpal ligaments. J Hand Surg Am 1993;18(2):226–31.

53. Neumann DA, Bielefeld T. The carpometacarpal joint of the thumb: stability, deformity, and therapeutic intervention. J Orthop Sports Phys Ther 2003; 33(7):386–99.

Acute Shoulder Injury

Andrew Cibulas, MD, MSME[a], Alexander Leyva, MD[a],
George Cibulas II, MD, PharmD[b], Michael Foss, BS[c], Agnieszka Boron, BS[d],
John Dennison, MD[a], Brett Gutterman, MD[a], Kimia Kani, MD[e], Jack Porrino, MD[f,g],
Laura W. Bancroft, MD[a],*, Kurt Scherer, MD[a]

KEYWORDS

- Proximal humerus fracture • Neer classification • Shoulder dislocation • Bankart lesion
- Hill-Sachs lesion • Rotator cuff tear • Biceps tendon rupture • Rockwood classification

KEY POINTS

- The management of proximal humeral fractures and acromioclavicular joint injuries are aided by accurate imaging description and classification.
- Careful imaging evaluation for concurrent bony injuries of the humeral head and glenoid should occur when a glenohumeral joint dislocation is diagnosed.
- Ultrasound examination is highly sensitive and specific for acute rotator cuff tear when performed appropriately.
- Injuries to the tendon of the long head of the biceps brachii are commonly seen in the setting of injuries to the glenoid labrum and/or rotator cuff.

INTRODUCTION

Imaging of the shoulder joint is frequently performed in the setting of trauma. The information conveyed by the radiologist to consulting physicians and surgeons is paramount in the management of acute injuries to the shoulder. Therefore, a firm grasp on the imaging findings that dictate a conservative versus operative treatment is of utmost importance. Imaging evaluation of acute injuries to the proximal humerus, glenohumeral joint, rotator cuff, long head of the biceps brachii tendon (LHBT), and acromioclavicular (AC) joint, in addition to key findings that impact orthopedic management, are detailed in this review.

PROXIMAL HUMERUS FRACTURES

Proximal humerus fractures account for 4% to 6% of all reported fractures in adults with a peak incidence in the sixth through ninth decades of life and a female predominance.[1–4] Proximal humerus fractures are typically seen with low-energy trauma in the elderly and osteoporotic patient populations and with high-energy trauma, such as motor vehicle accidents, in younger patients. Approximately 85% of proximal humeral fractures occur in those older than 50 years of age, commonly owing to falling on an outstretched hand.[1,2]

The Neer classification system of proximal humerus fractures is the most widely used system in clinical practice.[2,5] Fractures are classified by the number of displaced segments, including the greater tuberosity, lesser tuberosity, articular surface, and humeral diaphysis. Displacement of these segments is largely caused by the tensile forces produced by the rotator cuff muscles and their tendinous attachments to the proximal humerus and is present if there is either greater

[a] Department of Radiology, AdventHealth Orlando, 601 E Rollins St, Orlando, FL 32803, USA; [b] Department of Orthopaedic Surgery, University of Michigan, 1500 E Medical Center Dr, Ann Arbor, MI 48109, USA; [c] Lake Erie College of Osteopathic Medicine – Bradenton, 5000 Lakewood Ranch Blvd, Bradenton, FL 34211, USA; [d] University of Central Florida College of Medicine, 6850 Lake Nona Blvd, Orlando, FL 32827, USA; [e] University of Maryland, 22 S Greene St, Baltimore, MD 21201, USA; [f] University of Washington Medicine, Seattle, WA, USA; [g] Yale School of Medicine, 333 Cedar St, New Haven, CT 06510, USA
* Corresponding author.
E-mail address: laura.bancroft.MD@flhosp.org

Radiol Clin N Am 57 (2019) 883–896
https://doi.org/10.1016/j.rcl.2019.03.004
0033-8389/19/© 2019 Elsevier Inc. All rights reserved.

than 1 cm of separation between the fragment and the humerus or greater than 45° of angulation from its anatomic position.[5] Using these criteria, displacement fractures are categorized as either 1-part, 2-part, 3-part, or 4-part fractures and are further subdivided if dislocations or articular surface fractures are present **(Table 1)**.[3,5,6]

Table 1
The Neer classification system of proximal humerus fractures

	2 PART	3 PART	4 PART	
Anatomical Neck				
Surgical Neck				*Minimal Displacement*
Greater Tuberosity				
Lesser Tuberosity				
Fracture Dislocation *Anterior*				
Fracture Dislocation *Posterior*				*Articular surface*

Adapted from Neer CS, 2nd. Displaced proximal humeral fractures. I. Classification and evaluation. J Bone Joint Surg Am. 1970;52(6):1077-1089; with permission; and Illustrations by Valory Anne S. Vailoces, Orlando, FL; with permission.

Conventional Radiographs

Conventional radiographs are essential in the diagnosis of proximal humeral fractures, with the trauma series being the cornerstone for evaluation.[1,2] The trauma series of radiographs for the shoulder consists of 3 views: the scapular anteroposterior (AP) view, the lateral scapula view (Y) view, and the axillary view. At least 1 orthogonal view to the AP view is needed to evaluate angulation and displacement of fracture fragments; either the axillary view or the Y view is sufficient. The AP view combined with the axillary view has been shown to be superior in terms of classification accuracy.[7]

Computed Tomography Scans

Computed tomography (CT) scanning of the shoulder is sometimes indicated in the evaluation of proximal humeral fractures, particularly when the trauma series is indeterminate. Indications for CT scanning include complex fracture patterns and poor visualization of fracture lines.[1] CT scanning has also been recommended for the evaluation of rotation of fragments, the degree of tuberosity displacement, articular impression fractures, head-splitting fractures, and chronic fracture dislocations (**Figs. 1** and **2**). CT scanning has been advocated as being most useful for evaluating chronic fracture dislocations of the humeral head, allowing for the identification of the size and location of humeral head defects and secondary glenoid changes.[2]

Treatment Considerations

Management is partly guided by the Neer classification system, as well as other factors such as patient age, functional status, bone density, and other comorbidities.[1,3] Nonoperative management is typically used in 1-part, minimally displaced fractures.[2,3,8] Two-part and 3-part fractures may be treated operatively or nonoperatively depending on fracture displacement and angulation at the fracture site. It is important to make note of any concurrent glenohumeral dislocation in a 3-part fracture, because this factor will have implications for the type of surgery pursued.[3] Four-part fractures are the most severe and are generally treated with surgical intervention. They carry a high risk of avascular necrosis owing to disruption of the anterior humeral circumflex artery.[2,5] Valgus impaction in a 4-part fracture should also be noted owing to a decreased incidence of avascular necrosis compared with the classic 4-part fracture.[9]

SHOULDER DISLOCATION

The most commonly dislocated large joint in the human body is the glenohumeral joint. Acute dislocations of the glenohumeral joint are surgical

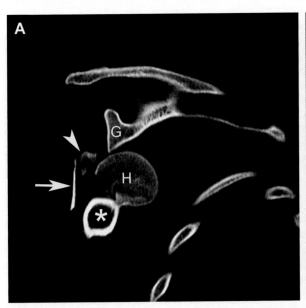
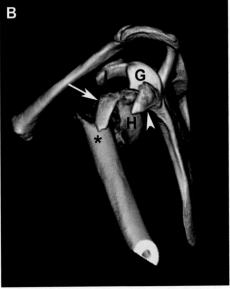

Fig. 1. A 32-year-old woman with a proximal humeral fracture dislocation after a motorcycle accident. A coronal oblique CT reformatted scan (*A*) and 3-dimensional surface rendered (*B*) images of the right shoulder demonstrate an acute Neer 3-part fracture of the proximal humerus with an anteroinferior, subcoracoid glenohumeral dislocation and displaced fragments of the greater tuberosity (*arrowhead*) and neck (*arrow*). G, glenoid; H, humerus. *Proximal diaphysis.

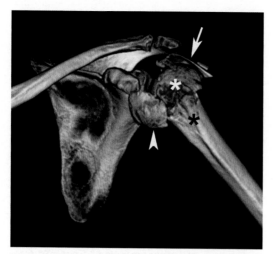

Fig. 2. A 48-year-old woman with a Neer 4-part fracture after a fall. A 3-dimensional surface rendered CT image of the left shoulder demonstrates an acute, Neer 4-part fracture of the proximal humerus. Fracture planes divide the humeral head (*white asterisk*) from the diaphysis (*black asterisk*), greater tuberosity (*arrow*), and lesser tuberosity (*arrowhead*).

emergencies which call for prompt management to increase the probability of achieving a stable reduction.[10] Glenohumeral joint dislocations are described based on the position of the humeral head in relation to the glenoid.

Anterior glenohumeral joint dislocations account for up to 95% of all glenohumeral joint dislocations and are most frequently caused by forceful abduction and external rotation of the shoulder secondary to trauma.[3,10,11] Posterior glenohumeral joint dislocations are responsible for 2% to 4% of glenohumeral joint dislocations and are the result of the humeral head being forced posteriorly while the humerus is internally rotated.[3,12] Inferior glenohumeral joint dislocation, known as luxatio erecta humeri, is the least common, occurring less than 1% of the time, and is caused by axial loading of an abducted humerus or traumatic hyperabduction.[13]

Conventional Radiographs

A standard AP radiograph is obtained in conjunction with an additional view, which may be axial, axial oblique, or Y view. Assessment of the degree and direction of dislocation is achieved using the Y view. Axial oblique images allow for the patient to keep the injured shoulder stationary; however, they do not provide a second view of the scapula, which may be indicated if scapular fracture is a concern.[10,11] Confirmation of glenohumeral joint dislocation is achieved by recognition of the

humeral head lying anterior, posterior, or inferior to the glenoid fossa.

Computed Tomography Scans

Additional trauma to the proximal humerus and glenoid tubercle is often seen on conventional radiography, which warrants further evaluation by CT scans. Fracture of the greater tuberosity of the humerus can be caused by shearing forces or avulsion as the humerus is displaced. Additionally, in anterior glenohumeral dislocation, a V-shaped impression deformity can be caused by impaction of the posterosuperior humeral head by the anterior aspect of the glenoid, known as a Hill-Sachs lesion, and fracture of the anteroinferior corner of the glenoid, known as a bony Bankart lesion, can also be seen (**Figs. 3–7**). Similarly, in patients who have suffered a posterior glenohumeral dislocation, impression of the anteromedial aspect of the humeral head by the posterior aspect of the glenoid is known as a reverse Hill-Sachs lesion, and fracture of the posteroinferior corner of the glenoid is known as a reverse bony Bankart lesion (**Figs. 8–10**).[3,11]

MR Imaging

MR imaging in the setting of glenohumeral dislocation is often of little clinical benefit, because concurrent rotator cuff and/or glenoid labral injuries may be unrelated to the glenohumeral dislocation given the prevalence of preexisting asymptomatic

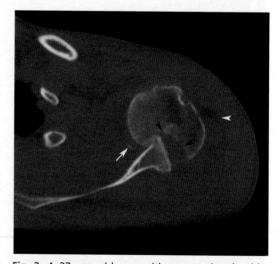

Fig. 3. A 27-year-old-man with an anterior shoulder dislocation. An axial CT scan of the left shoulder demonstrates an anterior glenohumeral dislocation with a large Hill-Sachs lesion (*black arrowheads*) engaged onto the glenoid rim and a small, linear medially displaced osseous Bankart lesion (*arrow*). Lipohemarthrosis is also visualized (*white arrowhead*).

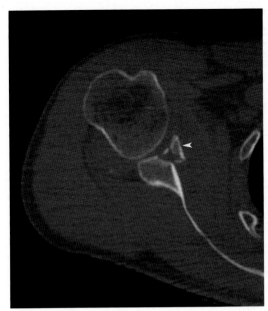

Fig. 4. A 38-year-old man with an anterior shoulder dislocation–relocation injury after a mountain biking accident. An axial CT scan of the right shoulder demonstrates a minimally displaced, comminuted osseous Bankart lesion (*arrowhead*).

rotator cuff and glenoid disease in the elderly and athletic patient populations.[3,10,12,13]

Treatment Considerations

Conventional radiographs of the shoulder must be obtained before reduction is attempted owing

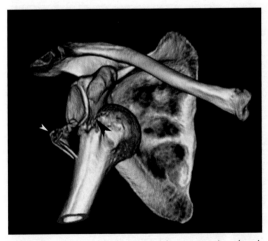

Fig. 5. A 58-year-old woman with an anterior shoulder fracture dislocation after fall. A 3-dimensional surface rendered CT reformation image shows an anterior shoulder dislocation with Hill-Sachs lesion (*black arrowhead*) and displaced lateral humeral head and greater tuberosity fragments (*white arrowhead*).

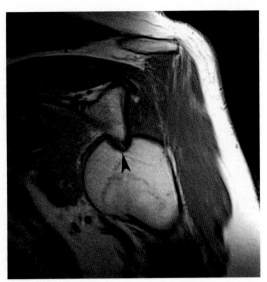

Fig. 6. A 67-year-old man with an anterior shoulder dislocation after a fall. A coronal T1-weighted MR image of the left shoulder shows an anterior shoulder dislocation with an engaged Hill-Sachs lesion (*arrowhead*) abutting the anteroinferior glenoid.

to the possibility of concurrent humeral head or glenoid fracture. Postreduction CT scans and/or MR imaging is often used to aid in surgical planning and evaluation of acute injuries to the rotator cuff, glenoid labrum, capsular glenohumeral ligaments, and neurovascular structures that impact the long-term stability of the glenohumeral joint.

When describing Hill-Sachs and reverse Hill-Sachs lesions, the involvement of the humeral head should be discussed. A Hill-Sachs lesion affecting less than 20% of the humeral head is usually not clinically significant; conversely, an injury affecting more than 40% of the humeral head is almost always clinically significant, which contributes to joint instability and recurrent injury. Reverse Hill-Sachs lesions that affect up to 25% of the humeral head are treated with closed reduction if stable and acute. When a reverse Hill-Sachs lesion affects more than 25% of the humeral head, operative management is considered with a preference for shoulder arthroplasty when more than 50% of the humeral head is involved.[3]

ACUTE ROTATOR CUFF TEAR

The rotator cuff is responsible for the stabilization and function of the shoulder joint and is composed of the muscles and tendons of the supraspinatus, infraspinatus, teres minor, and subscapularis muscles. Rotator cuff tears are a commonly seen injury of the shoulder, and chronic tears are more prevalent than acute tears.[14,15] Owing to the traumatic

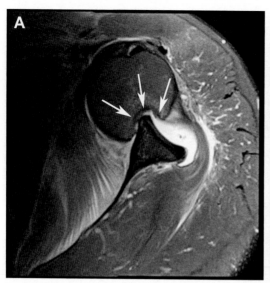

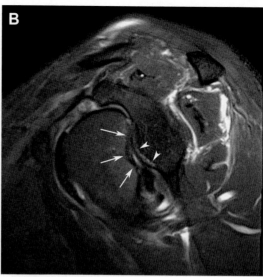

Fig. 7. A 44-year-old man with a new-onset seizure disorder and an anterior shoulder dislocation. Axial proton density (*A*) and sagittal T2-weighted (*B*) MR images demonstrate anterior shoulder dislocation with large, engaged Hill-Sachs lesion (*arrows*) abutting the anteroinferior glenoid lesion (*arrowheads*).

nature of acute rotator cuff tears they are often overlooked while excluding other injuries to the shoulder and most frequently remain unnoticed after a dislocated shoulder has been reduced. Pain often limits the complete clinical evaluation of the shoulder joint after traumatic injury; therefore, imaging is often needed for further assessment.[14]

Conventional Radiographs

Conventional radiographs of the shoulder are usually unremarkable in patients with an acute rotator cuff tear. If an active abduction view of the shoulder is taken, in which the patient abducts the shoulder to 90°, a decreased acromiohumeral distance (<2 mm) can be seen in acute rotator cuff tear.[15]

Ultrasound Examination

Ultrasound imaging of the shoulder is both a cost-efficient and cost-effective method of evaluation, with 91% sensitivity and 85% specificity for a diagnosis of rotator cuff tear when performed

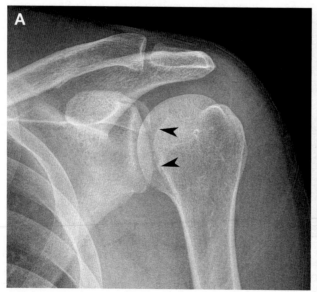

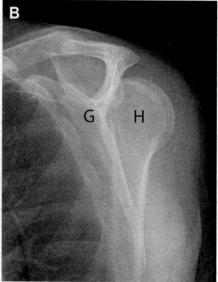

Fig. 8. A 36-year-old man with a posterior shoulder dislocation. AP (*A*) and Y-view (*B*) radiographs of the left shoulder demonstrate posterior glenohumeral dislocation with demonstration of the "trough sign" (*arrowheads*) owing to reverse Hill-Sachs lesion. G, glenoid; H, humeral head.

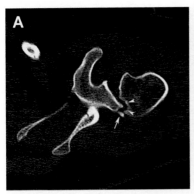
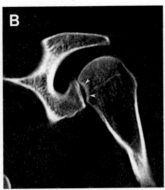
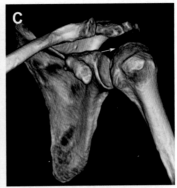

Fig. 9. A 46-year-old woman with a posterior shoulder dislocation. Axial (*A*) and coronal (*B*) 2-dimensional refor-matted and 3-dimensional surface-rendered (*C*) CT images demonstrate posterior glenohumeral dislocation (*arrow*) with an engaged reverse Hill-Sachs lesion (*arrowheads*).

appropriately. Ultrasound images of each of the rotator cuff tendons, the long head of the biceps tendon, and the posterior glenohumeral joint are obtained in a complete shoulder ultrasound examination.[14,15]

Rotator cuff tears are classified as full thickness or partial thickness. A complete tear is a full-thickness tear that is also full width. In full-thickness tears, fluid replaces the area of torn tendon extending from the bursal surface to the articular surface, causing a hypoechoic or anechoic defect and accentuation of the underlying cartilage (**Fig. 11**). Full-thickness tears of the supraspinatus can manifest in retraction of the

tendon under the AC joint, which results in nonvisualization. Partial thickness tears are seen as focal hypoechoic or anechoic lesions in the tendon that only involve the bursal or articular surface, which should be confirmed by imaging in 2 perpendicular planes.[15]

MR Imaging

MR imaging allows for reliable evaluation of the tendons and muscles of the rotator cuff, with 98% sensitivity and 79% specificity for acute rotator cuff tear (**Fig. 12**).[14,16] Complete tears are most readily identified using MR imaging compared with full-thickness tears. Areas of the tendon defect that have been replaced by fluid will be identified as hyperintense signal on T2-weighted, fat-suppressed, and gradient echo sequences, and represent the most direct finding of a rotator cuff tear.

If muscle atrophy and fatty replacement of the muscles are seen, they suggest chronic rotator cuff tear, and the amount of atrophy present

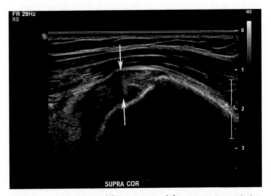

Fig. 10. A 62-year-old woman with a recurrent posterior shoulder dislocation. Axial proton density MR image demonstrates a right posterior glenohumeral dislocation with an engaged reverse Hill-Sachs lesion (*arrowheads*) and extensive surrounding soft tissue edema.

Fig. 11. A 77-year-old woman with an acute rotator cuff tear. A coronal gray scale ultrasound image of the right shoulder demonstrates a full-thickness supraspinatus tendon (*arrows*) involving the critical zone, without displacement of the fibers.

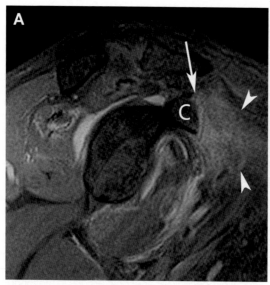

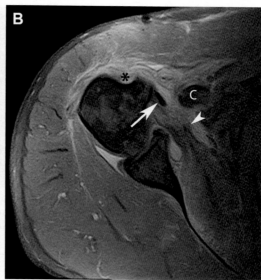

Fig. 12. A 57-year-old man with a coracoid fracture, dislocated biceps, and a subscapularis tendon tear. (*A*) A sagittal T2-weighted image shows a fracture (*arrow*) through the coracoid (C) with marked adjacent soft tissue swelling (*arrowheads*). (*B*) An axial proton density MR image demonstrates the displaced coracoid process fracture fragment (C), empty bicipital groove (*asterisk*), medially dislocated long head of the biceps tendon (*arrow*), and adjacent retracted full-thickness tear of the subscapularis tendon (*arrowhead*).

should be quantified.[17,18] Specific findings that favor an acute rotator cuff tear include muscular edema and a wavy or "kinked" appearance of the retracted, proximally torn tendon (**Fig. 13**). The extent of tendon retraction and/or the presence of bone bruising cannot reliably be used to determine the acuity of the injury.[16]

Treatment Considerations

The most important factors to discuss while evaluating rotator cuff tears include the size and location of the tear, associated rotator cuff muscle atrophy, concurrent dislocation or rupture of the LHBT, bony abnormalities of the coracoacromial arch, and arthrosis of the glenohumeral joint.[19] These factors have management implications and can aid in differentiating acute and chronic rotator cuff tears, which is often difficult owing to the prevalence of chronic rotator cuff tears in older patient populations.[15] Whenever possible, a review of the patient history and mechanism of injury is recommended while reviewing imaging.[16] This step is especially important in younger patients, because prompt surgical repair often leads to significant improvement in pain and function and return to normal occupation.[14]

TENDON OF THE LONG HEAD OF THE BICEPS BRACHII INJURY

Injuries of the LHBT are a common cause of shoulder pain and generally occur in concurrence

with additional shoulder injuries such as superior labral anterior and posterior tears of the glenoid labrum and supraspinatus tendon tears. This results in limited clinical evaluation and increases the difficulty of radiographic diagnosis.[20,21] LHBT rupture is much more common than ruptures of the short head or distal biceps tendon, representing up to 97% of all biceps brachii

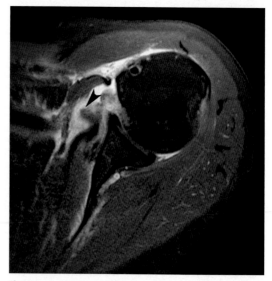

Fig. 13. A 69-year-old woman with a rotator cuff tear after a fall. Axial proton-density MR image of the left shoulder demonstrates acute rupture of the distal subscapularis tendon (*arrowhead*) with medial retraction to the level of the glenohumeral joint.

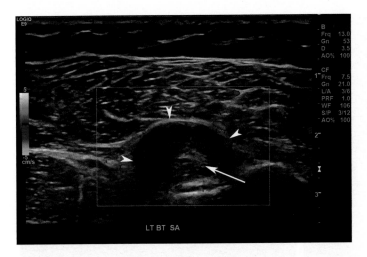

Fig. 14. A 59-year-old woman with LHBT tendinosis and tenosynovitis. Transverse ultrasound image of the left long head of the biceps tendon demonstrates fluid (*arrowheads*) surrounding the mildly thickened and heterogeneous long head of the biceps tendon (*arrow*), consistent with chronic tendinosis.

injuries. Patients older than the age of 50 are predisposed to LHBT tears owing to chronic biceps tendinitis (**Fig. 14**) leading to degeneration of the biceps tendon and subsequent rupture with little to no trauma.[21,22] Most imaging modalities have low sensitivity for properly evaluating LHBT injuries.[20,23]

Ultrasound Examination

The use of ultrasound imaging to detect LHBT tears is a cost-effective tool and is concomitantly performed during the evaluation of the rotator cuff. When performed appropriately, ultrasound examination has been found to be reliable for diagnosis of complete LHBT tears, biceps dislocation, and subluxation, but has not been found to be reliable for the diagnosis of partial-thickness tears or tendinosis.[22,24] The absence of a fibrillar pattern of the tendon on ultrasound imaging can be caused by degeneration, dislocation, or rupture. Acute rupture results in the empty

groove sign, which is an indication of retraction of the tendon (**Fig. 15**).[25]

MR Imaging

MR imaging is generally reserved for inconclusive ultrasound results. Both MR imaging and MR arthrography can used to evaluate the LHBT and other concurrent injuries. The advantage of MR arthrography is more accurate evaluation of the intraarticular LHBT, as well as an increased sensitivity for detection of additional pathology. Features that aid in the diagnosis of LHBT rupture include absence of the tendon secondary to retraction and the tendon sheath full of fluid signal intensity (**Fig. 16**).[24]

Treatment Considerations

Most LHBT ruptures are treated conservatively with pain relief, physical therapy, and exercise, because there is generally little loss of function. Surgery is considered if the patient has failed

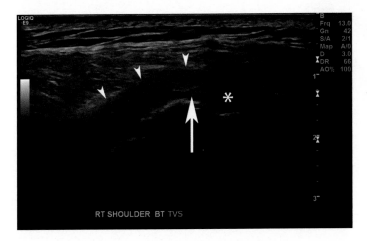

Fig. 15. A 69-year-old man with a medial biceps tendon subluxation. A transverse gray scale ultrasound image of the right shoulder demonstrates mild, medial subluxation of the biceps tendon (*arrow*) insinuating into the deep fibers of the subscapularis tendon (*arrowheads*) and an empty bicipital groove (*asterisk*).

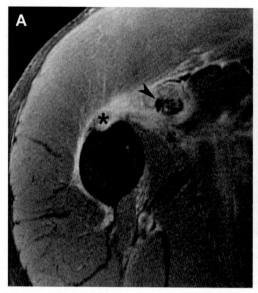 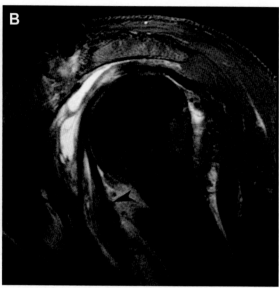

Fig. 16. A 62-year-old man with a biceps tendon dislocation and split tear. Axial proton density (*A*) and sagittal T2-weighted (*B*) MR images demonstrate a dislocated biceps tendon with longitudinal split tearing and tendinosis (*arrowheads*), empty bicipital groove (*asterisk*), and adjacent soft tissue swelling.

conservative treatment, is an athlete, performs manual labor, or if poor cosmetic outcome is a concern. It is important to fully evaluate the labrum for a coexisting superior labral anterior and posterior tears because surgical intervention will also be considered depending on the extent of the injury. If LHBT tears are left entirely untreated, bicep tendon tears can result in complete rupture.[21,24]

ACROMIOCLAVICULAR JOINT INJURY

Separations of the AC joint encompass up to 12% of dislocations involving the shoulder.[26,27] AC joint injuries are seen most commonly in males in the

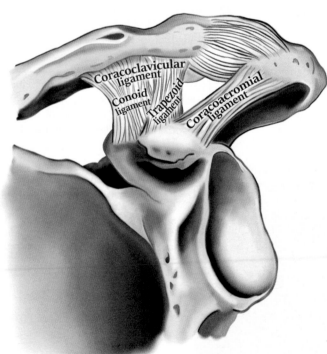

Fig. 17. CC and coracoacromial ligaments. Schematic depiction of the conoid and trapezoid ligaments, which combine to form the CC ligament (primary stabilizer of the AC joint). (*Courtesy of* Valory Anne S. Vailoces, Orlando, FL; with permission.)

Table 2
Summary of the Rockwood classification of AC separation

TYPE 1	**AC Ligament** Sprain or partial tear **CC Ligament** Intact **Trapezius & Deltoid Clavicular Attachments** Intact **Radiography** Often normal	**TYPE II**	**AC Ligament** Torn **CC Ligament** Sprain **Trapezius & Deltoid Clavicular Attachments** Intact or minimally detached **Radiography** Wide AC joint with normal or slightly increased CC distance
TYPE III	**AC Ligament** Torn **CC Ligament** Torn **Trapezius & Deltoid Clavicular Attachments** Distal trapezius & deltoid may be torn **Radiography** Wide AC & CC joints; superior position of distal clavicle; 25-100% increase in the coracoclavicular distance	**TYPE IV**	**AC Ligament** Torn **CC Ligament** Torn **Trapezius & Deltoid Clavicular Attachments** Torn trapezius or button-holed clavicle posteriorly **Radiography** Distal clavicle posterior to acromion on the axillary lateral view
TYPE V	**AC Ligament** Torn **CC Ligament** Torn **Trapezius & Deltoid Clavicular Attachments** Distal trapezius & deltoid torn **Radiography** Superiorly displaced clavicle; 100-300% increase in CC distance	**TYPE VI**	**AC Ligament** Torn **CC Ligament** Torn **Trapezius & Deltoid Clavicular Attachments** Distal trapezius & deltoid torn **Radiography** Distal clavicle inferior to acromion or coracoid

Data from Refs.[25,26,29]; and Illustrations by Valory Anne S. Vailoces, Orlando, FL; with permission.

third decade of life, typically with a history of contact sports or overhead manual labor. Acute injury results from forceful trauma to the acromion with the shoulder in the adducted position or a fall on an outstretched hand.[26–29]

A predictable pattern of injury to the structures that comprise the joint has been described beginning with disruption of the AC ligaments, followed by joint capsule, coracoclavicular (CC) ligaments, and finally the deltotrapezial fascia (**Fig. 17**).[26] Injury severity is most commonly graded with imaging using the Rockwood classification (**Table 2**).[27,30]

Conventional Radiographs

Simultaneous frontal views of both shoulders are acquired, and AC/CC interval measurements are compared between the injured and uninjured

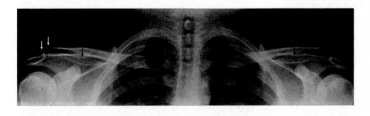

Fig. 18. A type II AC joint separation in 25-year-old man. AP radiograph of the AC joints reveals a type II separation of the left AC joint. There is mild asymmetric widening of the left AC joint and less than 50% superior displacement of the left distal clavicle, without widening of the left CC interval. Because the superior surface of a normal AC joint may be incongruent (*white arrows*), the congruency of the inferior surface of the AC joint is assessed on radiographs to rule out AC joint subluxation. The conoid tubercles (*black arrows*) are the sites of attachment for the conoid ligament.

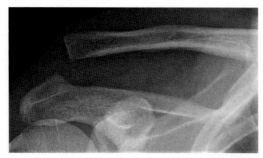

Fig. 19. A type V AC joint separation in a 21-year-old man. An AP radiograph of the right clavicle demonstrates more than 100% superior displacement of the distal clavicle, with tenting of the skin and widening of the CC interval.

side to assess for vertical instability. Imaging of the bilateral AC joints is preferable as a result of the anatomic variation inherent to this joint (**Fig. 18**).[26,27,29] The x-ray beam is positioned with a 10° to 15° cephalic tilt (Zanca view) providing optimal visualization of the AC joint by preventing superimposition of the joint with the adjacent proximal acromion/scapular spine.[26,27]

An AC interval that is greater than 6 to 7 mm or that is asymmetrically wider than the normal AC joint by 2 to 3 mm is considered abnormal (**Fig. 19**). The normal CC interval is considered to be 11 to 13 mm; a 5-mm discrepancy of the affected CC interval from the contralateral asymptomatic side is considered abnormal.[26-29]

The Rockwood classification relies on the Zanca view and an axillary view, with the axillary view obtained to assess for possible grade IV injury. The radiographic analysis of AC joint separations is reproducible in the vertical plane, which aids in the diagnosis of Rockwood grade II, III, and V injuries. Radiographic analysis of the AC joint in the horizontal plane does not have reliable

reproducibility and should not be used to make a diagnosis of Rockwood grade IV injuries.[30] Axillary or lateral views can be acquired to assess for posterior displacement of the clavicle and horizontal instability, seen with the Rockwood grade IV injury.[27,30]

The use of weighted stress views may theoretically be used to aid in distinguishing a Rockwood grade II and III injury by accentuating the AC and CC intervals; however, it is seldom useful in unmasking Rockwood grade III injuries that were not already apparent.[4,26-28] This method is also painful, more expensive, and requires additional radiation exposure.[4]

MR Imaging

Although not routinely performed in the context of AC joint separation, MR imaging has been shown to upgrade the clinical grade of injury. MR imaging will demonstrate varying degrees of edema and hemorrhage involving the soft tissue and bone marrow, as well as variable severity of injury to the AC and CC ligaments, as indicated by attenuation, disruption, edema, or hemorrhage of the ligaments (**Fig. 20**).[27]

Treatment Considerations

Treatment of AC separation is contingent on the grade of the injury. Generally, acute Rockwood grade I and II injuries are managed conservatively. There is no consensus management for grade III injury, with both conservative and surgical management used, and influential factors including failure of a trial of conservative therapy and patient activity level. Rockwood grades IV, V, and VI injuries typically require surgery. A Rockwood type IV injury can result in injury to the ipsilateral brachial plexus and adjacent vascular structures from posterior displacement of the clavicle.[26] The

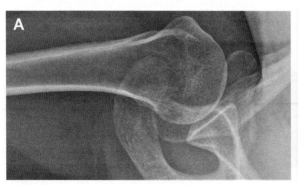
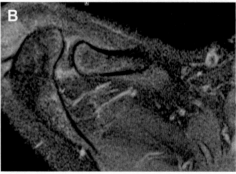

Fig. 20. Poor accuracy of the axillary view in the diagnosis of horizontal AC joint instability. An axillary view of the right AC joint (*A*) in a 38-year-old woman demonstrates an apparent type IV AC joint separation. (*B*) Axial proton density MR imaging, however, reveals a normal right AC joint.

preferred method of reconstruction varies based on surgeon and injury grade.[26,27]

SUMMARY

Acute shoulder injuries are commonly encountered by radiologists in everyday practice. The surgical approach and management varies between institutions and surgeons; therefore, it is imperative that radiologists accurately recognize and concisely report key findings that will aid in the stratification of patients between operative and conservative management.

ACKNOWLEDGMENTS

We would like to acknowledge the contribution of Valory Anne S. Vailoces for the illustrations.

REFERENCES

1. Schumaier A, Grawe B. Proximal humerus fractures: evaluation and management in the elderly patient. Geriatr Orthop Surg Rehabil 2018;9. 2151458517750516.

2. Zuckerman JD, Sahajpal DT. Fractures of the proximal humerus: classification, diagnosis, and nonoperative management. In: Iannotti JP, Williams GRJ, editors. Disorders of the shoulder: diagnosis and management. Philadelphia: Lippincott Williams & Wilkins; 2007. p. 841–68.

3. Sandstrom CK, Kennedy SA, Gross JA. Acute shoulder trauma: what the surgeon wants to know. Radiographics 2015;35(2):475–92.

4. Foroohar A, Tosti R, Richmond JM, et al. Classification and treatment of proximal humerus fractures: inter-observer reliability and agreement across imaging modalities and experience. J Orthop Surg Res 2011;6:38.

5. Carofino BC, Leopold SS. Classifications in brief: the Neer classification for proximal humerus fractures. Clin Orthop Relat Res 2013;471(1):39–43.

6. Neer CS 2nd. Displaced proximal humeral fractures. I. Classification and evaluation. J Bone Joint Surg Am 1970;52(6):1077–89.

7. Bahrs C, Rolauffs B, Sudkamp NP, et al. Indications for computed tomography (CT-) diagnostics in proximal humeral fractures: a comparative study of plain radiography and computed tomography. BMC Musculoskelet Disord 2009;10:33.

8. Slobogean GP, Johal H, Lefaivre KA, et al. A scoping review of the proximal humerus fracture literature. BMC Musculoskelet Disord 2015;16:112.

9. Brorson S, Bagger J, Sylvest A, et al. Diagnosing displaced four-part fractures of the proximal humerus: a review of observer studies. Int Orthop 2009; 33(2):323–7.

10. Cutts S, Prempeh M, Drew S. Anterior shoulder dislocation. Ann R Coll Surg Engl 2009;91(1):2–7.

11. Raby N, Hughes PM, Ricketts J. Appendicular and pelvic trauma. In: Grainger AJ, O'Connor P, editors. Grainger & Allison's diagnostic radiology: the musculoskeletal system. 6th edition. London: Elsevier; 2016. p. 183–6.

12. Gor DM. The trough line sign. Radiology 2002; 224(2):485–6.

13. Hassanzadeh E, Chang CY, Huang AJ, et al. CT and MRI manifestations of luxatio erecta humeri and a review of the literature. Clin Imaging 2015;39(5): 876–9.

14. Craig R, Holt T, Rees JL. Acute rotator cuff tears. BMJ 2017;359:j5366.

15. Moosikasuwan JB, Miller TT, Burke BJ. Rotator cuff tears: clinical, radiographic, and US findings. Radiographics 2005;25(6):1591–607.

16. Loew M, Magosch P, Lichtenberg S, et al. How to discriminate between acute traumatic and chronic degenerative rotator cuff lesions: an analysis of specific criteria on radiography and magnetic resonance imaging. J Shoulder Elbow Surg 2015; 24(11):1685–93.

17. Fuchs B, Weishaupt D, Zanetti M, et al. Fatty degeneration of the muscles of the rotator cuff: assessment by computed tomography versus magnetic resonance imaging. J Shoulder Elbow Surg 1999;8(6): 599–605.

18. Stoller DW, Fritz RC. Magnetic resonance imaging of impingement and rotator cuff tears. Magn Reson Imaging Clin N Am 1993;1(1):47–63.

19. Campbell RSD, Dunn AJ, McNally E, et al. Internal derangements of joints: upper and lower limbs. In: Grainger AJ, O'Connor P, editors. Grainger & Allison's diagnostic radiology: the musculoskeletal system. 6th edition. London: Elsevier; 2016. p. 24–9.

20. De Maeseneer M, Boulet C, Pouliart N, et al. Assessment of the long head of the biceps tendon of the shoulder with 3T magnetic resonance arthrography and CT arthrography. Eur J Radiol 2012;81(5):934–9.

21. Elser F, Braun S, Dewing CB, et al. Anatomy, function, injuries, and treatment of the long head of the biceps brachii tendon. Arthroscopy 2011;27(4): 581–92.

22. Gibbons L'. A torn shoulder': an emergency department case study. Int Emerg Nurs 2016;25:71–5.

23. Armstrong A, Teefey SA, Wu T, et al. The efficacy of ultrasound in the diagnosis of long head of the biceps tendon pathology. J Shoulder Elbow Surg 2006;15(1):7–11.

24. Mellano CR, Shin JJ, Yanke AB, et al. Disorders of the long head of the biceps tendon. Instr Course Lect 2015;64:567–76.

25. Ptasznik R, Hennessy O. Abnormalities of the biceps tendon of the shoulder: sonographic findings. AJR Am J Roentgenol 1995;164(2):409–14.

26. Kim AC, Matcuk G, Patel D, et al. Acromioclavicular joint injuries and reconstructions: a review of expected imaging findings and potential complications. Emerg Radiol 2012;19(5):399–413.

27. Alyas F, Curtis M, Speed C, et al. MR imaging appearances of acromioclavicular joint dislocation. Radiographics 2008;28(2):463–79 [quiz: 619].

28. Ha AS, Petscavage-Thomas JM, Tagoylo GH. Acromioclavicular joint: the other joint in the shoulder. AJR Am J Roentgenol 2014;202(2): 375–85.

29. Bossart PJ, Joyce SM, Manaster BJ, et al. Lack of efficacy of 'weighted' radiographs in diagnosing acute acromioclavicular separation. Ann Emerg Med 1988;17(1):20–4.

30. Gastaud O, Raynier JL, Duparc F, et al. Reliability of radiographic measurements for acromioclavicular joint separations. Orthop Traumatol Surg Res 2015; 101(8 Suppl):S291–5.

Overuse Injuries of the Shoulder

Hailey Allen, MD[a,*], Brian Y. Chan, MD[a], Kirkland W. Davis, MD[b],
Donna G. Blankenbaker, MD[b]

KEYWORDS

• Shoulder • Overuse • Impingement • Rotator cuff • Biceps tendon

KEY POINTS

- Shoulder overuse injuries are common and affect younger patients disproportionately; recognition of these injuries is important to maintain function and quality of life.
- The shoulder is supported by static and dynamic stabilizers, which allow a wide range of motion but make the joint prone to repetitive injury.
- Impingement syndromes are common in the overhead thrower, both due to motion at the extreme limits of normal and underlying predisposing anatomic factors.
- Skeletally immature patients are vulnerable to repetitive stress on a relatively weak proximal humeral physis, leading to unique patterns of injury.
- Overuse injuries represent a degenerative rather than inflammatory process; however, these may respond to conservative measures, such as image-guided corticosteroid injection and physical therapy.

INTRODUCTION

The glenohumeral joint is the most mobile joint in the body. The shoulder is stabilized by soft tissue structures, including the rotator cuff, joint capsule and glenohumeral ligaments, glenoid labrum, and the long head of the biceps brachii tendon (LHBT). Secondary structures, such as the bursae about the pectoral girdle, also assist with shoulder function. These soft tissue structures are uniquely susceptible to injury in athletes and normally active adults. In addition, the normal biomechanics of the shoulder expose the involved osseous structures to repetitive stresses that ultimately can manifest as shoulder pain.

This article discusses the various manifestations of overuse injuries in the shoulder, including those of the rotator cuff, LHBT, bursae, proximal humerus (Little Leaguer's shoulder), and distal clavicle. It discusses underlying structural abnormalities and biomechanics at the extreme ranges of normal motion that can lead to overuse injuries in the young athlete.

PRINCIPAL ANATOMY AND BIOMECHANICS OF THE SHOULDER

The shoulder is optimized for maximal range of motion, which comes at the expense of mechanical stability, depending primarily on tendinous and ligamentous underpinnings rather than osseous support structures. The glenoid provides a relatively small and shallow fossa for the humeral head.[1] The joint relies on coordination of both

Disclosure Statement: Dr K.W. Davis and Dr D.G. Blankenbaker are consultants for and receive royalties from Elsevier. Dr H. Allen and Dr B.Y. Chan have no disclosures.
[a] Department of Radiology and Imaging Sciences, University of Utah School of Medicine, 30 North 1900 East #1A071, Salt Lake City, UT 84132-2140, USA; [b] Department of Radiology, University of Wisconsin School of Medicine and Public Health, E3/366 Clinical Science Center, 600 Highland Avenue, Madison, WI 53792-3252, USA
* Corresponding author.
E-mail address: hailey.allen@hsc.utah.edu

Radiol Clin N Am 57 (2019) 897–909
https://doi.org/10.1016/j.rcl.2019.03.003
0033-8389/19/© 2019 Elsevier Inc. All rights reserved.

static and dynamic stabilizers. Static soft tissue stabilizers of the glenohumeral joint include the glenoid labrum, glenohumeral ligaments, and the joint capsule.[2] The fibrocartilaginous labrum extends around the glenoid rim and both deepens the glenoid and centers the humeral head with respect to the glenoid throughout its range of motion. The glenohumeral ligaments are focal thickenings of the glenohumeral joint capsule. The superior glenohumeral ligament stabilizes the anterosuperior aspect of the joint and the LHBT. The middle glenohumeral ligament resists anterior translation and abduction of the humerus. The inferior glenohumeral ligament (IGHL) is the most important passive stabilizer of the joint and resists humeral head dislocation with shoulder abduction and at the extremes of glenohumeral rotation.

The dynamic stabilizers of the shoulder include the rotator cuff tendons and the LHBT.[2] Coordinated contraction of the rotator cuff maintains humeral head centering and drives external and internal rotation of the shoulder.[3] The LHBT contributes to stability of the anterior and superior aspects of the joint.[2] The supraspinatus, subscapularis, and LHBT pass beneath the coracoacromial arch, which comprises the coracoid process, the acromion, and the intervening coracoacromial ligament. The structures of the coracoacromial arch and acromioclavicular joint are additional passive stabilizers of the superior glenohumeral joint.

LONG HEAD OF THE BICEPS TENDON INJURIES

The LHBT originates from the supraglenoid tubercle and superior labrum. It courses through the glenohumeral joint, supported by the biceps pulley complex within the rotator interval, before adopting an extraarticular position within the bicipital groove. The short head of the biceps has a relatively strong muscular attachment to the coracoid process,[4] and the weaker long head proximal attachment accounts for 96% of injuries to the biceps tendon.[5,6] The exact function of the LHBT remains unknown and has been postulated to be a humeral head depressor, a dynamic stabilizer of the glenohumeral joint, and a vestigial structure in humans.[2]

Injuries of the LHBT fall along a spectrum of tenosynovitis, tendinopathy, and partial or complete biceps tendon rupture. Overuse injuries of the LHBT usually occur in young athletes and older overhead manual laborers.[7] Baseball pitching is the most frequently associated activity, and other overhead sports such as tennis, swimming, and volleyball have also been implicated.

Degeneration of the LHBT is commonly associated with supraspinatus tendinopathy.[8] The LHBT can also subluxate or dislocate out of the bicipital groove, even in the absence of subscapularis tears if there is an injury to the biceps pulley complex.[9]

Tendinopathy may manifest as increased signal intensity or expansion of the LHBT, although the curved orientation of the LHBT introduces difficulties in interpretation secondary to magic angle and volume averaging artifacts (Fig. 1). Partial and longitudinal split tears demonstrate abnormal increased signal extending to the tendon surface, and an empty bicipital groove in the absence of prior tenotomy represents complete rupture.

Primary biceps tenosynovitis is uncommon and likely due to increased biomechanical stress provoked by variant anatomy of the bicipital groove.[10] Biceps tenosynovitis is more often secondary to other abnormalities such as rotator cuff tendinopathy or subacromial impingement. Fluid in the biceps tendon sheath, particularly if the tendon is morphologically normal, most often reflects decompression of glenohumeral joint fluid. MR imaging findings that suggest tenosynovitis include tendon thickening greater than 5 mm, increased intratendinous signal, fluid in the tendon sheath without concomitant glenohumeral joint fluid, and synovial enhancement.[11] Evidence of adhesions, such as intrasheath hypointense septa or eccentric positioning of the tendon within the sheath, also suggests tenosynovitis. Ultrasound (US) may show fluid and debris distending the tendon sheath or hyperemia on color Doppler imaging (Fig. 2).

Nonoperative treatment of symptoms attributed to the LHBT includes rest, physical therapy, and corticosteroid injection of the tendon sheath. Debridement can be performed if tendon fraying measures less than 30% to 50% in thickness.[12] Tenodesis is typically reserved for younger patients, with advantages including better cosmesis, increased strength in supination, and increased elbow flexion.[13,14] Tenotomy is easier to perform with rapid rehabilitation times; however, the loss of function must be considered in highly active patients.

SUBACROMIAL-SUBDELTOID BURSITIS

The subacromial-subdeltoid (SASD) bursa is a synovium-lined pouch that minimizes friction during supraspinatus movement along the undersurface of the deltoid muscle and coracoacromial arch. The bursa normally contains a trace volume of fluid and is surrounded by a thin layer of peribursal fat. The bursa extends medial to the coracoid

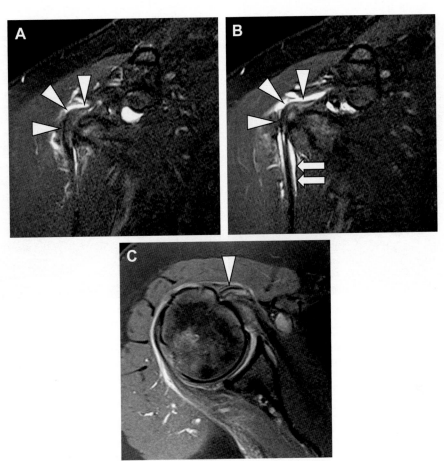

Fig. 1. A 65-year-old woman with right anterior shoulder pain. (*A, B*) Coronal T2 fat-suppressed and (*C*) axial proton density (PD) fat-suppressed MR images demonstrate marked thickening of the LHBT within the rotator interval and proximal bicipital groove (*white arrowheads*). Note trace fluid within the biceps tendon sheath (*white arrows* in *B*).

process, anteriorly over the bicipital groove, and inferolaterally along the outer margin of the greater tuberosity.[15] In the sagittal plane, the bursa adopts a horseshoe appearance draped over the subscapularis tendon and deep to the coracoid process. The SASD and subcoracoid bursae communicate in 11% to 55% of patients.[16,17]

SASD bursitis can be secondary to impingement or reactive to other pathologic conditions such as rotator cuff tendinopathy. Fluid within the SASD bursa can often occur with other overuse shoulder pathologic conditions, including acromioclavicular osteoarthritis and supraspinatus tendon tears, as well as other conditions, such as calcific tendinopathy, acute trauma, rheumatoid arthritis, infection, and pigmented villonodular synovitis.[18] Patients with SASD bursitis typically present with pain and limited range of motion.

Both US and MR imaging can reveal fluid and/or debris within the bursa. However, the quantity of fluid is likely more predictive of bursitis than the presence of fluid alone.[19,20] White and colleagues[21] assessed the SASD bursa on MR imaging in 36 asymptomatic volunteers and concluded that the normal bursa typically measures less than 2 mm in thickness. Factors predictive of abnormal bursal fluid included thickness greater than 3 mm or extension of fluid medial to the acromioclavicular joint or anterior to the humerus.[21] Other suggestive features include thickening of the bursal wall (**Fig. 3**).

First-line treatment is conservative and includes rest and nonsteroidal antiinflammatory medications. Persistent pain can be treated with intrabursal corticosteroid injection, often performed under US guidance. Recalcitrant cases may herald a concomitant shoulder pathologic condition and surgery, including subacromial decompression and bursectomy, may be performed.[22]

ROTATOR CUFF TENDINOPATHY

The rotator cuff comprises the supraspinatus, infraspinatus, teres minor, and subscapularis.

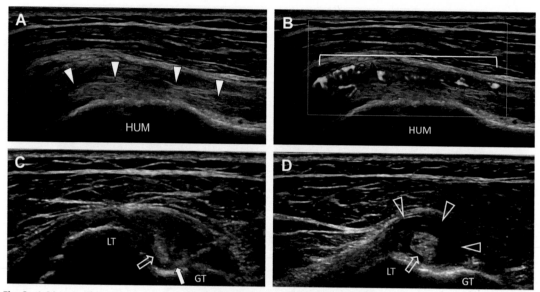

Fig. 2. A 39-year-old man with right anterior shoulder pain. (*A, B*) Longitudinal grayscale and power Doppler images of the bicipital groove demonstrate a thickened LHBT with loss of the normal fibrillar pattern (*white arrowheads in A*), and hyperemia within the tendon sheath (*bracket in B*). (*C*) Transverse grayscale image during US-guided corticosteroid injection shows the needle in plane with the transducer with tip positioned within the tendon sheath (*white arrow*) deep to the LHBT (*open arrow*). (*D*) Postprocedural transverse grayscale image demonstrates anechoic injectate within the tendon sheath (*open arrowheads*) and around the LHBT (*open arrow*). GT, greater tuberosity; HUM, humerus; LT, lesser tuberosity.

These myotendinous structures operate as an interconnected unit, and injury to any of these structures may predispose to injuries elsewhere in the rotator cuff.[23] The rotator cuff enables the shoulder to function over a wide range of internal rotation, external rotation, and abduction. The supraspinatus tendon attaches primarily to the superior facet of the greater tuberosity, as well as to the superior half of the middle facet, where its fibers interleave with those of the infraspinatus tendon.[24] The infraspinatus tendon attaches primarily to the middle facet. The teres minor attaches to the inferior facet of the greater tuberosity and to the surgical neck of the posterior humerus. The subscapularis attaches to the lesser tuberosity, with continuation of fibers over the bicipital groove as the transverse humeral ligament. There is notable individual variation of the tendon attachments with respect to the humerus, with significant interdigitation of fibers between adjacent tendons.[25] Each tendon is composed of articular and bursal surfaces, which are on the deep and superficial sides of the tendon, respectively.

Tendon degeneration and tearing are most commonly sequelae of overuse, whether in the overhead athlete or from chronic wear and tear in older individuals. One meta-analysis revealed

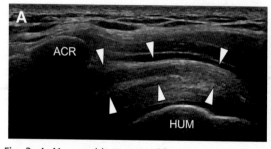
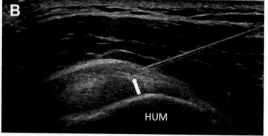

Fig. 3. A 41-year-old woman with pain on right arm abduction. (*A*) Longitudinal grayscale US image of the subacromial-subdeltoid bursa reveals intermediate echogenicity distending a thick-walled bursa (*white arrowheads*). (*B*) Longitudinal grayscale image during US-guided therapeutic corticosteroid injection demonstrates the needle in plane with the transducer and tip positioned within the bursa (*white arrow*). ACR, acromion.

an association between hand dominance and older age with rotator cuff tears, supporting the role of overuse in rotator cuff injury.[26] Theories on the pathogenesis of rotator cuff injuries have commonly been categorized into 1 of 2 mechanisms: extrinsic, or related to impingement from external structures, versus intrinsic, secondary to primary tendon degeneration over time.[27,28] However, a rotator cuff pathologic condition is likely multifactorial with contributions from both intrinsic and extrinsic mechanisms.[29] Specific patterns of pathologic rotator cuff conditions in impingement syndromes are discussed further in the following section.

Imaging findings of tendon degeneration include tendon thickening and signal change, with intermediate (less than fluid) T2 signal on MR imaging or hypoechogenicity on US with loss of the normal echogenic fibrillar pattern on US (**Fig. 4**). Tears on both MR imaging and US appear as fluid within the tendon, which may extend to articular or bursal surfaces or be confined within the tendon substance (interstitial tears) (**Fig. 5**). Articular surface

tears are at least twice as common as bursal surface tears,[30] possibly secondary to increased collagen of the bursal side of the tendon, which provides higher resistance to tensile stress. Full-thickness tendon tears demonstrate fluid extending from the articular to the bursal surface.

Rotator cuff tears are initially treated with physical therapy to increase strength and range of motion. Patients with persistent symptoms can undergo tendon debridement for low-grade (<50% thickness) partial-thickness tears and primary repair for full-thickness tears. In chronic cases in which the torn retracted tendon fibers cannot be reapproximated, synthetic or cadaver interposition grafts can be used.[31]

IMPINGEMENT

Impingement syndromes of the shoulder are a heterogeneous group of conditions that vary in cause and clinical presentation. External shoulder impingement includes subacromial impingement, which is the most common,[27] and subcoracoid

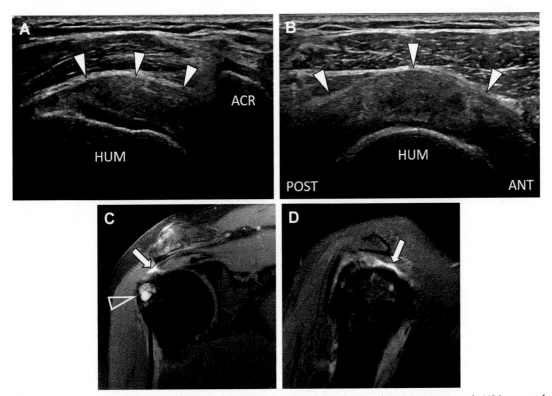

Fig. 4. A 57-year-old woman with right shoulder pain. (*A*, *B*) Longitudinal and transverse grayscale US images of the rotator cuff demonstrate diffuse thickening and hypoechogenicity of the supraspinatus tendon with loss of the normal fibrillar pattern (*white arrowheads*), consistent with tendinopathy. The patient experienced worsening pain and an magnetic resonance (MR) arthrogram was performed subsequently. (*C*) Coronal T1 fat-suppressed and (*D*) sagittal T2 fat-suppressed MR arthrogram images demonstrate a gadolinium-filled cleft in the distal supraspinatus tendon (*white arrows*), consistent with progression to full-thickness tear. There is associated cyst formation in the greater tuberosity (*open arrowhead* in *C*). ANT, anterior; POST, posterior.

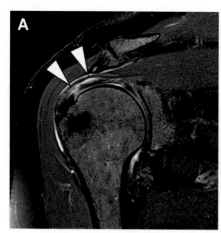
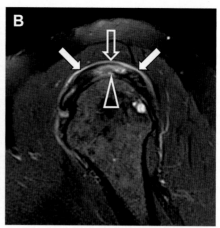

Fig. 5. A 45-year-old woman with progressive right shoulder pain. (*A*) Coronal T2 fat-suppressed MR image demonstrates fluid and intermediate signal intensity in the interstitial fibers of the supraspinatus tendon proximal to the insertion (*white arrowheads*). (*B*) Double oblique sagittal T2 fat-suppressed MR image demonstrates fluid signal intensity extending to the articular surface of the central supraspinatus tendon (*open arrowhead*). Intact fibers are located along the bursal surface (*open arrow*) and both anteriorly and posteriorly (*white arrows*). These findings are compatible with partial thickness, partial width articular-sided tearing with intrasubstance delamination of the tendon superimposed on tendinopathy.

impingement, which affects the anterior cuff and capsule. Internal impingement can be subdivided into posterosuperior and anterosuperior subtypes, and most commonly occurs in overhead throwing athletes.

SUBACROMIAL IMPINGEMENT

Subacromial impingement describes the entrapment of the rotator cuff and superior glenohumeral capsular structures between the greater tuberosity of the humerus and the coracoacromial arch with arm abduction and elevation. Normally, the soft tissue structures glide smoothly underneath the coracoacromial arch. Loss of the gliding mechanism is the characteristic feature of subacromial impingement and can lead to pain, rotator cuff tendinopathy, and (eventually) tendon tears.[32]

There are 2 types of subacromial impingement that occur in different patient populations with distinct contributing factors. Secondary subacromial impingement occurs in younger patients and athletes, who are predisposed to decentering of the humeral head during abduction and overhead activities owing to relative ligamentous laxity and weakness or discoordination of the dynamic joint stabilizers.

Primary subacromial impingement is more common and more commonly affects older patients and nonathletes.[33] Historically, subacromial impingement has been attributed to structural variants or abnormalities that narrow the subacromial space, such as subacromial spurs, a laterally downsloping acromion, hooked (Bigliani type III)

acromion process, persistent os acromiale, or undersurface acromioclavicular osteophyte. More recent studies, however, have questioned the likelihood of these characteristics to cause impingement in the absence of concomitant glenohumeral instability.[34,35] More recent studies implicate a growing role for rotator cuff dysfunction in the development of primary impingement.[2,36]

Patients with subacromial impingement present with pain and limited range of motion with shoulder abduction between 40° and 120°.[37] Although subacromial impingement is a clinical diagnosis, radiographs are important in the initial diagnostic evaluation of patients with suspected impingement and can reveal potential primary causes.[37] Early sequelae of impingement include fluid distention of the SASD bursa and supraspinatus tendinopathy.[38–40] Tendon fibrosis and enlargement from tendinopathy contribute to further narrowing of the subacromial space, exacerbating and potentially accelerating tendon degeneration and tearing (**Fig. 6**).

Treatment of subacromial impingement depends on the cause and the extent of the cuff abnormality. Patients with impingement related to joint laxity may improve with physical therapy and strengthening exercises,[41] with capsular plication reserved for patients with refractory symptoms. Subacromial decompression, distal clavicle resection, bursectomy, and os acromiale resection are surgical options targeting the underlying structural cause of impingement[27,36,37,42] and are often combined with rotator cuff repair or debridement.

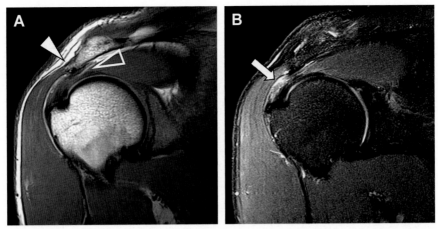

Fig. 6. A 29-year-old man with pain on right upper extremity abduction. (*A*) Coronal T1 MR image of the shoulder demonstrates lateral downsloping of the acromion (*white arrowhead*). There is mild effacement of the subacromial fat and mass effect on the underlying supraspinatus tendon (*open arrowhead*). (*B*) Coronal T2 fat-suppressed MR image demonstrates bursal-surface high signal and tendon thickening (*white arrow*), consistent with tendinopathy.

SUBCORACOID IMPINGEMENT

In subcoracoid impingement, an uncommon form of impingement, patients present with pain with shoulder adduction and internal rotation, thought to be secondary to entrapment of the subscapularis tendon between the coracoid process and the lesser tuberosity of the humeral head.[43] It is primarily a clinical diagnosis; however, imaging findings may include an elongated or angulated coracoid process, narrowing of the coracohumeral interval (<1 cm), or a prominent lesser tuberosity.[44] MR imaging can characterize coracoid morphology and directly demonstrate coracohumeral narrowing and/or impingement of the subscapularis, although this depends on patient positioning and is best assessed with internal rotation (**Fig. 7**). MR imaging may reveal indirect findings of subscapularis tendinopathy and tendon tears. US also can demonstrate coracohumeral narrowing and direct findings of impingement with internal rotation during real-time evaluation.[45]

INTERNAL IMPINGEMENT

Internal impingement typically refers to posterosuperior impingement, a condition in which the supraspinatus tendon, infraspinatus tendon, or both are pathologically interposed between the greater tuberosity and the posterior glenoid with the shoulder in extreme abduction and external rotation.[46,47] It affects baseball pitchers in the late cocking phase of the pitch and also can occur in swimmers, volleyball players, javelin throwers, and tennis players.[48] With excessive contact in repeated overhead activities, the entrapped

superior rotator cuff can become tendinopathic or tear. The posterosuperior labrum and posterior humeral head can also be affected. Anterior instability is also associated with posterosuperior impingement, with laxity of the anterior glenohumeral joint capsule considered a significant factor in the development of impingement.[49]

On MR imaging, findings of posterosuperior impingement include abnormal signal intensity, fraying, or tearing of the undersurface of the supraspinatus or infraspinatus tendons. Blunting, fraying, or tears of the posterosuperior labrum and cystic changes of the posterior humeral head more posteriorly than with common rotator cuff abnormalities are other characteristic findings. Abduction external rotation MR imaging can directly demonstrate impingement.[50] Of note, physiologic interposition of the cuff between the glenoid and humeral head is common and does not indicate impingement if the patient is asymptomatic and the cuff and labrum are morphologically normal.[51]

Current treatment includes correction of the underlying glenohumeral laxity with capsular plication, surgical treatment of the labrum or rotator cuff, and strengthening of the muscles of the pectoral girdle to minimize translation of the humerus with muscle fatigue.[47]

A significantly less common type of internal impingement, termed anterosuperior impingement, occurs when the anterior supraspinatus tendon, subscapularis tendon, the LHBT, and anterosuperior joint capsule are entrapped between the anterosuperior glenoid with shoulder adduction and internal rotation.[52] Preceding injury

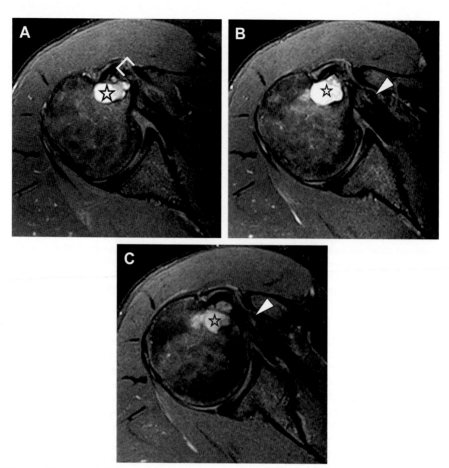

Fig. 7. A 48-year-old man with right anterior shoulder pain on adduction and internal rotation. (*A–C*) Serial axial PD fat-suppressed images of the shoulder demonstrate narrowing of the coracohumeral interval (*bracket in A*). There is tendinopathy of the traversing subscapularis tendon (*white arrowheads* in *B* and *C*) and cystic change (*stars*) in the adjacent lesser tuberosity.

to the biceps pulley allows medial subluxation of the LHBT, progressive degeneration of the subscapularis insertion, and eventual abnormal anterosuperior translation of the humeral head.[53] Affected patients are typically older nonathletes presenting with anterior shoulder pain and weakness. MR imaging findings in anterosuperior impingement include primary injury to the biceps pulley, subluxation of the LHBT, tendinopathy or tearing of the anterior supraspinatus and cranial subscapularis tendons, and fraying or tearing of the anterosuperior labrum.[49,51,53]

BENNETT LESION

An additional finding in the shoulders of throwing athletes is ossification of the posterior band of the IGHL, termed the Bennett lesion of the shoulder (**Fig. 8**). This was originally posited to be related to traction on the inferior glenoid by the long head of the triceps tendon; however, subsequent arthroscopic and imaging studies determined the lesion was extraarticular and within the capsule itself.[54,55] The formation of reactive bone within the capsule is believed to be a result of impaction of the posterior humeral head on the posteroinferior glenoid at the attachment of the posterior band of the IGHL, which resists translation of the humeral head either inferiorly or posteriorly, depending on whether the arm is externally or internally rotated.[56] Maximum contact between the capsule and the posteroinferior glenoid occurs during the late cocking phase of the baseball pitch, when the arm is maximally abducted and externally rotated. Patients present with pain during the late cocking phase, during the follow-through or deceleration phase, which also asymmetrically impacts the posterior capsule, or during both phases. The Bennett lesion is thought to be associated with posterosuperior labral tears and articular-sided fibrillation or tearing of the infraspinatus tendon,

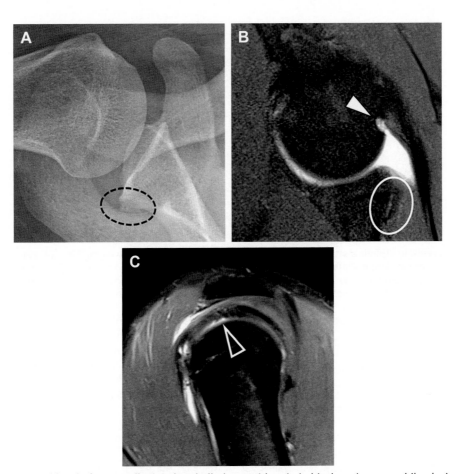

Fig. 8. A 33-year-old male former collegiate baseball player with pain in his throwing arm while playing recreational softball. (*A*) Axillary radiograph of the shoulder demonstrates mineralization adjacent to the posterior glenoid (*dashed circle*). (*B*) Oblique axial T1 fat-suppressed MR arthrogram image with the shoulder abducted and externally rotated demonstrates a small cyst in the posterosuperior humeral head adjacent to the infraspinatus attachment (*white arrowhead*). Note the low signal intensity adjacent to the posterior glenoid corresponding to the aforementioned mineralization on radiographs (*solid circle*). (*C*) Sagittal PD fat-suppressed MR image shows gadolinium filling very subtle articular surface partial thickness tears in the distal posterosuperior supraspinatus tendon (*open arrowhead*).

and can be seen concomitantly with posterosuperior impingement.[56]

DISTAL CLAVICULAR OSTEOLYSIS

Stress-induced distal clavicular osteolysis was originally described as an overuse injury affecting athletes and weightlifters.[57] Patients present with chronic acromioclavicular joint pain exacerbated by activity. Weakness, joint subluxation, and a history of a specific traumatic event should be absent.[58] Radiographs reveal lucency or tapering of the distal clavicle and resorption of the distal clavicular cortex. MR imaging findings include distal clavicular bone marrow edema, cortical thinning, and subchondral cysts (**Fig. 9**).[59] Differential considerations for the imaging findings of

osteolysis include prior trauma, hyperparathyroidism, infection, rheumatoid arthritis, and gout, although osteolysis related to overuse is usually distinguished based on clinical history and physical examination.

Proposed etiologic factors include repetitive microtrauma resulting in microfractures of the distal clavicle and weakening of the trabecular bone. Weight training bench press type maneuvers in particular exert significant traction on the acromioclavicular joint and may be implicated in the development of osteolysis.[57]

Initial symptom management includes the cessation or modification of provocative activities, antiinflammatory medications, and ice. For cases in which cessation of activities is either ineffective or impractical, resection of the distal clavicle has

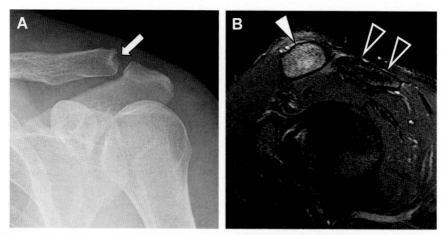

Fig. 9. A 38-year-old athletic man with left acromioclavicular joint pain while weightlifting. (*A*) Anteroposterior shoulder radiograph demonstrates focal erosion of the distal clavicle subchondral bone (*white arrow*) with a normal-appearing acromion. (*B*) Sagittal T2 fat-suppressed MR image demonstrates bone marrow edema in the distal clavicle (*white arrowhead*) in contrast to the normal acromion (*open arrowheads*).

been shown to alleviate symptoms and facilitate return to activities.[60]

LITTLE LEAGUER'S SHOULDER

Little Leaguer's shoulder is a stress injury of the proximal humeral physis. It is a result of repetitive overhead throwing, typically in the baseball pitcher aged 11 to 16 years.[61] It has also been reported in cricket, volleyball, and badminton players.[62] Most patients present with pain over the proximal humerus, with more than a quarter of patients reporting weakness during external rotation.[61]

The favored mechanism is repeated stress on a relatively weak physis during a period of rapid growth.[61] During normal skeletal maturation,

chondrocytes on the metaphyseal side of the physis die and mineralize, leading to longitudinal growth of the humerus. Torque and distraction forces on the physis during throwing are hypothesized to disrupt the metaphyseal vasculature,[63] leading to prolonged survival of nonmineralized, hypertrophic chondrocytes along the metaphyseal side of the physis.

Radiographic findings include physeal irregularity or widening[61,62,64]; however, radiographs are usually normal if patients are imaged within 10 days of symptom onset.[64] The lateral physis is affected more often, which is presumed to be secondary to a thicker posteromedial periosteum.[65] Comparison with radiographs of the unaffected shoulder may be helpful to confirm physeal widening (**Fig. 10**). Other reported findings include

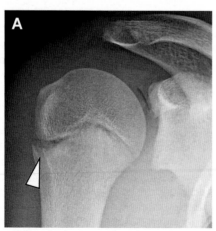
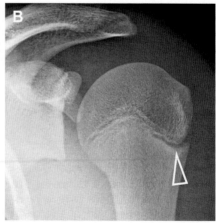

Fig. 10. A 13-year-old male baseball player with right shoulder pain when throwing. (*A*) A Grashey external rotation radiograph demonstrates irregularity and widening of the lateral proximal humeral physis (*white arrowhead*). (*B*) Radiograph of the asymptomatic contralateral shoulder demonstrates the expected normal appearance of the physis (*open arrowhead*).

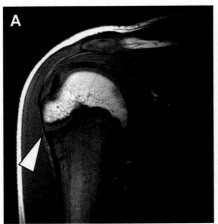
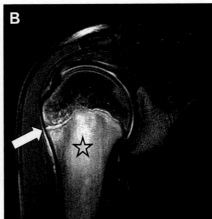

Fig. 11. A 11-year-old male baseball pitcher with right arm pain during pitching. (*A*) Coronal T1 MR image of the shoulder demonstrates widening of the proximal humeral physis (*white arrowhead*). (*B*) Coronal T2 fat-suppressed MR image demonstrates fluid signal within the physis (*arrow*) and marked juxtaphyseal marrow edema in the proximal humeral metaphysis (*star*).

fragmentation and demineralization or sclerosis of the juxtaphyseal metaphysis.[61] On MR imaging, there is focal extension of physeal low T1 signal into the metaphysis, with hyperintense T2 signal in the adjacent metaphysis (**Fig. 11**). The epiphysis is typically spared.[66]

Treatment involves rest followed by gradual return to activity after resolution of pain.[67] Kanematsu and colleagues[62] studied 19 baseball players and found that the mean time to resolution of physeal widening on radiographs was 4.7 months. Continued activity can progress to formation of a physeal bar and subsequent limb length discrepancies[65] or angulation deformities.[68]

SUMMARY

The shoulder is uniquely predisposed to overuse injuries given its ability to accommodate a wide range of motion. Many of these overuse injuries commonly affect younger and active individuals, and early diagnosis of these entities has a disproportionately large effect on maintaining function and quality of life. Recognizing the predisposing anatomic factors and extent of the pathologic condition on various imaging modalities is crucial to guiding appropriate conservative or surgical management.

REFERENCES

1. Howell SM, Galinat BJ. The glenoid-labral socket. A constrained articular surface. Clin Orthop Relat Res 1989;(243):122–5.
2. Lugo R, Kung P, Ma CB. Shoulder biomechanics. Eur J Radiol 2008;68(1):16–24.
3. Halder AM, Itoi E, An KN. Anatomy and biomechanics of the shoulder. Orthop Clin North Am 2000;31(2):159–76.
4. Crichton JC, Funk L. The anatomy of the short head of biceps - not a tendon. Int J Shoulder Surg 2009; 3(4):75–9.
5. Carter AN, Erickson SM. Proximal biceps tendon rupture: primarily an injury of middle age. Phys Sportsmed 1999;27(6):95–101.
6. Gilcreest EL. Dislocation and elongation of the long head of the biceps brachii: an analysis of six cases. Ann Surg 1936;104(1):118–38.
7. Snyder SJ, Banas MP, Karzel RP. An analysis of 140 injuries to the superior glenoid labrum. J Shoulder Elbow Surg 1995;4(4):243–8.
8. Redondo-Alonso L, Chamorro-Moriana G, Jimenez-Rejano JJ, et al. Relationship between chronic pathologies of the supraspinatus tendon and the long head of the biceps tendon: systematic review. BMC Musculoskelet Disord 2014;15:377.
9. Werner A, Ilg A, Schmitz H, et al. Tendinitis of the long head of biceps tendon associated with lesions of the "biceps reflection pulley". Sportverletz Sportschaden 2003;17(2):75–9 [in German].
10. Curtis AS, Snyder SJ. Evaluation and treatment of biceps tendon pathology. Orthop Clin North Am 1993; 24(1):33–43.
11. Tuckman GA. Abnormalities of the long head of the biceps tendon of the shoulder: MR imaging findings. AJR Am J Roentgenol 1994;163(5): 1183–8.
12. Nho SJ, Strauss EJ, Lenart BA, et al. Long head of the biceps tendinopathy: diagnosis and management. J Am Acad Orthop Surg 2010;18(11):645–56.
13. Mariani EM, Cofield RH, Askew LJ, et al. Rupture of the tendon of the long head of the biceps brachii.

Surgical versus nonsurgical treatment. Clin Orthop Relat Res 1988;(228):233–9.

14. Sturzenegger M, Beguin D, Grunig B, et al. Muscular strength after rupture of the long head of the biceps. Arch Orthop Trauma Surg 1986;105(1):18–23.

15. Kennedy MS, Nicholson HD, Woodley SJ. Clinical anatomy of the subacromial and related shoulder bursae: a review of the literature. Clin Anat 2017; 30(2):213–26.

16. Horwitz MT, Tocantins LM. An anatomical study of the role of the long thoracic nerve and the related scapula bursae in the pathogenesis of local paralysis of the serratus anterior muscle. Anat Rec 1938; 71:375–81.

17. Schraner AB, Major NM. MR imaging of the subcoracoid bursa. AJR Am J Roentgenol 1999;172(6): 1567–71.

18. Draghi F, Scudeller L, Draghi AG, et al. Prevalence of subacromial-subdeltoid bursitis in shoulder pain: an ultrasonographic study. J Ultrasound 2015; 18(2):151–8.

19. Mirowitz SA. Normal rotator cuff: MR imaging with conventional and fat-suppression techniques. Radiology 1991;180(3):735–40.

20. Farooki S, Seeger LL. MR imaging of sports injuries of the shoulder. Semin Musculoskelet Radiol 1997; 1(1):51–63.

21. White EA, Schweitzer ME, Haims AH. Range of normal and abnormal subacromial/subdeltoid bursa fluid. J Comput Assist Tomogr 2006;30(2):316–20.

22. Henkus HE, de Witte PB, Nelissen RG, et al. Bursectomy compared with acromioplasty in the management of subacromial impingement syndrome: a prospective randomised study. J Bone Joint Surg Br 2009;91(4):504–10.

23. Andarawis-Puri N, Ricchetti ET, Soslowsky LJ. Rotator cuff tendon strain correlates with tear propagation. J Biomech 2009;42(2):158–63.

24. Minagawa H, Itoi E, Konno N, et al. Humeral attachment of the supraspinatus and infraspinatus tendons: an anatomic study. Arthroscopy 1998;14(3): 302–6.

25. Chang EY, Chung CB. Current concepts on imaging diagnosis of rotator cuff disease. Semin Musculoskelet Radiol 2014;18(4):412–24.

26. Sayampanathan AA, Andrew TH. Systematic review on risk factors of rotator cuff tears. J Orthop Surg (Hong Kong) 2017;25(1). 2309499016684318.

27. Neer CS 2nd. Anterior acromioplasty for the chronic impingement syndrome in the shoulder: a preliminary report. J Bone Joint Surg Am 1972;54(1):41–50.

28. Codman EA. Complete rupture of the supraspinatus tendon. Operative treatment with report of two successful cases. 1911. J Shoulder Elbow Surg 2011; 20(3):347–9.

29. Seitz AL, McClure PW, Finucane S, et al. Mechanisms of rotator cuff tendinopathy: intrinsic, extrinsic,

or both? Clin Biomech (Bristol, Avon) 2011;26(1): 1–12.

30. Ellman H. Diagnosis and treatment of incomplete rotator cuff tears. Clin Orthop Relat Res 1990;(254): 64–74.

31. Seker V, Hackett L, Lam PH, et al. Evaluating the outcomes of rotator cuff repairs with polytetrafluoroethylene patches for massive and irreparable rotator cuff tears with a minimum 2-year follow-up. Am J Sports Med 2018;46(13):3155–64.

32. Flatow EL, Soslowsky LJ, Ticker JB, et al. Excursion of the rotator cuff under the acromion. Patterns of subacromial contact. Am J Sports Med 1994;22(6): 779–88.

33. Cone RO 3rd, Resnick D, Danzig L. Shoulder impingement syndrome: radiographic evaluation. Radiology 1984;150(1):29–33.

34. Bigliani LU, Ticker JB, Flatow EL, et al. The relationship of acromial architecture to rotator cuff disease. Clin Sports Med 1991;10(4):823–38.

35. Chang EY, Moses DA, Babb JS, et al. Shoulder impingement: objective 3D shape analysis of acromial morphologic features. Radiology 2006;239(2): 497–505.

36. Harrison AK, Flatow EL. Subacromial impingement syndrome. J Am Acad Orthop Surg 2011;19(11): 701–8.

37. Hardy DC, Vogler JB 3rd, White RH. The shoulder impingement syndrome: prevalence of radiographic findings and correlation with response to therapy. AJR Am J Roentgenol 1986;147(3):557–61.

38. Seeger LL, Gold RH, Bassett LW, et al. Shoulder impingement syndrome: MR findings in 53 shoulders. AJR Am J Roentgenol 1988;150(2):343–7.

39. Read JW, Perko M. Shoulder ultrasound: diagnostic accuracy for impingement syndrome, rotator cuff tear, and biceps tendon pathology. J Shoulder Elbow Surg 1998;7(3):264–71.

40. Tuite MJ. Magnetic resonance imaging of rotator cuff disease and external impingement. Magn Reson Imaging Clin N Am 2012;20(2):187–200, ix.

41. Lippitt S, Harryman D. Diagnosis and management of AMBRI syndrome. Tech Orthop 1991;6:61–73.

42. Gebremariam L, Hay EM, Koes BW, et al. Effectiveness of surgical and postsurgical interventions for the subacromial impingement syndrome: a systematic review. Arch Phys Med Rehabil 2011;92(11): 1900–13.

43. Dines DM, Warren RF, Inglis AE, et al. The coracoid impingement syndrome. J Bone Joint Surg Br 1990; 72(2):314–6.

44. Giaroli EL, Major NM, Lemley DE, et al. Coracohumeral interval imaging in subcoracoid impingement syndrome on MRI. AJR Am J Roentgenol 2006; 186(1):242–6.

45. Tracy MR, Trella TA, Nazarian LN, et al. Sonography of the coracohumeral interval: a potential technique

for diagnosing coracoid impingement. J Ultrasound Med 2010;29(3):337–41.

46. Giaroli EL, Major NM, Higgins LD. MRI of internal impingement of the shoulder. AJR Am J Roentgenol 2005;185(4):925–9.

47. Davidson PA, Elattrache NS, Jobe CM, et al. Rotator cuff and posterior-superior glenoid labrum injury associated with increased glenohumeral motion: a new site of impingement. J Shoulder Elbow Surg 1995;4(5):384–90.

48. Jobe FW, Pink M. Classification and treatment of shoulder dysfunction in the overhead athlete. J Orthop Sports Phys Ther 1993;18(2):427–32.

49. Cowderoy GA, Lisle DA, O'Connell PT. Overuse and impingement syndromes of the shoulder in the athlete. Magn Reson Imaging Clin N Am 2009; 17(4):577–93, v.

50. Tirman PF, Bost FW, Garvin GJ, et al. Posterosupe-rior glenoid impingement of the shoulder: findings at MR imaging and MR arthrography with arthro-scopic correlation. Radiology 1994;193(2):431–6.

51. McFarland EG, Hsu CY, Neira C, et al. Internal impingement of the shoulder: a clinical and arthro-scopic analysis. J Shoulder Elbow Surg 1999;8(5): 458–60.

52. Struhl S. Anterior internal impingement: an arthro-scopic observation. Arthroscopy 2002;18(1):2–7.

53. Habermeyer P, Magosch P, Pritsch M, et al. Antero-superior impingement of the shoulder as a result of pulley lesions: a prospective arthroscopic study. J Shoulder Elbow Surg 2004;13(1):5–12.

54. Bennett GE. Shoulder and elbow lesions distinctive of baseball players. Ann Surg 1947;126(1):107–10.

55. Lombardo SJ, Jobe FW, Kerlan RK, et al. Posterior shoulder lesions in throwing athletes. Am J Sports Med 1977;5(3):106–10.

56. Ferrari JD, Ferrari DA, Coumas J, et al. Posterior ossification of the shoulder: the Bennett lesion. Etiol-ogy, diagnosis, and treatment. Am J Sports Med 1994;22(2):171–5 [discussion: 175–6].

57. Cahill BR. Osteolysis of the distal part of the clavicle in male athletes. J Bone Joint Surg Am 1982;64(7): 1053–8.

58. Schwarzkopf R, Ishak C, Elman M, et al. Distal clavicular osteolysis: a review of the literature. Bull NYU Hosp Jt Dis 2008;66(2):94–101.

59. de la Puente R, Boutin RD, Theodorou DJ, et al. Post-traumatic and stress-induced osteolysis of the distal clavicle: MR imaging findings in 17 patients. Skeletal Radiol 1999;28(4):202–8.

60. Roedl JB, Nevalainen M, Gonzalez FM, et al. Fre-quency, imaging findings, risk factors, and long-term sequelae of distal clavicular osteolysis in young patients. Skeletal Radiol 2015;44(5):659–66.

61. Carson WG Jr, Gasser SI. Little Leaguer's shoulder. A report of 23 cases. Am J Sports Med 1998; 26(4):575–80.

62. Kanematsu Y, Matsuura T, Kashiwaguchi S, et al. Radiographic follow-up study of Little Leaguer's shoulder. Skeletal Radiol 2015;44(1):73–6.

63. Lyman S, Fleisig GS, Waterbor JW, et al. Longitudi-nal study of elbow and shoulder pain in youth base-ball pitchers. Med Sci Sports Exerc 2001;33(11): 1803–10.

64. Fleming JL, Hollingsworth CL, Squire DL, et al. Little Leaguer's shoulder. Skeletal Radiol 2004;33(6): 352–4.

65. Bae DS. Humeral shaft and proximal humerus, shoulder dislocation. In: Flynn JM, Skaggs DL, Waters PM, editors. Rockwood & Wilkins fractures in children. 8th edition. Philadelphia: Wolters Kluwer Health; 2015. p. 751–806.

66. Obembe OO, Gaskin CM, Taffoni MJ, et al. Little Leaguer's shoulder (proximal humeral epiphysioly-sis): MRI findings in four boys. Pediatr Radiol 2007;37(9):885–9.

67. Taylor DC, Krasinski KL. Adolescent shoulder in-juries: consensus and controversies. Instr Course Lect 2009;58:281–92.

68. Hosokawa Y, Mihata T, Itami Y, et al. Little Leaguer's shoulder can cause severe three-dimensional hu-meral deformity. Clin Orthop Surg 2017;9(4):537–41.

The Acutely Injured Elbow

Teck Yew Chin, MBChB, MSc, FRCR*, Hong Chou, MBBS, FRCR,
Wilfred C.G. Peh, MBBS, MD, FRCP (Glasg), FRCP (Edin), FRCR

KEYWORDS

- Acute elbow injuries • Elbow fractures • Elbow dislocations • Elbow soft tissue injuries

KEY POINTS

- Elbow injuries are common and require an understanding of the relevant anatomy, pathophysiologic mechanisms, and injury patterns for accurate diagnoses.
- Injuries to the various osseous and soft tissue components are evaluated through multimodality imaging, which include radiography, computed tomography scans, MR imaging, and ultrasound imaging.
- Recognizing common fracture and/or dislocation classifications allows communication of information efficiently to clinical colleagues.

INTRODUCTION

Acute elbow injuries constitute a common subset of musculoskeletal joint and bone injuries in both athletes and the general adult population. Together with the forearm, elbow injuries constitute up to 15% of emergency visits for upper extremity injuries.[1] These injuries have a large spectrum of clinical presentation and imaging findings. The radiologist plays a crucial role in identifying both major and subtle injuries that direct patient management and prognosticate outcomes. This article examines the patterns, mechanisms, and imaging considerations of common acute elbow injuries across the various structures of the elbow, providing key concepts in the interpretation of these injuries.

ELBOW ANATOMY AND STABILITY

The elbow is a highly stable joint owing to its inherent osteoarticular anatomy and the dynamic–static interactions of the capsuloligamentous and musculotendinous soft tissue stabilizing structures surrounding it. It is a trocho-ginglymoid joint composed of 3 synovial articulations between the humerus, radius, and ulna, and

encapsulated within a common synovial capsule. The radiocapitellar and ulnotrochlear (ginglymoid) hinge joints allow movement in one plane along the flexion–extension arc from 0° to 150°. The proximal radioulnar (trochoid) joint provides a 180° rotational axis for supination and pronation.[2–4] The elbow ligaments comprise the medial and lateral collateral ligamentous complexes. Together with the ulnotrochlear joint, they form the primary stabilizers of the elbow joint. The secondary stabilizers comprise the rest of the other joint articulations and soft tissues, which include the radiocapitellar joint, the common flexor and common extensor musculotendinous units, and the joint capsule.

IMAGING APPROACH AND FINDINGS

Despite rapid advancement in multimodality imaging, conventional radiography remains the first-line imaging investigation for screening and baseline assessment of the elbow in acute situations. It is inexpensive, easily accessible, and understood by both radiologists and nonradiology colleagues in excluding gross osseous injury and dislocations, after physical examination. Standard anteroposterior (AP) and lateral views are obtained in most

Disclosure Statement: Nothing to disclose.

Department of Diagnostic Radiology, Khoo Teck Puat Hospital, 90 Yishun Central, Singapore 768828, Republic of Singapore

* Corresponding author.

E-mail address: chin.teck.yew@ktph.com.sg

Radiol Clin N Am 57 (2019) 911–930

https://doi.org/10.1016/j.rcl.2019.03.006

institutions. The AP view is acquired with the central beam directed perpendicular to the fully extended elbow with the hand in supination, although this optimal position may be limited owing to the patient's injuries. This view allows an assessment of the medial and lateral epicondyles, the radiocapitellar joint, the trochlear articular surface, and the carrying angle.

The lateral view is acquired 90° to the AP view with the shoulder in abduction, the forearm resting on the table with the thumb directed upward, and the elbow flexed at 90°. The central beam is positioned over the radial head. The olecranon, coronoid process, anterior half of the radial head, and ulnohumeral joint congruency are assessed on this view. Additional important soft tissue evaluation of the anterior and posterior fat pads, along with the geometric relationships of the joints via the radiocapitellar and anterior humeral lines, are obtained.

In a normal elbow, the anterior fat pad resides in the coronoid fossa and is seen as a closely apposed slim triangle with straight anterior margins (**Fig. 1**). The posterior fat pad resides in the olecranon fossa and is not normally visualized. In trauma, the presence of a joint effusion displaces the fat pads from their recesses and can be secondary signs of an underlying intraarticular fracture.[5] The anterior humeral line, drawn from the anterior cortex of the humeral diaphysis, passes through the central third of the capitellum. Disruption of this line is associated with supracondylar and capitellar fractures. The radiocapitellar line

assesses the radiocapitellar alignment, with a central line through the radial diaphysis bisecting through the capitellum regardless of projection (see **Fig. 1**). Malalignment is associated with radiocapitellar dislocation.

Complementary specialized views such as the radial head, coronoid, medial oblique, and lateral oblique views may be performed based on clinical requirements, but are now uncommon in general practice given the availability of superior cross-sectional imaging. These additional views may still have a larger role in pediatric imaging than in the adult population.[6]

Computed tomography (CT) scanning is used in complex fractures to characterize the injuries in detail. It is useful in situations where the ability to obtain optimal radiographs is hindered from impaired range of movement. Three-dimensional CT reconstructions provide a visual adjunct that is helpful to surgical colleagues, particularly for preoperative planning. In the context of dislocation, a CT scan is nearly always recommended to determine further osseous injuries not apparent on radiographs.[7,8] The optimal position is with the arm extended over the head with the wrist in supination. If there are patient constraints owing to pain and reduced range of movement from the injury, the arm can be placed anteriorly over the body, though this positioning increases streak artifacts and requires postprocessing to obtain orthogonal planes.

MR imaging is less often indicated in acute trauma, being more suitable for assessing

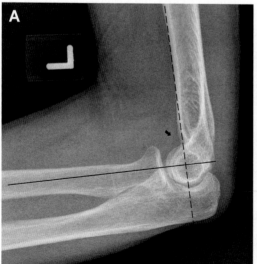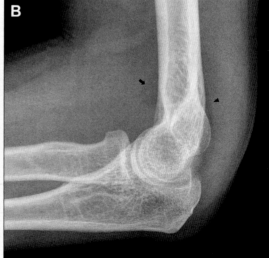

Fig. 1. Lateral radiograph of the elbow shows the (*A*) anterior humeral line (*dashed line*), the radiocapitellar line (*solid line*) and the normal anterior fat pad (*arrow*). (*B*) Elevation of the anterior (*arrow*) and posterior (*arrowhead*) fat pads indicate an underlying effusion and possible intraarticular fracture in acute trauma.

subacute to chronic injuries, but depends on local context and availability. It is useful in problem solving situations, such as identifying suspected occult or stress fractures. High-performance athletes and younger active adults are a subset of patients who benefit from early MR imaging for the detailed assessment of soft tissue damage that can alter management, function preservation, and overall recovery,[9] particularly in complex fracture–dislocation injuries.

Most bone or soft tissue injuries are accompanied by localized edema and joint effusions. The primary MR sequences in trauma therefore revolve around fluid sensitive T2-weighted and/or proton density sequences with fat saturation, or short tau inversion recovery sequences. These sequences are useful for localizing the injuries and allow a distinction of ligamentous and tendinous structures. T1-weighted and proton density non–fat saturation sequences contribute to anatomic evaluation of both the soft tissue and bone marrow. Achieving a balance between these sequences in the 3 orthogonal planes varies among different institutions, and consideration of the various anatomic structures that are optimally visualized in each plane (eg, ligaments and common flexor/extensor tendon attachments in coronal, distal triceps, and biceps tendons in sagittal planes).

CT/MR arthrographic studies have little role in the context of acute trauma and are used mainly in the evaluation of subtle subacute to chronic joint and soft tissues injuries not apparent on standard imaging. This would include subtle osteochondral and capsuloligamentous injuries,[10] as well as underlying persistent joint instability. Targeted ultrasound examination of isolated superficial soft tissue injuries is largely confined to the evaluation of the distal biceps or triceps muscles and tendon attachments, and the common flexor and extensor tendons and underlying respective collateral ligaments.

FRACTURES

Fractures involving the elbow occur with an incidence of approximately 7 to 8 in 10,000 in the adult population[11] and represent 5% of all fractures sustained.[2] Of this, radial head fractures account for one-third to one-half of all elbow fractures,[12,13] with distal humerus fractures accounting for another 30%. Recognizing fracture patterns and the extent of the injuries helps to direct management and prognosticate outcome. Many orthopedic fracture classification systems exist in the literature and are unique and specific to anatomic locations. These systems are useful in providing a standardized method of describing fractures, guiding surgical and nonsurgical options, but can have a pitfall of mixed interoperator and intraoperator reproducibility.[14,15] If in doubt, a description of key findings should suffice.

Distal Humeral Fractures

The distal humerus includes the medial and lateral column, which constitute the axial load-bearing capabilities of the humerus,[16] bridged centrally by the trochlea, which acts as a tie arch (**Fig. 2**). The medial epicondyle is composed of the medial column from which the common flexor tendon and the medial collateral ligament (MCL) complex originates. The lateral column comprises of both the lateral epicondyle and capitellum, to which the lateral collateral ligament (LCL) complex and common extensor tendon have proximal attachments at the lateral epicondyle. The main osseous static osseous stabilizer of the elbow joint is the ulnohumeral joint, constituted by the trochlea articulation within the trochlea notch. Additionally, the trochlea central groove interlocks with a sagittal ridge within the semilunar notch, further emphasizing its primary role in elbow joint stability;

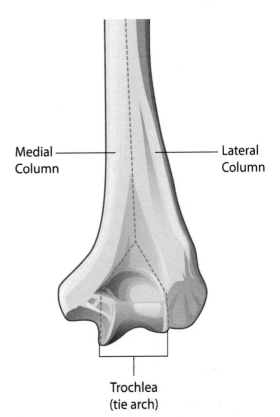

Medial Column — Lateral Column

Trochlea (tie arch)

Fig. 2. The distal humerus comprises of the medial and lateral columns bridged by the trochlea, which acts as a tie arch.

hence, any fracture extending into the trochlea is therefore unstable.[17,18]

Distal humerus fractures usually occur from high energy direct trauma in younger adults, or a fall on an outstretched hand (FOOSH) more commonly associated with the elderly and osteoporotic population.[19] There are several classifications for distal humeral fractures. The Jupiter and Mehne classification is traditionally more recognized within the radiologic community (**Fig. 3**) and provides information on articular involvement and the orientation of the fracture lines. However, the revised and largely accepted orthopedic classification currently used widely is the Swiss Arbeitsgemeinschaft fur Osteosynthesefragen-Association for the Study of Internal Fixation (AO-ASIF) group. This offers more precise radiological descriptions and considers 3 main variables of articular involvement, column location and degree of comminution (**Fig. 4**), with increasing complexity from A1 through to C3 (**Fig. 5**). Regardless of the classification, the decision for surgical versus nonsurgical management considers many other factors, including age, bone condition, and patient morbidity.

The AO-ASIF classification can encompass further divisions, which can reach up to 27

Fig. 3. Jupiter and Mehne classification of distal humerus fractures with 6 main fracture patterns.

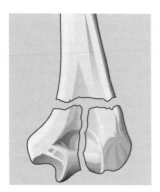

1. High T intercondylar

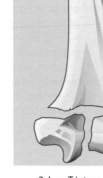

2. Low T intercondylar

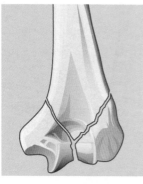

3. Y intercondylar

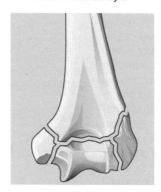

4. H intercondylar

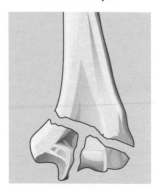

5. Lambda pattern (medial)

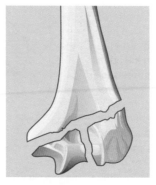

6. Lambda pattern (lateral)

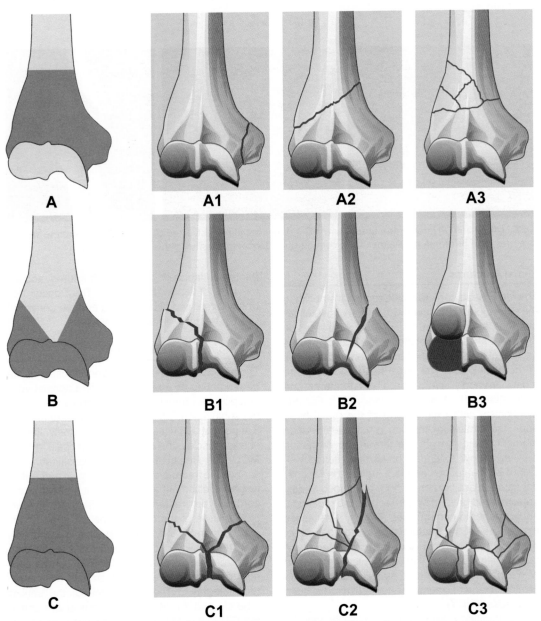

Fig. 4. AO-ASIF classification of distal humeral fractures. The top row (*A*) comprises the extraarticular fractures: A1 (medial or lateral apophyseal avulsion), A2 (simple metaphyseal fracture), and A3 (comminuted metaphyseal fractures). The middle row (*B*) comprises the partial articular fractures with or without column involvement: B1 (lateral condyle sagittal fractures), B2 (medial condyle sagittal fractures), and B3 (frontal articular fracture in the coronal plane). The bottom row (*C*) comprises the complete articular fractures with involvement of both columns: C1 (metaphyseal and articular column simple fractures), C2 (simple articular fracture with metaphyseal comminution), and C3 (comminuted metaphyseal and articular fractures).

subvariants and may be cumbersome in application. A simplified classification proffered by Sanchez-Sotelo[19] aims to address this from a practical surgical perspective. It recognizes 4 main fracture patterns that stratifies complexity, management, and outcome: 1, supraintercondylar/column fractures; 2, articular fractures; 3, low transcondylar fractures; and 4, partial articular fractures.

What the referring physician needs to know

No fracture classification is perfect, and it should consider local context with application to surgical colleagues to offer practical utility.

If in doubt, a description of intraarticular involvement, location, comminution, and displacement should suffice in most situations.

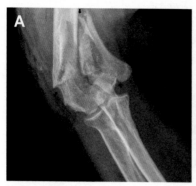 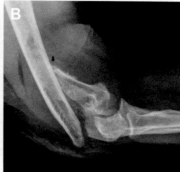 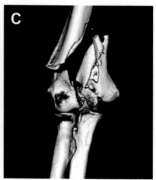

Fig. 5. (*A*) AP and (*B*) lateral radiographs with (*C*) 3-dimensional reconstructed CT image show complete articular fractures with bicolumn involvement and comminution (*arrows*), classifying this as a C3 fracture.

Radial Fractures

The radial head confers multidirectional stability to the elbow joint. In tandem with lateral capsuloligamentous structures, it resists valgus stresses in the coronal plane,[20] posterior dislocation in the sagittal plane, and cranial translation of the radius in the axial plane. The radial head and neck are most commonly involved in elbow fractures and dislocations. The typical mechanism is a FOOSH mechanism with axial loading of the radial head upon the capitellum through a valgus–pronation moment, typically with the forearm in pronation and the elbow extended or partially flexed.[12,21] Out of all the various methodologies, the Mason-Johnston classification[22,23] is the most widely implemented grading system across the radiologic and orthopedic communities (**Fig. 6**). It assesses the severity of the fracture(s) based on degree of displacement, comminution, and associated dislocation, with type I and II injuries typically managed with a trial of conservative therapy, and type III and IV injuries requiring surgery often with a radial head prosthesis (**Fig. 7**).

The modified Mason-Johnston classification by Hotchkiss includes the clinical presence of a mechanical block or incongruous motion which qualifies an injury as a type II injury requiring open reduction and internal fixation or the excision of unstable bone fragments.[24–26] MR imaging assessment may be useful in such instances to assess the integrity of the MCL complex as excision of a large radial head fragment requires an intact anterior oblique MCL band. Otherwise the procedure may lead to further elbow instability, given their combined roles in resisting valgus stress.

Ulnar Fractures

The ulnar coronoid process and olecranon are the 2 main anatomic areas involved in elbow ulnar fractures. Isolated olecranon fractures account for 10% of elbow fractures.[27] They occur from both indirect and direct trauma and are commonly seen in fracture–dislocation injuries.

Coronoid Process Fractures

The coronoid process is an important osseous stabilizer, acting as a strut that buffers against varus and posterior translation forces, preventing posterior subluxation.[28] It is also the attachment point of 3 important soft tissue stabilizers, namely, the brachialis muscles, the anterior joint capsule, and the MCL. The Regan and Morrey classification describes the fracture severity in terms of percentage height involvement in the horizontal shear plane–coronoid tip fracture (type I), fracture involving 50% or less of the coronoid height (type II), and greater than 50% (type III; **Fig. 8**). It is established that the stability of the elbow joint is significantly compromised when more than 50% of the coronoid process is involved, regardless of ligamentous integrity.[29] The importance of the sublime tubercle and the MCL attachment at the anteromedial facet of the coronoid process in preserving varus and rotational stability has led to the O'Driscoll classification,[30] in which involvement of the anteromedial facet (see **Fig. 8**) in type II and type III fractures requires surgical intervention (**Fig. 9**). This classification is widely used by the orthopedic community.

Pearls and pitfalls

Isolated coronoid process fractures are rare accounting for less than 2% of elbow fractures.[31]

They are often indicative of more serious underlying injuries associated with other elbow injuries such as dislocations[32] and should prompt further CT imaging because radiographs may not demonstrate the full extent of injury.[30]

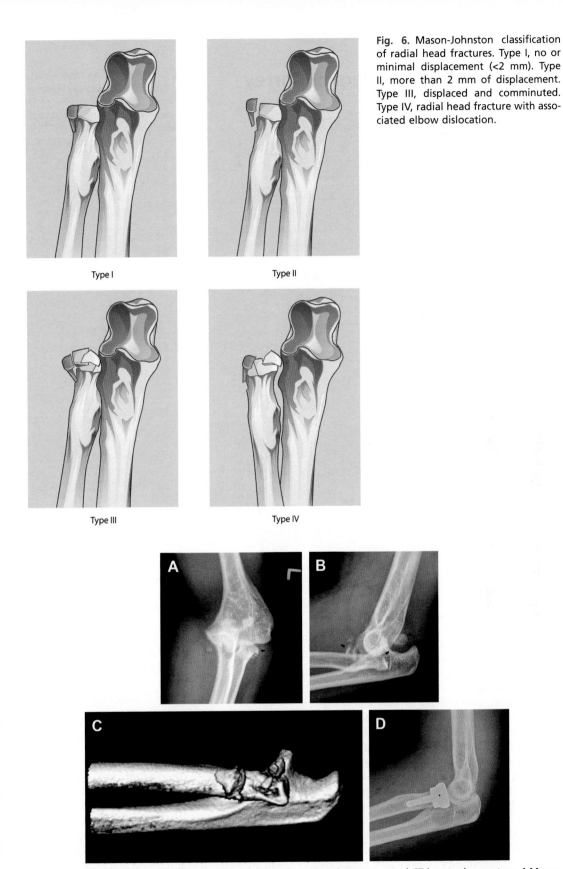

Type I

Type II

Type III

Type IV

Fig. 6. Mason-Johnston classification of radial head fractures. Type I, no or minimal displacement (<2 mm). Type II, more than 2 mm of displacement. Type III, displaced and comminuted. Type IV, radial head fracture with associated elbow dislocation.

Fig. 7. (*A*) AP and (*B*) lateral radiographs with (*C*) 3-dimensional reconstructed CT image show a type 4 Mason-Johnston injury (*arrows*) (*D*) requiring a radial head prosthesis (*asterisk*). The intraarticular fragment (*arrowhead*) was excised intraoperatively.

O'Driscoll

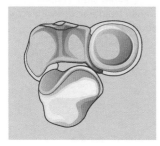

Type I

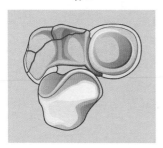

Type II

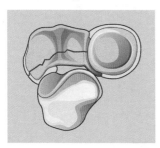

Type III

Regan-Morrey

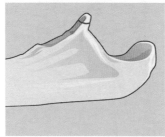

Type I

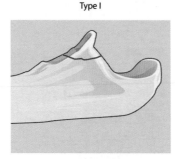

Type II

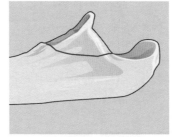

Type III

Fig. 8. Comparison between the O'Driscoll and Regan-Morrey classifications of coronoid fractures. The main difference is the recognition of antero-medial facet involvement in the O'Driscoll classification, which constitutes a type II injury.

Olecranon Fractures

The olecranon articulates with the trochlea mainly through the trochlear notch, forming the bulk of the ulnohumeral articulation, with contribution from the coronoid process. This provides a strong brace against anterior translative forces and is also a significant contributor to rotational stability, resisting varus and valgus torques. The olecranon process is the posterior summit of the elbow joint, providing the attachment for the triceps muscle. Complex multidirectional forces often occur in olecranon fractures. These can occur from direct impact injuries such as falls or road traffic accidents, or from paradoxic contractures of the surrounding muscles usually involving the triceps and brachialis.[33,34] Several classification systems exist in characterizing olecranon fractures, which include the Schatzkers, Colon and colleagues, and Mayo classification systems, none of which are preferred universally. Of these, the Mayo classification system is more recognized with its emphasis on the degree of displacement, comminution, and presence of instability,[35] with surgical fixation recommended if there is more than 3 mm of fracture distraction (**Fig. 10**).

DISLOCATION

The elbow is the second most commonly dislocated joint in the body, after the shoulder.[36,37] A FOOSH is the typical mechanism, with high-impact sports injuries, direct trauma, and road traffic accidents accounting for most other causes. Most adult dislocations occur posterior and posterolaterally (**Fig. 11**), and the description is based on the position of the radius and ulna relative to the humerus after the injury. This involves an axial load on the hyperextended elbow with the forearm in supination and a valgus stress applied at the elbow during internal rotation.[38,39] Dislocations in other planes (eg, anterior, lateral,

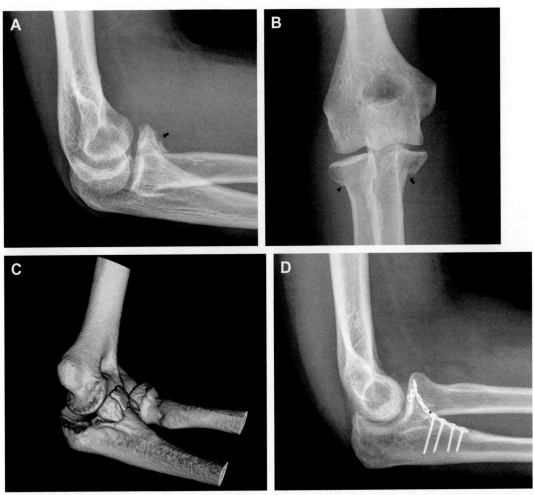

Fig. 9. (*A*) Lateral and (*B*) AP radiographs with (*C*) 3-dimensional reconstructed CT image show a type III coronoid process fracture (*arrows*) that requires (*D*) plate fixation (*asterisk*). A concomitant radial neck fracture is also present (*arrowhead*).

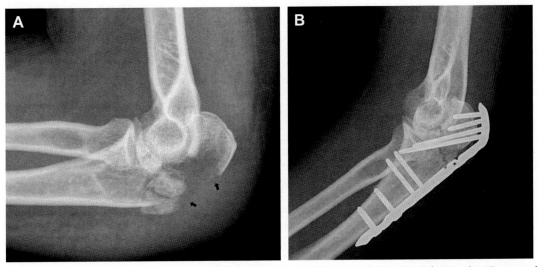

Fig. 10. Lateral radiographs show olecranon fractures (*arrows*). (*A*) Fracture distraction of more than 3 mm and comminuted fragments requires (*B*) plate and screw fixation (*asterisk*) rather than tension band or Kirschner wire fixation.

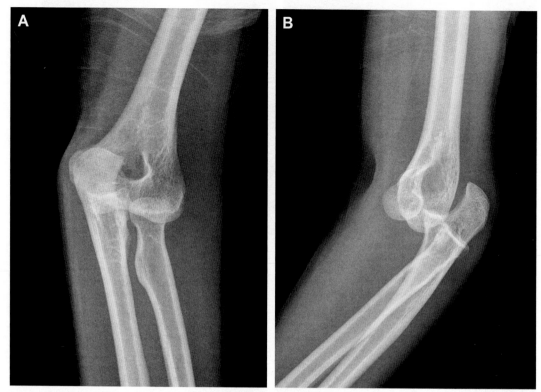

Fig. 11. (A) AP and (B) lateral radiographs show posterior dislocation of the elbow.

medial) are uncommon. Anterior dislocation may rarely occur from a rebound mechanism secondary to a prior posterior dislocation.[40] Another rare variant is the divergent dislocation, which leads to the separation of the radius and ulna as the distal humerus impacts inferiorly with disruption to the interosseous membrane. Anterior and divergent dislocations are more likely associated with neurovascular injuries.[41,42] As with any other joint, elbow dislocations need to be distinguished between simple (no associated fracture) and complex (associated with underlying fractures) variants, with the latter being far more difficult to treat.

Simple Dislocation

Traditionally, the well-established pathogenesis of a simple dislocation is likened to a sequential compromise of the soft tissue structures from a lateral to medial direction, termed the Horii circle.[38] The current staging of elbow dislocation follows this sequence of events, beginning with a tear of the lateral ulnar collateral ligament (stage 1) through complete disruption of the MCL (stage 3b). However, some recent studies suggest that the medial soft tissues, beginning with the MCL, are the first structures to be injured or avulsed,

leading to the ladder cascade of other soft tissue injuries toward the anterior joint capsule and finally, the lateral stabilizers. This finding is evidenced by imaging and surgical studies demonstrating that the majority of the sample patients had predominant and more severe medial-sided ligamentous injuries in comparison to the lateral sided stabilizers after simple dislocations.[43–45] Regardless of pathogenesis, attaining closed reduction aiming to provide stability is necessary for conservative healing and restoration of function. The key is ulnotrochlear articulation congruency. The outcomes of this patient group managed nonsurgically is usually excellent, with only 1% to 2% presenting with recurrent instability.[46,47] Immediate surgical intervention is controversial and subject to the attending clinical team.

Radiography with AP and lateral views enables an accurate diagnosis of most cases of simple dislocation. CT scans can be performed if there is suspicion of an occult fracture. MR imaging is indicated in postreduction joints, which remain highly unstable, to determine the extent of soft tissue disruption that may necessitate surgical intervention for example, a ruptured common extensor origin, which requires surgical repair[45] (Fig. 12). Care is needed, however, because MR imaging

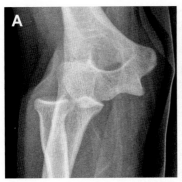
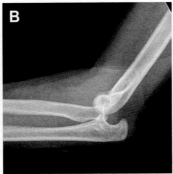
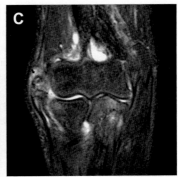

Fig. 12. (*A*) AP and (*B*) lateral radiographs show a simple posterolateral dislocation. Despite reduction, the joint remained highly unstable owing to (*C*) complete rupture of the common extensor origin (*arrow*) and radial collateral ligament (*asterisk*) on the coronal T2-weighted fat-saturated MR image. These are indications for surgical repair.

appearances can overstate the severity of injuries and the findings ultimately need to be correlated with the clinical findings.

Complex Dislocation

Complex dislocations involve both osseous and soft tissue structures and are, therefore, highly challenging to manage. Complications such as posttraumatic arthritis, chronic instability, recurrent dislocations, stiffness, and pain are common in this patient subgroup, but can be negated with prudent care. Many complex dislocations will have a combination of various fracture types across several bones, as detailed elsewhere in this article. There are, however, some common fracture patterns, such as the "terrible triad" and the Monteggia fracture–dislocation, which are useful in identifying associated pathology. Imaging approach involves a combination of radiography with greater emphasis on cross-sectional imaging.

Terrible Triad

Complex dislocations of the elbow have associations with fractures of the radial head and coronoid process. When all 3 are present, it is known as the terrible triad and signifies the presence of severe underlying capsuloligamentous derangement (**Fig. 13**) with a high potential for complications such as chronic instability, posttraumatic arthritis, and loss of function.[48] In most cases, corrective surgery is warranted. More recently, some studies have trialed conservative approaches to this injury, based on a combination of both clinical and imaging findings. The main imaging criteria to recognize on CT scans and radiographs for consideration of nonsurgical management would be the presence of a good concentric reduction of the ulnohumeral and radiocapitellar joints, an absence of the drop sign[49] on the lateral radiograph (ulnohumeral joint distance <4 mm [**Fig. 14**]), and a low-grade coronoid fracture.[50–52]

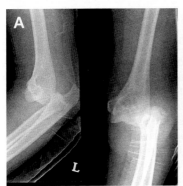
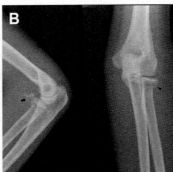
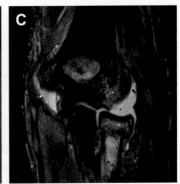

Fig. 13. AP and lateral radiographic views of a posterolateral dislocation (*A*) before and (*B*) after reduction show the coronoid process (*arrow*) and radial head (*arrowhead*) fractures constituting the terrible triad. (*C*) Coronal T2-weighted fat-saturated MR image shows rupture of the LCL (*arrow*) and MCL (*arrowhead*) with accompanying joint effusion (*black asterisk*) and bone marrow edema (*white asterisks*).

Monteggia Fracture–Dislocation

The Monteggia fracture–dislocation is the combination of an ulnar fracture with a radiocapitellar dislocation. The mechanism is through a direct blow onto the ulna or a FOOSH with a hyperextended or supinated forearm.[53,54] These injuries are classified by the Bado system,[55] based on ulnar fracture apex angulation, direction of radiocapitellar dislocation, and the presence or absence of a radial diaphyseal fracture (**Fig. 15**). Although radiographs often demonstrate most of the injuries, CT scanning is recommended to identify and further characterize fractures not apparent radiographically.

Pearls and pitfalls

Monteggia fracture–dislocations may be missed owing to spontaneous radiocapitellar relocation. High clinical suspicion is required and MR imaging is useful to evaluate osseous and ligamentous integrity in such cases.

LIGAMENTOUS INJURIES

The MCL complex is composed of 3 bands—the anterior oblique, posterior oblique, and transverse bundles—of which the anterior oblique is the primary restraint against valgus stresses on the elbow. In acute trauma, MCL injuries can occur with fractures and dislocations from direct and high impact forces. The association of MCL tears in athletes involved in overhead ball-throwing sports is typically that of chronic and repetitive overuse injury rather than a sudden rupture or avulsion. The LCL complex has 3 distinct structures, namely: the radial collateral ligament, lateral ulnar collateral ligament, and the annular ligament. The LCL complex functions to resist varus forces and if injured, leads to posterolateral rotatory instability.[56,57] Acute LCL injuries often occur in tandem with elbow dislocations.

Evaluation is best done on MR imaging obtained using coronal fluid-sensitive sequences and shows increased signal within and around the ligaments. Other findings include a loss of the normal striations of the ligamentous architecture, fluid clefts, laxity, and discontinuation of the ligament (**Fig. 16**). Midsubstance tears are more common in acute traumatic tears than in distal or proximal attachment injuries for MCL injuries, whereas LCL injuries tend to occur at the proximal lateral epicondyle origin. Ultrasound examination is more relevant in assessing subacute to chronic injuries because there are often concomitant joint and osseous injuries in the acute situation.

MUSCULOTENDINOUS INJURIES

Acute injuries to the muscle and tendons of the elbow are uncommon, when compared with those incurred by chronic repetitive etiologies. Both the distal attachments of the biceps and triceps tendons may incur injuries from a single traumatic acute episode owing to uncoordinated muscle contractions and eccentric loading.[58] For the common flexor and extensor tendon, pathologies are much more associated with chronicity, for example, lateral and medial epicondylitis. Acute tendon disruptions can occur but often in tandem with dislocations (**Fig. 17**) as discussed elsewhere in this article.

Biceps Tendon Injuries

Rupture of the distal portion of the biceps myotendinous structures are associated with male smokers and steroid usage.[59,60] Apart from direct trauma, the injury occurs from a forced extension of the 90° flexed elbow owing to a resistive load, with weightlifters being a classic example. They mostly occur 1 to 2 cm proximal to the radial tuberosity insertion, with proposed mechanisms related to a combination of a relatively hypovascular region and mechanical impingement by the radial tuberosity during forearm rotation.[61] A palpable gap and Popeye sign may be observed in cases of tendon retraction.

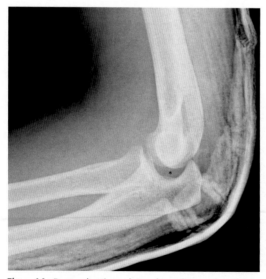

Fig. 14. Postreduction lateral radiograph shows persistent joint instability with increased ulnotrochlear distance of more than 4 mm (*asterisk*) consistent with the drop sign.

Pearls, pitfalls and variants

Biceps tendon retraction in ruptures requires concurrent disruption to the aponeurotic biceps sheath (or lacertus fibrosis), because the tendon may otherwise remain tethered in place.

A common variant is the bifurcation of the distal biceps tendon into the distal long and short heads. This can be mistaken for a partial tear of a single biceps tendon unit when it is actually a complete tear of one of these distinct, bifurcated units, most often the short head.[62]

Bicipital bursitis is a differential of a ruptured distal biceps tendon, particularly if there is background tendinosis.

MR imaging is accurate in diagnosing distal biceps tendon ruptures. Fluid-sensitive sequences show tendon discontinuity with fluid in the empty sheath in complete rupture and is best appreciated on sagittal and axial planes (**Fig. 18**). There is often edema, sometimes with hemorrhage, in the remaining tendon substance and the adjacent muscle and soft tissues. Targeted ultrasound imaging has high sensitivity and specificity, rivalling MR imaging in the evaluation of the distal biceps tendon and can be offered as a first-line investigation.[63,64] This imaging modality, however, requires careful technique with trained operators to minimize misdiagnosis. The long axis image is best to visualize the injury, which manifests as hypoechoic to anechoic tendon disruption accompanied by fluid in or around the tendon sheath (**Fig. 19**). Isolated injuries to the lacertus fibrosus are rare (**Fig. 20**)

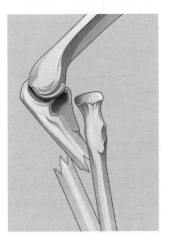

Type I

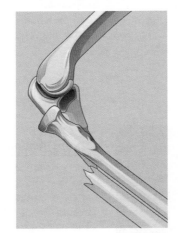

Type II

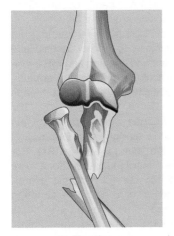

Type III

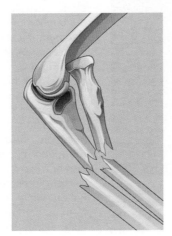

Type IV

Fig. 15. Bado classification of Monteggia fracture–dislocation. Type I, anterior radial head dislocation with anterior angulation of ulnar apex. Type II, posterior radial head dislocation with posterior angulation of ulnar apex. Type III, lateral radial head dislocation with ulnar fracture. Type IV, anterior radial head dislocation with ulnar and radial shaft fractures.

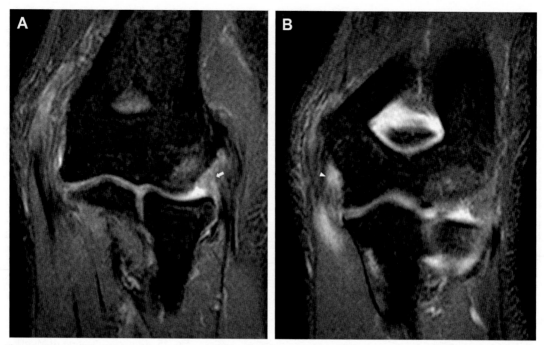

Fig. 16. Coronal T2-weighted fat-saturated MR images show a (*A*) high-grade partial tear of the radial collateral ligament (*arrow*) and (*B*) rupture of the MCL (*arrowhead*) after elbow dislocation.

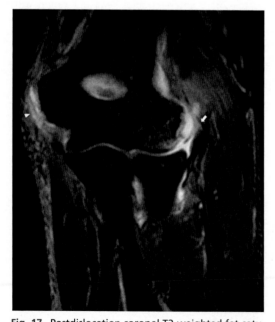

Fig. 17. Postdislocation coronal T2-weighted fat-saturated MR image shows complete uncovering of the humeral epicondyles from complete rupture of the common flexor (*arrowhead*) and extensor (*arrow*) tendon origins. The underlying MCL and LCL are also disrupted.

and unlikely to have significant long-term impact on function.

Triceps Tendon Injuries

Triceps tendon avulsions occur from chronic overuse in sporting athletes, but can present acutely after eccentric loading through single impact events like a fall or a road traffic accident.[65,66] The same group of patients involved in distal biceps tendon injuries are also predisposed for triceps avulsions, which can occur from contraction of the muscle against a flexed elbow. Radiographs show avulsive bone fragments from the olecranon summit in up to 80% of cases (Flake sign; **Fig. 21**).[67] Ultrasound imaging and MR imaging are both highly accurate and maybe equal in sensitivity and specificity in diagnosing triceps tendon tears.[68]

On ultrasound images, there may be an anechoic fluid with tendon disruption and retraction in complete tears (see **Fig. 21**). For partial tears, the tendinous striations are partially preserved and careful dynamic examination while scanning can aid differentiation from a complete tear. MR imaging will show fluid within the injured area and the sagittal plane is most useful for determining the extent of injury (**Fig. 22**).

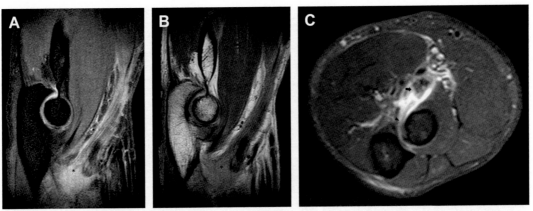

Fig. 18. Sagittal (*A*) proton density fat-saturated (FS) and (*B*) proton density MR images show the ruptured and retracted tendon stump (*asterisks*) with surrounding debris and fluid. (*C*) Additional axial T2-weighted FS MR image shows the tendon stump (*arrow*) and expected insertion site on the radial tuberosity (*arrowhead*).

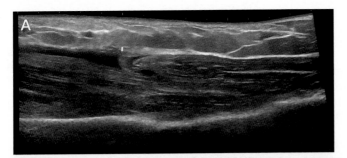

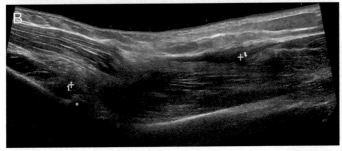

Fig. 19. Ultrasound longitudinal image shows (*A*) the ruptured and retracted distal biceps tendon stump (*arrow*) with anechoic fluid filling the empty tendon sheath. (*B*) The stump retraction distance (*between the cursors*) is measured from the tendon stump (*arrow*) to the radial tuberosity (*asterisk*).

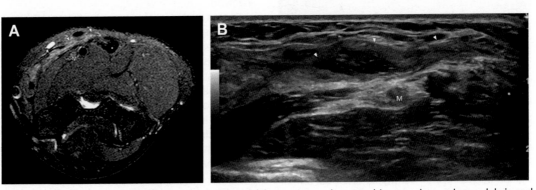

Fig. 20. (*A*) Axial T2-weighted fat-saturated MR and (*B*) transverse ultrasound images show edema, debris and thickening of the lacertus fibrosus (*arrowheads*) in relation to the median nerve (M) and biceps tendon (*asterisk*).

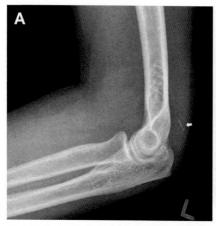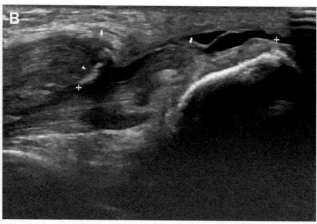

Fig. 21. (*A*) Lateral radiograph shows the Flake sign of a triceps avulsion fracture (*arrow*). (*B*) Ultrasound longitudinal image shows the corresponding osseous fragment (*arrowhead*) with rupture of the triceps tendon insertion with 2 distinct stumps (*arrows*) and surrounding anechoic fluid. The distance from the most retracted stump is measured to the expected olecranon insertion (*between the cursors*).

OSTEOCHONDRAL INJURIES

Osteochondral fractures occur from chronic overuse and repetitive trauma, but can occasionally present acutely in the elbow, usually at the capitellum, through mechanisms that include impaction, dislocations, and shear-type injuries.[69] Radiographs may depict subarticular lucencies and a joint effusion. MR imaging shows a corresponding articular bone defect, depending on the severity of the injury, often with marrow edema and a joint effusion (**Fig. 23**). Identifying displaced intraarticular bodies may warrant surgical intervention for removal or reattachment.

NEUROVASCULAR INJURIES

Neurovascular injuries are associated with complex dislocations, particularly with open or penetrating injuries. Nerve injuries are more common, with neuropraxias occurring in up to 20% of elbow dislocations.[70] The ulnar nerve is most often involved, with ulnar neuropathy being present in 11% to 14% of elbow dislocations.[71] This condition is usually transient and occurs from a stretching mechanism as it traverses the cubital tunnel. The anterior interosseous nerve is less commonly injured, and the median nerve itself is rarely involved.

For arterial vascular injuries, the incidence is estimated between 5% to 13%, but is rare in the absence of an open injury.[72,73] In dislocations, vascular compromise can occur from compression rather than direct disruption/laceration of the vessel and may even occur after reduction. The brachial artery is the main vessel involved in such cases. Imaging is limited in either acute situations, because clinical examination usually suffices, and, if vascular compromise is established, rapid intervention is warranted. MR imaging may show neuropathy with high T2-weighted signal changes and swelling of the afflicted nerves (**Fig. 24**), but this is highly

Fig. 22. Sagittal proton density fat-saturated MR image shows an acute partial tear (*arrow*) involving 50% of the tendon substance at the triceps insertion.

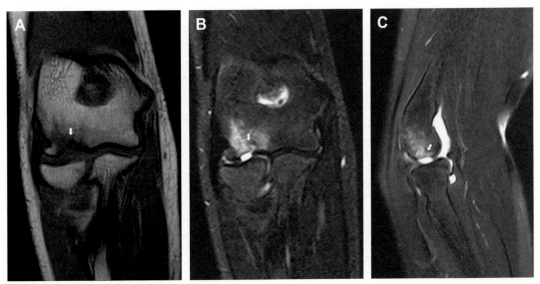

Fig. 23. (*A*) Coronal T1-weighted, (*B*) coronal short tau inversion recovery, and (*C*) sagittal T2-weighted fat-saturated MR images show an acute osteochondral fracture and defect in the capitellum (*arrows*) with surrounding bone marrow edema, sustained in a young adult during a national badminton tournament.

nonspecific and often does not correlate with any pertinent clinical symptoms.

SUMMARY

Acute elbow injuries are common, with a wide and challenging spectrum of imaging findings. Comprehensive diagnostic assessment can involve combinations of standard radiographs, cross-sectional imaging and dynamic ultrasound evaluation. Recognizing the osseous and soft tissue injury patterns across these various modalities, with an understanding of the biomechanics and pathophysiology, enables the radiologist to make an accurate diagnosis and provide a crucial role in optimizing the patient's outcome. The utilization of commonly accepted classifications also enables efficient communication of findings to our clinical colleagues to facilitate management.

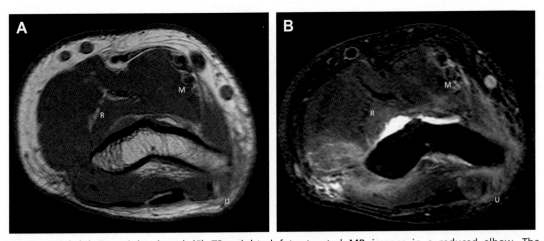

Fig. 24. Axial (*A*) T1-weighted and (*B*) T2-weighted fat-saturated MR images in a reduced elbow. The patient had parasthesia and weakness in the ring and little fingers. The ulnar nerve (U) seems to be swollen and edematous compared with the radial (R) and median (M) nerves, just before it enters the cubital tunnel.

REFERENCES

1. Pitts SR, Niska RW, Xu J, et al. National hospital ambulatory medical care survey: 2006 emergency department summary. Natl Health Stat Report 2008;7:1–38.

2. Rosas HG, Lee KS. Imaging acute trauma of the elbow. Semin Musculoskelet Radiol 2010;14:394–411.

3. Frick MA. Imaging of the elbow: a review of imaging findings in acute and chronic traumatic disorders of the elbow. J Hand Ther 2006;19:98–112.

4. Fowler KA, Chung CB. Normal MR imaging anatomy of the elbow. Magn Reson Imaging Clin N Am 2004; 12:191–206.

5. Bohrer SP. The fat pad sign following elbow trauma: its usefulness and reliability in suspecting "invisible" fractures. Clin Radiol 1970;21:90–4.

6. Crosby NE, Greenberg JA. Radiographic evaluation of the elbow. J Hand Surg Am 2014;39:1408–14.

7. Bohndorf K, Kilcoyne RF. Traumatic injuries: imaging of peripheral musculoskeletal injuries. Eur Radiol 2002;12:1605–16.

8. Sormaala MJ, Sormaala A, Mattila VM, et al. MDCT findings after elbow dislocation: a retrospective study of 140 patients. Skeletal Radiol 2014;43:507–12.

9. Bucknor MD, Stevens KJ, Steinbach LS. Elbow imaging in sport: sports imaging series. Radiology 2016;279:12–28.

10. Waldt S, Bruegel M, Ganter K, et al. Comparison of multislice CT arthrography and MR arthrography for the detection of articular cartilage lesions of the elbow. Eur Radiol 2005;15:784–91.

11. Kodde IF, Kaas L, Flipsen M, et al. Current concepts in the management of radial head fractures. World J Orthop 2015;6:954–60.

12. Mckee MD, Jupiter JB. Trauma to the adult elbow and fractures of the distal humerus. In: Browner BD, editor. Skeletal trauma: basic science, management, and reconstruction. 3rd edition. Philadelphia: Saunders; 2003. p. 1404–80.

13. Harrison JWK, Chitre A, Lammin K, et al. Radial head fractures in adults. Curr Orthop 2007;21:59–64.

14. Swiontkowski MF, Agel J, McAndrew MP, et al. Outcome validation of the AO/OTA fracture classification system. J Orthop Trauma 2000;14:534–41.

15. Pignataro GS, Junqueira AE, Matsunaga FT, et al. Evaluation of the reproducibility of the AO/ASIF classification for humeral shaft fractures. Rev Bras Ortop 2015;50:378–82.

16. Jupiter JB, Mehne DK. Fractures of the distal humerus. Orthopedics 1992;15:825–33.

17. Bazzocchi A, Gomez MPA, Bartoloni A, et al. Emergency and trauma of the elbow. Semin Musculoskelet Radiol 2017;21:257–81.

18. Morrey BF. Anatomy of the elbow joint. In: Morrey BF, editor. The elbow and its disorders. Philadelphia: WB Saunders; 1993. p. 16–52.

19. Sanchez-Sotelo J. Distal humerus fractures. In: Antuña S, Barco R, editors. Essentials in elbow surgery. London: Springer; 2014. p. 47–60.

20. Morrey BF, Tanaka S, An KN. Valgus stability of the elbow: a definition of primary and secondary constraints. Clin Orthop Relat Res 1991;265: 187–95.

21. Amis AA, Miller JH. The mechanisms of elbow fractures: an investigation using impact tests in vitro. Injury 1995;26:163–8.

22. Mason ML. Some observations on fractures of the head of the radius with a review of one hundred cases. Br J Surg 1954;42:123–32.

23. Johnston GW. A follow-up of one hundred cases of fracture of the head of the radius with a review of the literature. Ulster Med J 1962;31:51–6.

24. Hotchkiss RN. Fractures and dislocations of the elbow. In: Rockwood CA Jr, Green DP, Bucholz RW, et al, editors. Rockwood and Green's fractures in adults. 4th edition. Philadelphia: Lippincott-Raven; 1996. p. 929–1024.

25. Hotchkiss RN. Displaced fractures of the radial head: internal fixation or excision? J Am Acad Orthop Surg 1997;5:1–10.

26. Iannuzzi NP, Leopold SS. In brief: the Mason classification of radial head fractures. Clin Orthop Relat Res 2012;470:1799–802.

27. Rommens PM, Kühle R, Schneider RU, et al. Olecranon fractures in adults: factors influencing outcome. Injury 2004;35:1149–57.

28. Closkey RF, Goode JR, Kirschenbaum D, et al. The role of the coronoid process in elbow stability. A biomechanical analysis of axial loading. J Bone Joint Surg Am 2000;82-A:1749–53.

29. Beingessner DM, Dunning CE, Stacpoole RA, et al. The effect of coronoid fractures on elbow kinematics and stability. Clin Biomech (Bristol, Avon) 2007;22: 183–90.

30. O'Driscoll SW, Jupiter JB, Cohen MS, et al. Difficult elbow fractures: pearls and pitfalls. Instr Course Lect 2003;52:113–34.

31. Regan W, Morrey B. Fractures of the coronoid process of the ulna. J Bone Joint Surg Am 1989;71: 1348–54.

32. O'Driscoll SW. Classification and evaluation of recurrent instability of the elbow. Clin Orthop Relat Res 2000;370:34–43.

33. Linscheid RL, Wheeler DK. Elbow dislocations. JAMA 1965;194:1171–6.

34. Ring D. Fractures and dislocations of the elbow. In: Rockwood CA, Green DP, Bucholz RW, editors. Rockwood and Green's fractures in adults. 6th edition. Philadelphia: Lippincott Williams & Wilkins; 2006. p. 989–1049.

35. Wiegand L, Bernstein J, Ahn J. Fractures in brief: olecranon fractures. Clin Orthop Relat Res 2012; 470:3637–41.

36. Stoneback JW, Owens BD, Sykes J, et al. Incidence of elbow dislocations in the United States population. J Bone Joint Surg Am 2012;94:240–5.

37. Cohen MS, Hastings H 2nd. Acute elbow dislocation: evaluation and management. J Am Acad Orthop Surg 1998;6:15–23.

38. O'Driscoll SW, Morrey BF, Korinek S, et al. Elbow subluxation and dislocation. A spectrum of instability. Clin Orthop Relat Res 1992;280:186–97.

39. O'Driscoll SW. Elbow dislocations. In: Morrey BF, Sanchez-Sotelo J, editors. The elbow and its disorders. 4th edition. Philadelphia: Saunders/Elsevier; 2009. p. 436–49.

40. Venkatram N, Wurm V, Houshian S. Anterior dislocation of the ulnar-humeral joint in a so-called 'pulled elbow'. Emerg Med J 2006;23:e37.

41. Slowik GM, Fitzimmons M, Rayhack JM. Closed elbow dislocation and brachial artery damage. J Orthop Trauma 1993;7:558–61.

42. Limb D, Hodkinson SL, Brown RF. Median nerve palsy after posterolateral elbow dislocation. J Bone Joint Surg Br 1994;76:987–8.

43. Schreiber JJ, Potter HG, Warren RF, et al. Magnetic resonance imaging findings in acute elbow dislocation: insight into mechanism. J Hand Surg Am 2014;39:199–205.

44. Rhyou IH, Kim YS. New mechanism of the posterior elbow dislocation. Knee Surg Sports Traumatol Arthrosc 2012;20:2535–41.

45. Robinson PM, Griffiths E, Watts AC. Simple elbow dislocation. Shoulder Elbow 2017;9:195–204.

46. Mehlhoff TL, Noble PC, Bennett JB, et al. Simple dislocation of the elbow in the adult: results after closed treatment. J Bone Joint Surg Am 1998;70:244–9.

47. Modi CS, Wasserstein D, Mayne IP, et al. The frequency and risk factors for subsequent surgery after a simple elbow dislocation. Injury 2015;46:1156–60.

48. Ring D, Jupiter JB, Zilberfarb J. Posterior dislocation of the elbow with fractures of the radial head and coronoid. J Bone Joint Surg Am 2002;84-A:547–51.

49. Coonrad RW, Roush TF, Major NM, et al. The drop sign, a radiographic warning sign of elbow instability. J Shoulder Elbow Surg 2005;14:312–7.

50. Mathew PK, Athwal GS, King GJ. Terrible triad injury of the elbow: current concepts. J Am Acad Orthop Surg 2009;17:137–51.

51. Chan K, MacDermid JC, Faber KJ, et al. Can we treat select terrible triad injuries nonoperatively? Clin Orthop Relat Res 2014;472:2092–9.

52. Doornberg JN, van Duijn J, Ring D. Coronoid fracture height in terrible-triad injuries. J Hand Surg Am 2006;31:794–7.

53. Jupiter JB, Kellam JF. Diaphyseal fractures of the forearm. In: Browner BD, editor. Skeletal trauma: basic science, management, and reconstruction.

3rd edition. Philadelphia: Saunders; 2003. p. 1363–403.

54. Hertel R, Rothenfluh DA. Fractures of the shafts of the radius and ulna. In: Rockwood CA, Green DP, Bucholz RW, editors. Rockwood and Green's fractures in adults. 6th edition. Philadelphia: Lippincott Williams & Wilkins; 2006. p. 965–88.

55. Bado JL. The Monteggia lesion. Clin Orthop Relat Res 1967;50:71–86.

56. McAdams TR, Masters GW, Srivastava S. The effect of arthroscopic sectioning of the lateral ligament complex of the elbow on posterolateral rotatory stability. J Shoulder Elbow Surg 2005;14:298–301.

57. Dunning CE, Zarzour ZD, Patterson SD, et al. Ligamentous stabilizers against posterolateral rotatory instability of the elbow. J Bone Joint Surg Am 2001;83-A:1823–8.

58. Tom JA, Kumar NS, Cerynik DL, et al. Diagnosis and treatment of triceps tendon injuries: a review of the literature. Clin J Sport Med 2014;24:197–204.

59. Safran MR, Graham SM. Distal biceps tendon ruptures: incidence, demographics, and the effect of smoking. Clin Orthop Relat Res 2002;404:275–83.

60. Schneider A, Bennett JM, O'Connor DP, et al. Bilateral ruptures of the distal biceps brachii tendon. J Shoulder Elbow Surg 2009;18:804–7.

61. Seiler JG 3rd, Parker LM, Chamberland PD, et al. The distal biceps tendon: two potential mechanisms involved in its rupture: arterial supply and mechanical impingement. J Shoulder Elbow Surg 1995;4:149–56.

62. Koulouris G, Malone W, Omar IM, et al. Bifid insertion of the distal biceps brachii tendon with isolated rupture: magnetic resonance findings. J Shoulder Elbow Surg 2009;18:e22–5.

63. Fuente JDL, Blasi M, Martinez S, et al. Ultrasound classification of traumatic distal biceps brachii tendon injuries. Skeletal Radiol 2018;47:519–32.

64. Lobo Lda G, Fessell DP, Miller BS, et al. The role of sonography in differentiating full versus partial distal biceps tendon tears: correlation with surgical findings. AJR Am J Roentgenol 2013;200:158–62.

65. Sollender JL, Rayan GM, Barden GA. Triceps tendon rupture in weight lifters. J Shoulder Elbow Surg 1998;7:151–3.

66. Nocerino EA, Cucchi D, Arrigoni P, et al. Acute and overuse elbow trauma: radio-orthopaedics overview. Acta Biomed 2018;89:124–37.

67. Vidal AF, Drakos MC, Allen AA. Biceps tendon and triceps tendon injuries. Clin Sports Med 2004;23:707–22.

68. Tagliafico A, Gandolfo N, Michaud J, et al. Ultrasound demonstration of distal triceps tendon tears. Eur J Radiol 2012;81:1207–10.

69. Bancroft LW, Pettis C, Wasyliw C, et al. Osteochondral Lesions of the Elbow. Semin Musculoskelet Radiol 2013;17:446–54.

70. Carter SJ, Germann CA, Dacus AA, et al. Orthopedic pitfalls in the ED: neurovascular injury associated with posterior elbow dislocations. Am J Emerg Med 2010;28:960–5.

71. Nelson AJ, Izzi JA, Green A, et al. Traumatic nerve injuries about the elbow. Orthop Clin North Am 1999;30:91–4.

72. Kuhn MA, Ross G. Acute elbow dislocations. Orthop Clin North Am 2008;39:155–61.

73. Baulot E, Giroux A, Ciry-Gomez M, et al. Brachialis arteria rupture following closed posterior elbow dislocation. Case report and literature review. Ann Chir Main Memb Super 1997;16:258–62.

Overuse Injuries of the Elbow

Arvin B. Kheterpal, MD, Miriam A. Bredella, MD*

KEYWORDS

- Elbow • MR imaging • Tendinopathy • Ulnar collateral ligament • Lateral collateral ligament
- Valgus extension overload syndrome • Apophysitis

KEY POINTS

- Chronic overuse injuries of the elbow can affect tendons, ligaments, and bones.
- Overuse of tendons results in tendinopathy, which can lead to partial- or full-thickness tears.
- Repetitive microtrauma to the ulnar collateral ligament can be seen in the overhead throwing athlete, which can also lead to partial- or full-thickness tears.
- Osseous changes from overuse include reactive bone marrow edema, osteophyte formation, enthesopathy, heterotopic ossification, osteochondral lesions, and stress injuries.

INTRODUCTION

Repetitive microtrauma in the elbow from chronic overuse occurs in both athletes and nonathletes. Although the diagnosis is often made clinically, imaging is helpful to confirm the diagnosis, grade the injury, and guide treatment. Tendons, ligaments, and bones can be affected, and the radiologist must be able to identify commonly seen patterns of injury.

MR imaging is particularly helpful in evaluating overuse injuries in the elbow, as tendons, ligaments, bones, and cartilage can be assessed. Tendinopathy can be distinguished from partial- or full-thickness tears, and reactive changes in the bone marrow can be easily identified. Ultrasound is also a useful modality for focused evaluation of tendons and ligaments in the elbow, but there are limitations in osseous evaluation. Although reactive changes along the surface of the bone can be seen, the bone marrow cannot be evaluated with ultrasound. Radiographs and computed tomography (CT) scans allow for excellent evaluation of the bones due to the high spatial resolution, but evaluation of tendons and ligaments is more limited. This article focuses on the MR imaging appearance of overuse injuries of the elbow involving tendons, ligaments, and bones.

TENDONS

Tendinopathy in the Elbow

Tendinopathy is commonly encountered in the elbow. Although clinicians often refer to tendinopathies at the medial and lateral elbow as "epicondylitis," reactive changes in the bone may or may not be present. Furthermore, there are usually no inflammatory cells microscopically.[1,2] As a result, most radiologists prefer the terms tendinopathy and tendinosis over epicondylitis and tendinitis.[2-4]

Repetitive overuse leading to microtears that incompletely heal is thought to be the underlying cause of tendinopathy.[2,5,6] Tendinopathy can progress to partial-thickness or full-thickness tears. The diagnosis is usually made with history and physical examination, sometimes in combination with imaging. Treatment is usually conservative, including physical therapy, bracing, rest, and avoiding provoking activities.[7,8] Oral

Disclosure Statement: The authors have nothing to disclose.
Division of Musculoskeletal Imaging and Intervention, Department of Radiology, Massachusetts General Hospital, Harvard Medical School, 55 Fruit Street Yawkey Suite 6E, Boston, MA 02114, USA
* Corresponding author.
E-mail address: mbredella@mgh.harvard.edu

Radiol Clin N Am 57 (2019) 931–942
https://doi.org/10.1016/j.rcl.2019.03.005

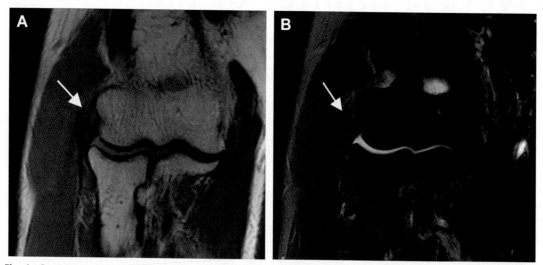

Fig. 1. Common extensor tendinopathy. Coronal proton-density (*A*) and fat-suppressed T2-weighted (*B*) images show thickening of the common extensor origin with increased signal intensity (*arrows*).

nonsteroidal anti-inflammatory drugs or targeted peritendinous corticosteroid injections can be helpful to manage pain. Ultrasound-guided tendon fenestration and injection of autologous blood or platelet-rich plasma are also among other treatment options; however, recent studies have advised against the use of platelet-rich plasma injection for chronic epicondylar tendinopathy.[9] If conservative measures fail, surgery may be required whereby the tendon can be debrided or released.[2,8,10–12]

Common Extensor Tendinopathy

Common extensor tendinopathy is commonly called "tennis elbow" because it is often seen in patients who play racket sports where there is overuse of the forearm extensor muscles and tendons, but the condition is not limited to athletes. It affects men and women equally, predominantly in the fifth and sixth decades. Patients report lateral elbow pain, and on physical examination, have point tenderness over the common extensor tendon origin.[8,13–16]

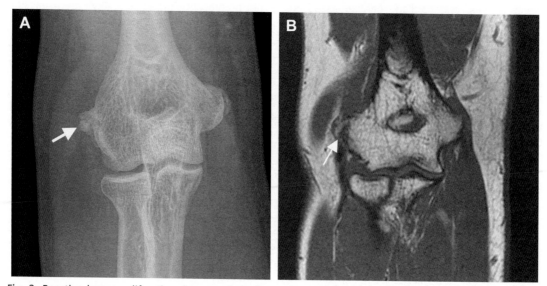

Fig. 2. Reactive bony proliferative changes of the lateral epicondyle on frontal radiograph (*A*) and coronal T1-weighted MR imaging (*B*) (*arrows*) associated with common extensor tendinopathy.

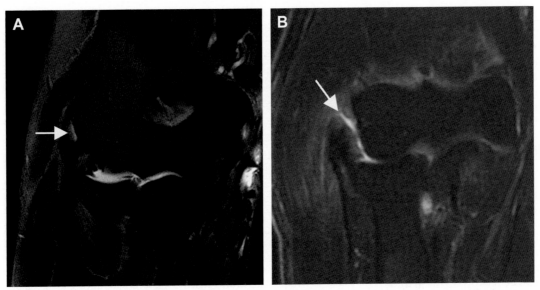

Fig. 3. Coronal fat-suppressed T2-weighted images show partial tear (*A*) and full-thickness tear (*B*) of common extensor origin with abnormal fluid signal within the tendon (*arrows*).

The common extensor tendon consists of the extensor carpi radialis brevis, extensor digitorum, extensor digiti minimi, and extensor carpi ulnaris. On MR imaging, tendinopathy is characterized by high intrasubstance signal alteration on both T1- and T2-weighted, proton-density-weighted sequences with or without tendon thickening (**Fig. 1**). The extensor carpi radialis brevis component of the tendon is usually most prominently involved. There can be surrounding soft tissue edema and associated bone marrow edema or bony proliferative changes[7,16–20] (**Fig. 2**). Tendinopathy can progress to partial- or full-thickness tearing, which can be distinguished on MR imaging by fluid-intensity signal (**Fig. 3**). Abnormalities of the lateral ulnar collateral ligament (LUCL) are often associated with common extensor tendinopathy/tearing (**Fig. 4**), and this must be carefully interrogated.[21]

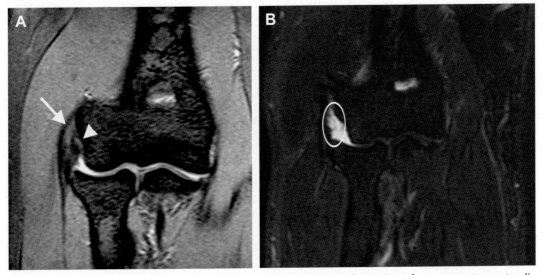

Fig. 4. Lateral ulnar collateral ligament (LUCL) pathologic condition in the setting of common extensor tendinopathy/tear. Coronal gradient echo image (*A*) demonstrates partial tear of the proximal LUCL (*arrowhead*) and common extensor tendinopathy (*arrow*). Coronal fat-suppressed T2-weighted image (*B*) demonstrates full-thickness tear of the LUCL and common extensor origin (*circle*).

Common Flexor Tendinopathy

Common flexor tendinopathy is often called "golfer's elbow," but, like common extensor tendinopathy, it affects both athletes and nonathletes. Common flexor tendinopathy is less common than common extensor tendinopathy.[22] The common flexor tendon provides stability to valgus and flexion forces at the elbow, which are commonly sustained in sports. Chronic symptoms can result from overuse or incomplete healing of avulsion injuries. Patients report medial elbow pain, and on physical examination, have point tenderness over the common flexor tendon origin. Tendinopathy with increased intrasubstance signal alteration with or without thickening and associated edema is seen on MR imaging (**Fig. 5**). Associated bony reactive changes are often present (**Fig. 6**). In more severe cases, partial- or full thickness tears can be seen[5–7,17,23–25] (**Fig. 7**).

Biceps Tendinopathy

Overuse injury of the distal biceps tendon, such as seen in weightlifters, can result in tendinopathy. On MR imaging, the distal biceps tendon has increased intrasubstance signal with or without thickening.[26,27] The flexed elbow, abducted shoulder, supinated forearm (FABS) view allows a longitudinal assessment along the entire length of the distal biceps tendon. The FABS view is obtained with the patient prone with the shoulder abducted

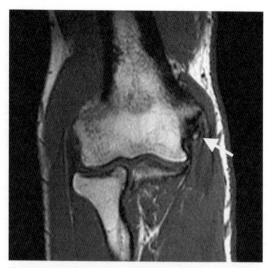

Fig. 6. Coronal proton-density-weighted image demonstrates reactive bony proliferative changes along the medial epicondyle (*arrow*) associated with common flexor tendinopathy.

180°, the elbow flexed 90°, and the forearm supinated[28] (**Fig. 8**). Repetitive microtrauma can also result in a partial-thickness tear. Full-thickness tears however are usually associated with an acute injury.[29,30]

The distal biceps tendon does not have a tendon sheath. Instead, the bicipitoradial bursa is interposed between the distal tendon and anterior humeral cortex in order to reduce friction between

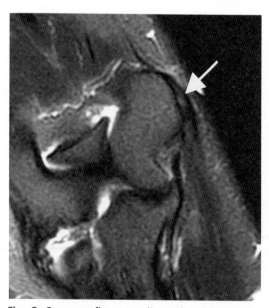

Fig. 5. Common flexor tendinopathy. Coronal fat-suppressed T2-weighted image shows thickening of the common flexor origin with increased signal intensity (*arrow*).

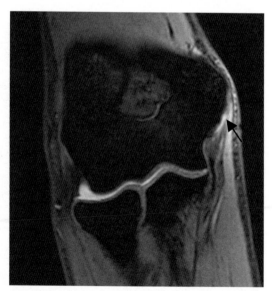

Fig. 7. Coronal fat-suppressed proton-density-weighted image demonstrates thickening and increased fluid signal in the substance of the common flexor origin (*arrow*), consistent with partial tear.

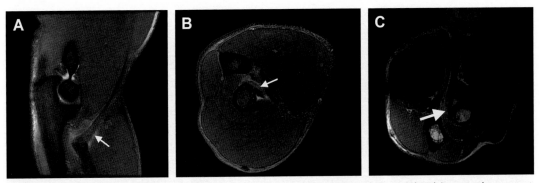

Fig. 8. Distal biceps tendinopathy. Sagittal (*A*) and axial (*B*) fat-suppressed T2-weighted images demonstrate thickening of the distal biceps tendon with increased signal intensity (*arrows*). FABS view (*C*) shows the entire length of the distal biceps tendon (*arrow*).

the tendon and bone. Reactive fluid can accumulate in the bicipitoradial bursa resulting in a bursitis[17,31] (**Fig. 9**). Chronic bicipitoradial bursitis may weaken the biceps tendon and predispose it to tearing.[17,30]

Triceps Tendinopathy

Triceps tendinopathy can be a cause of posterior elbow pain but is much less common than the aforementioned tendinopathies in the elbow. It can occur as a result of repetitive forceful or rapid extension, such as in weight training.[32] The tendinous attachment will show increased intrasubstance signal alteration, with or without thickening. Enthesopathy and/or reactive osseous or soft tissue changes can be seen at the attachment site[33] (**Fig. 10**). Full-thickness tears are usually associated with an acute injury.[29,34,35]

LIGAMENTS
Ulnar Collateral Ligament

The LUCL is composed of the anterior, transverse, and posterior bands or bundles. The anterior band of the LUCL is the primary soft tissue stabilizer to valgus forces at the elbow.[24,36] Repetitive microtrauma to the LUCL predominantly occurs in overhead throwing athletes, particularly in baseball pitchers. During the late cocking and early acceleration phase of pitching in baseball, the LUCL experiences repetitive tensile forces that result in laxity and tears over time.[24,37,38] Clinically, it can be difficult to characterize the severity of injury, so MR imaging is paramount in the workup.[13]

Even in asymptomatic high-performance baseball pitchers, morphologic changes can be seen in the LUCL on MR imaging.[39] Thickening of the LUCL with or without intrasubstance signal

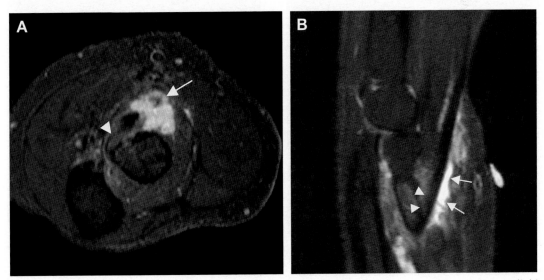

Fig. 9. Radiobicipital bursitis. Axial (*A*) and sagittal (*B*) fat-suppressed T2-weighted images demonstrate radiobicipital bursitis (*arrows*) in a patient with insertional biceps tendinopathy (*arrowheads*).

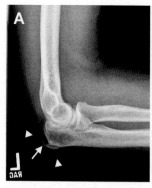
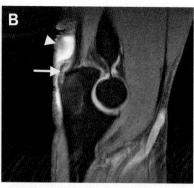
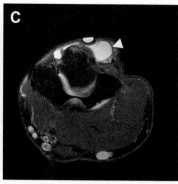

Fig. 10. Triceps tendinopathy with enthesopathy and associated soft tissue reactive changes. Lateral radiograph of the elbow (*A*) demonstrates triceps enthesopathy (*arrow*). There is associated soft tissue swelling (*arrowheads*). Sagittal (*B*) and axial (*C*) fat-suppressed T2-weighted images demonstrate thickening and increased signal intensity of the distal triceps insertion, consistent with tendinopathy (*arrow*). Associated olecranon bursitis is present (*arrowheads*).

alteration has been described[39,40] (**Fig. 11**). These findings are usually considered adaptive change in the high-performance pitcher. However, degeneration, attenuation, and superimposed acute injuries (**Fig. 12**), partial- or full-thickness tears, can also occur over time. Tears can occur proximally at the humeral attachment, in the midsubstance, or distally at the sublime tubercle attachment. Chronic injuries can result in heterotopic ossification within the substance of the tendon (**Fig. 13**).

Ossification within the tendon should be distinguished from an acute avulsion injury, which can occur at the sublime tubercle.[37,38]

Morphologic changes in the LUCL can also be seen on ultrasound, including thickening, heterogeneity, hypoechoic foci, and/or calcifications.[41] True hypoechoic foci must be distinguished from anisotropy. Dynamic ultrasound with valgus stress can also provide valuable information about the integrity of the LUCL, by assessing the degree of ulnohumeral joint space gapping and comparing it with the contralateral side.[41–43]

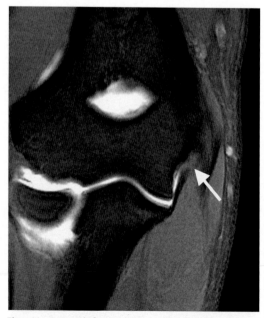

Fig. 11. Coronal fat-suppressed T2-weighted image from an elbow MR arthrogram demonstrates chronic overuse with thickening and increased signal intensity of the proximal portion of the LUCL (*arrow*) in a baseball pitcher.

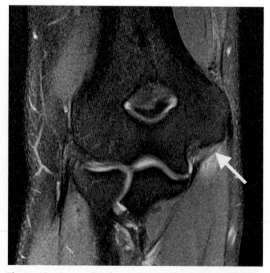

Fig. 12. Coronal fat-suppressed proton-density-weighted image in a baseball pitcher demonstrates chronic overuse of the LUCL with thickening of the proximal portion with superimposed acute injury, manifested by increased signal intensity of the ligament and surrounding soft tissues (*arrow*).

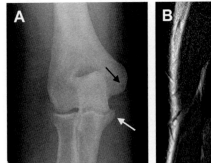
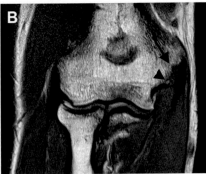
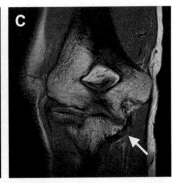

Fig. 13. Chronic osseous changes associated with LUCL overuse in a professional baseball pitcher. Frontal radiograph (*A*) demonstrates bony proliferative changes along the sublime tubercle of the ulna (*white arrow*). Erosion of medial epicondyle at the proximal attachment of the LUCL is noted (*black arrow*). Coronal proton-density-weighted image (*B*) demonstrates erosion (*black arrow*) and bony proliferative change (*arrowhead*) at the proximal attachment of the LUCL. Coronal proton-density-weighted image (*C*) demonstrates thickening of the distal LUCL at its attachment to the sublime tubercle from chronic overuse (*arrow*).

Lateral Collateral Ligament Complex

The lateral collateral ligament complex consists of the radial collateral ligament, LUCL, and annular ligament. Lateral collateral ligament injuries secondary to chronic varus stress are less common than medial sided injuries. As previously described, common extensor tendinopathy/tears are often associated with abnormalities of the LUCL.[21] This association is important because the LUCL stabilizes the elbow against varus and rotatory stress, and insufficiency of the ligament can lead to posterolateral rotatory instability.[5,32,44]

On MR imaging, chronic overuse of the lateral collateral ligament complex is manifested by thickening of the components of the lateral collateral ligament complex with or without intrasubstance signal alteration. These changes can propagate to partial- and full-thickness tears[16,17,45] (**Fig. 14**).

BONES
Valgus Extension Overload Syndrome

Valgus stress at the elbow during rapid elbow extension results in shearing forces along the olecranon. This has been described as "valgus

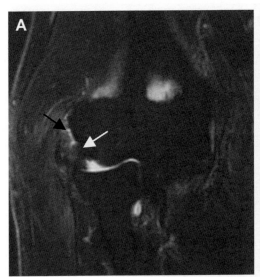
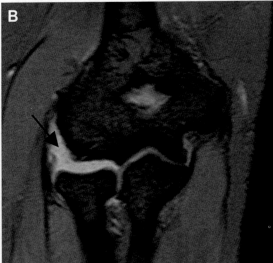

Fig. 14. Chronic overuse of the lateral collateral ligament complex. Coronal fat-suppressed T2-weighted image (*A*) demonstrates thickening and increased signal intensity of the proximal lateral collateral ligament (*white arrow*). Associated common extensor tendinopathy and partial tear are also present (*black arrow*). Coronal gradient-echo image (*B*) demonstrates full-thickness tear of the lateral collateral ligament (*black arrow*) in a patient with posterolateral rotatory instability.

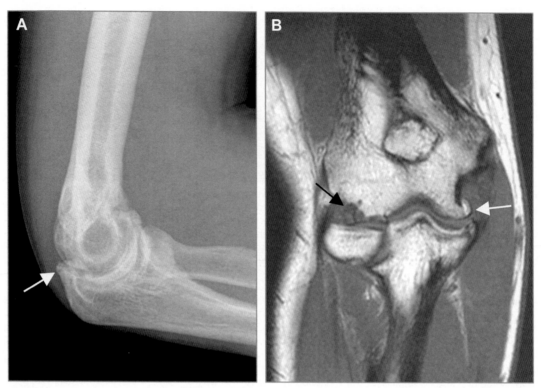

Fig. 15. Lateral radiograph (*A*) demonstrates osteophyte formation of the olecranon (*arrow*) in a professional baseball pitcher. Coronal proton-density-weighted image (*B*) shows medial osteophytes (*white arrow*) and associated osteochondral lesion of the capitellum (*black arrow*).

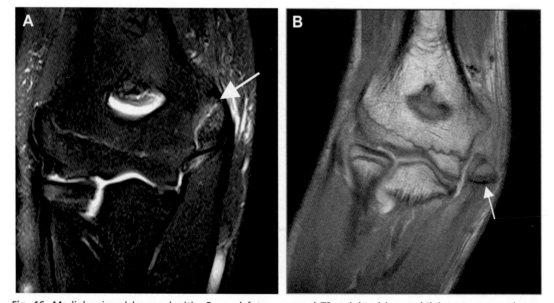

Fig. 16. Medial epicondyle apophysitis. Coronal fat-suppressed T2-weighted image (*A*) in a teenager demonstrates fluid signal in the area of the medial physis with associated marrow edema (*arrow*). Coronal proton-density-weighted image (*B*) in a different patient demonstrates avulsion and displacement of the medial physis (*arrow*).

extension overload syndrome" in baseball pitchers. Shearing forces posteromedially result in osteophyte formation, which can be painful, can cause impingement, and in some cases, can fracture resulting in loose bodies.[37,38,46] The osteophytes are best seen on CT scan, but an anteroposterior radiograph of the elbow in acute flexion can also be helpful for osteophyte detection, because the posteromedial joint becomes profiled. In addition to marginal osteophytes, articular cartilage defects over the trochlea and olecranon with or without underlying bone marrow edema, and posteromedial synovitis can be seen with MR imaging[47] (**Fig. 15**). Insertional tendinopathy at the medial border of the triceps has also

been described.[47] Surgical treatment includes arthroscopic debridement, osteophyte excision, and removal of loose bodies.[47,48]

Apophysitis

Medial epicondyle apophysitis is common in skeletally immature patients in the setting of chronic valgus stress because the growth plate at the apophysis is weaker than the LUCL. This condition is commonly called "little leaguer's elbow" because it is commonly seen in young baseball pitchers, but it can affect any overhead throwing athlete. On radiographs, the apophysis can be fragmented, overgrown, and/or displaced. On

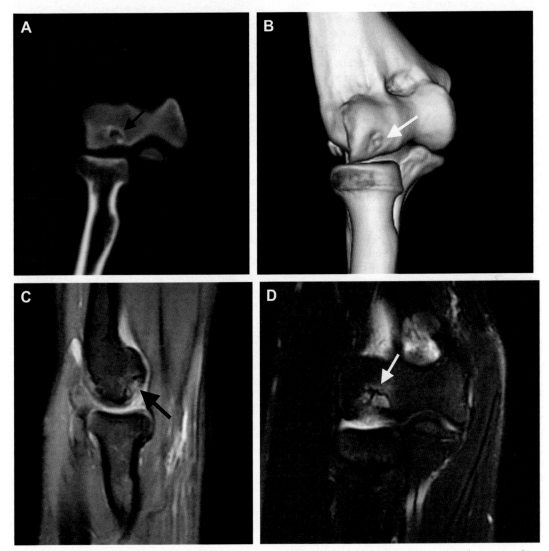

Fig. 17. Osteochondral defect of the capitellum. Coronal (*A*) and 3D (*B*) reformatted CT images show osteochondral defect of the capitellum (*arrows*). Sagittal (*C*) and coronal (*D*) fat-suppressed T2-weighted images demonstrate marrow edema of the capitellum underlying the cartilage defect (*arrows*).

MR imaging, the apophysis has increased signal on fluid-sensitive sequences, and the physis appears widened with periphyseal edema. In advanced stages, the physis can be displaced[13,37,49] (**Fig. 16**). Traction apophysitis can also occur elsewhere in the elbow, such as the olecranon, but this is less common. Treatment in most cases includes rest, activity modification, and physical therapy.

Osteochondral Lesions

Chronic valgus stress also results in compressive forces at the radiocapitellar joint. This can cause osteochondral lesions, most commonly involving the anterior and lateral aspect of the capitellum.[20,37,38,49] The greatest compressive and valgus forces in overhead throwing occur when the elbow is flexed, so the lesions usually occur along the anterior and lateral aspect of the capitellum. Early on, the diagnosis may be difficult to make on radiographs alone. However, as the condition progresses, subchondral lucency can be seen radiographs. In more advanced cases, there can be sclerosis, remodeling, fragmentation, and formation of loose bodies on radiographs and CT. Initially on MR imaging, there is hypointense subchondral signal abnormality on T1-weighted sequences with surrounding bone marrow edema. There may also be overlying cartilage defects (**Fig. 17**). The lesion should be interrogated for any undercutting fluid signal, which can be a sign of an unstable fragment.[20,50] The radiologist must be sure to distinguish capitellar osteochondral lesions from the normal pseudodefect of the capitellum, which is located more posteriorly than the usual osteochondral lesion.[51]

Treatment of the stable lesion is usually conservative, with rest and activity modification. Treatment of the unstable lesion is usually surgical and can include fixation, debridement, microfracture, and in some cases either osteochondral autograft or allograft transfer.[52]

Stress Fractures

Stress fractures of the olecranon from chronic valgus overload have been described in many athletes, including javelin throwers, gymnasts, and baseball pitchers.[32,53–55] Radiographs may show linear sclerosis or an incomplete fracture line. MR imaging is the most sensitive for detection, where bone marrow edema in combination with a linear fracture line can make the diagnosis[56] (**Fig. 18**). Stress fractures involving other bones of the elbow, such as the radial neck, are less common. Treatment is conservative, with rest and activity modification. However, if a stress

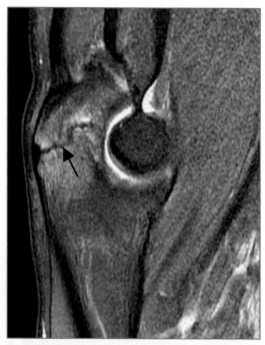

Fig. 18. Olecranon stress fracture. Sagittal fat-suppressed T2-weighted image in a baseball pitcher demonstrates marrow edema with hypointense fracture line (*arrow*).

fracture progresses to complete fracture with a displaced fragment, surgical fixation may be necessary.[32,53–55]

SUMMARY

Chronic overuse injuries in the elbow occur in athletes and nonathletes and affect a wide range of ages. Tendons, ligaments, and bones can be affected. MR imaging is usually the most helpful in distinguishing the offending structure and grading the severity of injury. Other modalities, including ultrasound, CT, and radiographs, can also give valuable information in the appropriate setting.

REFERENCES

1. Regan W, Wold LE, Coonrad R, et al. Microscopic histopathology of chronic refractory lateral epicondylitis. Am J Sports Med 1992;20(6):746–9.
2. Walz DM, Newman JS, Konin GP, et al. Epicondylitis: pathogenesis, imaging, and treatment. Radiographics 2010;30(1):167–84.
3. Nirschl RP. Elbow tendinosis/tennis elbow. Clin Sports Med 1992;11(4):851–70.
4. Nirschl RP. Muscle and tendon trauma: tennis elbow. In: Morrey BF, editor. The elbow. 2nd edition. Philadelphia: Saunders; 2000. p. 537–52.

5. Bucknor MD, Stevens KJ, Steinbach LS. Elbow imaging in sport: sports imaging series. Radiology 2016;280(1):328.

6. Ciccotti MC, Schwartz MA, Ciccotti MG. Diagnosis and treatment of medial epicondylitis of the elbow. Clin Sports Med 2004;23(4):693–705, xi.

7. Rineer CA, Ruch DS. Elbow tendinopathy and tendon ruptures: epicondylitis, biceps and triceps ruptures. J Hand Surg Am 2009;34(3):566–76.

8. Tarpada SP, Morris MT, Lian J, et al. Current advances in the treatment of medial and lateral epicondylitis. J Orthop 2018;15(1):107–10.

9. De Smet AA, Winter TC, Best TM, et al. Dynamic sonography with valgus stress to assess elbow ulnar collateral ligament injury in baseball pitchers. Skeletal Radiol 2002;31(11):671–6.

10. Gabel GT, Morrey BF. Operative treatment of medical epicondylitis. Influence of concomitant ulnar neuropathy at the elbow. J Bone Joint Surg Am 1995;77(7):1065–9.

11. Mishra A, Pirolo JM, Gosens T. Treatment of medial epicondylar tendinopathy in athletes. Sports Med Arthrosc Rev 2014;22(3):164–8.

12. Nirschl RP, Pettrone FA. Tennis elbow. The surgical treatment of lateral epicondylitis. J Bone Joint Surg Am 1979;61(6A):832–9.

13. Cain EL Jr, Dugas JR, Wolf RS, et al. Elbow injuries in throwing athletes: a current concepts review. Am J Sports Med 2003;31(4):621–35.

14. Field LD, Savoie FH. Common elbow injuries in sport. Sports Med 1998;26(3):193–205.

15. Gabel GT, Morrey BF. Tennis elbow. Instr Course Lect 1998;47:165–72.

16. Kotnis NA, Chiavaras MM, Harish S. Lateral epicondylitis and beyond: imaging of lateral elbow pain with clinical-radiologic correlation. Skeletal Radiol 2012;41(4):369–86.

17. Kijowski R, Tuite M, Sanford M. Magnetic resonance imaging of the elbow. Part II: Abnormalities of the ligaments, tendons, and nerves. Skeletal Radiol 2005;34(1):1–18.

18. Martin CE, Schweitzer ME. MR imaging of epicondylitis. Skeletal Radiol 1998;27(3):133–8.

19. Potter HG, Hannafin JA, Morwessel RM, et al. Lateral epicondylitis: correlation of MR imaging, surgical, and histopathologic findings. Radiology 1995;196(1):43–6.

20. Sampath SC, Sampath SC, Bredella MA. Magnetic resonance imaging of the elbow: a structured approach. Sports Health 2013;5(1):34–49.

21. Bredella MA, Tirman PF, Fritz RC, et al. MR imaging findings of lateral ulnar collateral ligament abnormalities in patients with lateral epicondylitis. AJR Am J Roentgenol 1999;173(5):1379–82.

22. Shiri R, Viikari-Juntura E, Varonen H, et al. Prevalence and determinants of lateral and medial epicondylitis: a population study. Am J Epidemiol 2006;164(11):1065–74.

23. Alcid JG, Ahmad CS, Lee TQ. Elbow anatomy and structural biomechanics. Clin Sports Med 2004;23(4):503–17, vii.

24. Rossy WH, Oh LS. Pitcher's elbow: medial elbow pain in the overhead-throwing athlete. Curr Rev Musculoskelet Med 2016;9(2):207–14.

25. Safran MR, Baillargeon D. Soft-tissue stabilizers of the elbow. J Shoulder Elbow Surg 2005;14(1 Suppl S):179S–85S.

26. Chew ML, Giuffre BM. Disorders of the distal biceps brachii tendon. Radiographics 2005;25(5):1227–37.

27. Fitzgerald SW, Curry DR, Erickson SJ, et al. Distal biceps tendon injury: MR imaging diagnosis. Radiology 1994;191(1):203–6.

28. Giuffre BM, Moss MJ. Optimal positioning for MRI of the distal biceps brachii tendon: flexed abducted supinated view. AJR Am J Roentgenol 2004;182(4):944–6.

29. Stucken C, Ciccotti MG. Distal biceps and triceps injuries in athletes. Sports Med Arthrosc Rev 2014;22(3):153–63.

30. Williams BD, Schweitzer ME, Weishaupt D, et al. Partial tears of the distal biceps tendon: MR appearance and associated clinical findings. Skeletal Radiol 2001;30(10):560–4.

31. Skaf AY, Boutin RD, Dantas RW, et al. Bicipitoradial bursitis: MR imaging findings in eight patients and anatomic data from contrast material opacification of bursae followed by routine radiography and MR imaging in cadavers. Radiology 1999;212(1):111–6.

32. Hayter CL, Giuffre BM. Overuse and traumatic injuries of the elbow. Magn Reson Imaging Clin N Am 2009;17(4):617–38, v.

33. Donaldson O, Vannet N, Gosens T, et al. Tendinopathies around the elbow part 2: medial elbow, distal biceps and triceps tendinopathies. Shoulder Elbow 2014;6(1):47–56.

34. Farrar EL 3rd, Lippert FG 3rd. Avulsion of the triceps tendon. Clin Orthop Relat Res 1981;(161):242–6.

35. Koplas MC, Schneider E, Sundaram M. Prevalence of triceps tendon tears on MRI of the elbow and clinical correlation. Skeletal Radiol 2011;40(5):587–94.

36. Patten RM. Overuse syndromes and injuries involving the elbow: MR imaging findings. AJR Am J Roentgenol 1995;164(5):1205–11.

37. Ouellette H, Bredella M, Labis J, et al. MR imaging of the elbow in baseball pitchers. Skeletal Radiol 2008;37(2):115–21.

38. Ouellette HA, Palmer W, Torriani M, et al. Throwing elbow in adults. Semin Musculoskelet Radiol 2010;14(4):412–8.

39. Kooima CL, Anderson K, Craig JV, et al. Evidence of subclinical medial collateral ligament injury and posteromedial impingement in professional baseball players. Am J Sports Med 2004;32(7):1602–6.

40. Del Grande F, Aro M, Jalali Farahani S, et al. High-resolution 3-T magnetic resonance imaging of the shoulder in nonsymptomatic professional baseball pitcher draft picks. J Comput Assist Tomogr 2016; 40(1):118–25.

41. Nazarian LN, McShane JM, Ciccotti MG, et al. Dynamic US of the anterior band of the ulnar collateral ligament of the elbow in asymptomatic major league baseball pitchers. Radiology 2003;227(1):149–54.

42. Ciccotti MC, Hammoud S, Dodson CC, et al. Stress ultrasound evaluation of medial elbow instability in a cadaveric model. Am J Sports Med 2014;42(10): 2463–9.

43. Ciccotti MG, Atanda A Jr, Nazarian LN, et al. Stress sonography of the ulnar collateral ligament of the elbow in professional baseball pitchers: a 10-year study. Am J Sports Med 2014;42(3):544–51.

44. Olsen BS, Vaesel MT, Sojbjerg JO, et al. Lateral collateral ligament of the elbow joint: anatomy and kinematics. J Shoulder Elbow Surg 1996;5(2 Pt 1): 103–12.

45. Desharnais L, Kaplan PA, Dussault RG. MR imaging of ligamentous abnormalities of the elbow. Magn Reson Imaging Clin N Am 1997;5(3):515–28.

46. Wilson FD, Andrews JR, Blackburn TA, et al. Valgus extension overload in the pitching elbow. Am J Sports Med 1983;11(2):83–8.

47. Cohen SB, Valko C, Zoga A, et al. Posteromedial elbow impingement: magnetic resonance imaging findings in overhead throwing athletes and results of arthroscopic treatment. Arthroscopy 2011; 27(10):1364–70.

48. Koh JL, Zwahlen BA, Altchek DW, et al. Arthroscopic treatment successfully treats posterior elbow impingement in an athletic population. Knee Surg Sports Traumatol Arthrosc 2018;26(1):306–11.

49. Delgado J, Jaramillo D, Chauvin NA. Imaging the injured pediatric athlete: upper extremity. Radiographics 2016;36(6):1672–87.

50. Sampaio ML, Schweitzer ME. Elbow magnetic resonance imaging variants and pitfalls. Magn Reson Imaging Clin N Am 2010;18(4):633–42.

51. Rosenberg ZS, Beltran J, Cheung YY. Pseudodefect of the capitellum: potential MR imaging pitfall. Radiology 1994;191(3):821–3.

52. Smith MV, Bedi A, Chen NC. Surgical treatment for osteochondritis dissecans of the capitellum. Sports Health 2012;4(5):425–32.

53. Hulkko A, Orava S, Nikula P. Stress fractures of the olecranon in javelin throwers. Int J Sports Med 1986;7(4):210–3.

54. Maffulli N, Chan D, Aldridge MJ. Derangement of the articular surfaces of the elbow in young gymnasts. J Pediatr Orthop 1992;12(3):344–50.

55. Maffulli N, Chan D, Aldridge MJ. Overuse injuries of the olecranon in young gymnasts. J Bone Joint Surg Br 1992;74(2):305–8.

56. Kijowski R, Tuite M, Sanford M. Magnetic resonance imaging of the elbow. Part I: normal anatomy, imaging technique, and osseous abnormalities. Skeletal Radiol 2004;33(12):685–97.

The Acutely Injured Wrist

Federico Bruno, MD[a], Francesco Arrigoni, MD[a], Pierpaolo Palumbo, MD[a], Raffaele Natella, MD[b], Nicola Maggialetti, MD[c], Alfonso Reginelli, MD[b], Alessandra Splendiani, MD[a], Ernesto Di Cesare, MD[a], Alberto Bazzocchi, MD, PhD[d], Giuseppe Guglielmi, MD[e], Carlo Masciocchi, MD[a], Antonio Barile, MD[a],*

KEYWORDS

• Trauma • Wrist fractures • Carpal instability • TFCC injuries • Pediatric wrist fractures

KEY POINTS

• An accurate clinical and radiological evaluation of wrist traumas is fundamental for the best clinical outcome of the patient.
• Understanding of the mechanisms of injury and injury patterns can help in alerting to the possibility of associated injuries and provide precise treatment management.
• The evaluation of direct and indirect signs of injury on radiographic examination is essential to diagnose bone fractures and associated soft tissue injuries.
• Among other imaging modalities for the evaluation of the acutely injured wrist, CT has a fundamental role for assessing occult and comminuted fractures, whereas MRI is superior in the evaluation of ligament injuries and for some bony injuries, especially in pediatric patients.

INTRODUCTION

The wrist is one of the main functional joints in daily life activities, and is particularly susceptible to traumatic injuries.[1,2] Wrist injuries represent about 28% of all musculoskeletal injuries, accounting for 14.0% to 30.0% of all traumas in the emergency department and 28.0% of all musculoskeletal injuries.[3] Wrist traumas require prompt treatment of the structures involved, so a precise diagnosis of the type of injury is essential.[2]

Clinical evaluation is not always sufficient to estimate the type of damage, and radiological instrumental examinations are essential to complete the diagnosis. Radiographic examination is the first-line method of imaging, even if false-negative rates are reported to be up to 40%.[4] Tomographic imaging methods, such as computed tomography (CT)

and MR imaging, are therefore the tools of study that are often used, especially in the case of occult fractures, and for the diagnosis of ligament and soft tissue lesions.[5–16] Ultrasound (US), although with some limitations, also can have a complementary role.[17]

Bony Injuries

Bone traumas of the wrist more frequently follow a fall onto an outstretched hand, and the forces applied to the distal of the radius cause fractures at this level.[3]

Conventional radiography

The assessment of radiograms in posteroanterior and lateral projection must include, in addition to the recognition of cortical interruption as a direct sign of fractures, several indirect signs[18]:

Disclosure: The authors have nothing to disclose.
[a] Department of Biotechnological and Applied Clinical Sciences, University of L'Aquila, Via Vetoio 1, Coppito, L'Aquila (AQ) 67100, Italy; [b] Department of Precision Medicine, University of Campania "L.Vanvitelli", Via Santa Maria di Costantinopoli 104, 80138 Naples, Italy; [c] Department Life and Health "V. Tiberio", University of Molise, Via Francesco De Sanctis, 86100 Campobasso, Italy; [d] Diagnostic and Interventional Radiology, IRCCS Istituto Ortopedico Rizzoli, Via C. Pupilli 1, 40136 Bologna, Italy; [e] Department of Radiology, University of Foggia, Viale Luigi Pinto 1, Foggia 71100, Italy
* Corresponding author.
E-mail address: antonio.barile@cc.univaq.it

Radiol Clin N Am 57 (2019) 943–955
https://doi.org/10.1016/j.rcl.2019.05.003

- Uniformly, the space between the carpal bones and the carpometacarpal space must be approximately 1–2 mm
- The alignment of the carpal bones must follow the Gilula lines, represented by 3 arches described along the proximal surface of the proximal row of carpal bones, the distal articular surface of carpal bones, and the proximal curvature of the capitate and hamate, respectively. In the event of irregularities, interruptions, or steps on these lines there is a strong suspicion of fracture or ligament injury
- The metacarpals must be aligned with the distal row of carpal bones (in particular the third metacarpal with the capitate). The loss of this alignment very often indicates dislocation
- On the lateral film, the distal radial angle should be evaluated. The distal radius has a volar tilt (the angle between a line drawn along the long axis of the radius and a line drawn from the dorsal to the volar rim of the radius) of about 10°. Alterations of this angle are an indirect sign of fracture
- Radiographic alterations of the soft tissues, in particular of the pronator fat stripe, can identify subtle radius fracture

Computed tomography

The CT examination is an excellent complement to the radiographic examination thanks to the high resolution, and the possibility of obtaining multiplanar and 3D reconstructions. Individual cases in which CT is used are complex fracture-dislocations, fractures of the articular surface, and small isolated fractures of the carpal bones (particularly hamate and capitate), and for presurgical planning.[19]

MR imaging

MR imaging is not routinely used in emergency, but is the examination of choice in cases of occult fractures (in particular of the scaphoid). It is also fundamental in detecting bone contusion (or bone bruise) resulting from subcortical trabecular microfractures with intraosseous hemorrhage and edema.[20–22]

Distal radial fractures Colles fracture is the most common type of fracture, especially in adult women with osteoporosis. The pattern includes (i) fracture of the distal radius, without the involvement of the articular surface, (ii) dorsal angulation of distal fragment, (iii) dorsal displacement of the fragment, and (iv) associated fracture of the ulnar styloid process[18,23] (**Fig. 1**).

Barton injury is defined as a fracture line through the articular surface of the carpal extremity of the radius with dorsal subluxation. The bone fragment can be of different size, involving up to 50% of the articular surface, but is usually small. The lunate remains together with the displaced radial fragment, a feature that distinguishes this type of fracture from a radiocarpal dislocation[24] (**Fig. 2**). In cases of volar subluxation, the injury is termed a reverse Barton fracture (**Fig. 3**).

Hutchinson or Chauffeur fracture is an isolated fracture of the radial styloid process. The fracture line is intra-articular and runs obliquely from the cortical surface. The radial styloid process is more involved due to the resistance of the radioscapholunate and the radiolunotriquetal ligament on the styloid side.[23]

Die punch injury is a depressed comminuted (up to 4 fragments) intra-articular fracture of the radial articular surface caused by the impaction of the lunate on the lunate fossa of the radius. The entire extension of the fracture lines can be challenging to asses with conventional radiograms, having both sagittal and coronal components, but is accurately depicted with CT. This type of fracture usually is associated with more complex osseous and ligamentous injuries[14,19] (**Fig. 4**).

Ulnar fractures Fractures of the ulna, particularly of the styloid, are frequently associated with distal radius injuries. Two patterns of distal ulnar fractures: type I, involving the distal tip of the ulnar styloid, and type II, involving the base. These latter injuries are frequently associated with disruption of the triangular fibrocartilage (TFC) insertion and distal radioulnar joint (DRUJ) instability.[18]

Carpal bone fractures Scaphoid fractures are the most frequent in the bony traumas of the carpus, representing an incidence of about 60%. The high incidence of scaphoid involvement is because the scaphoid acts as a bridge between the proximal and distal bones of the carpus, and is more easily put under stress. The waist area of the scaphoid is also crossed by the radiocapitate ligament. Finally, in dorsiflexion trauma the scaphoid impacts with the dorsal profile of the radius.[18,25]

The evaluation of suspected scaphoid fractures requires special radiographic projections, because, in standard anteroposterior (AP) and lateral view, the X-ray beam crosses the scaphoid obliquely and not perpendicularly, thus subtle fractures can be easily missed. Dedicated radiographic projections are usually obtained with the wrist in ulnar deviation and the tube angled at 45° toward the elbow.[26]

A major complication, occurring in about 30% of scaphoid fractures is avascular necrosis of the

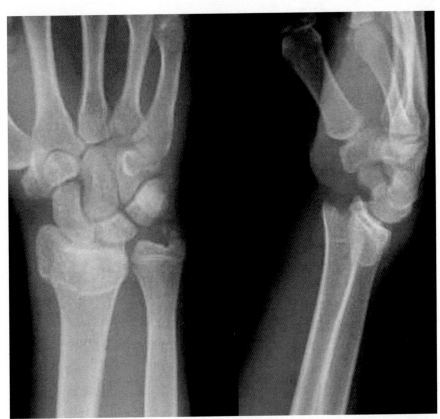

Fig. 1. Wrist anteroposterior (AP) and lateral view showing a Colles fracture of the distal radius. Note the dorsal angulation of the distal radius fragment and the associated fracture of the ulnar styloid. Radial articular surface is not involved.

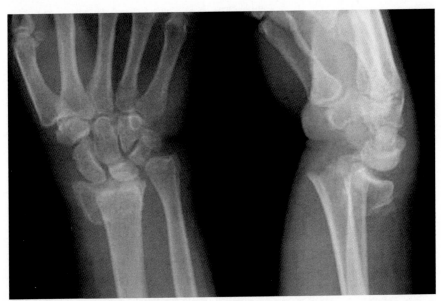

Fig. 2. Wrist AP and lateral view showing a Barton fracture of the distal radius. Note the fracture line through the articular surface with dorsal subluxation. The lunate remains together with the displaced radial fragment.

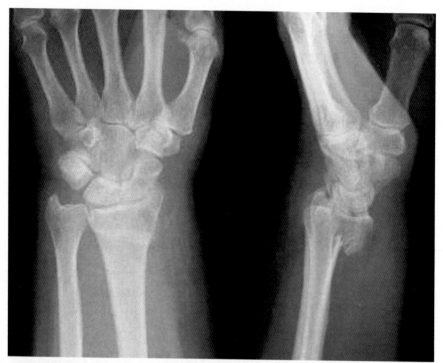

Fig. 3. Wrist AP and lateral view showing a Barton fracture of the distal radius.

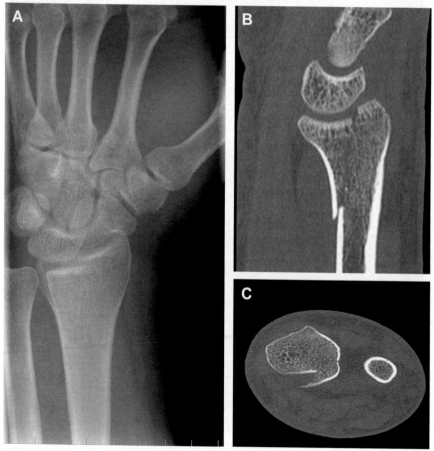

Fig. 4. Wrist AP view (*A*) showing a die punch injury of the distal radius. Note the depression of the articular surface fragment. CT coronal (*B*) and axial (*C*) reconstructions better depict the extension of the fracture lines.

scaphoid, especially in the waist and lower pole fractures, because the blood supply, provided from the distal pole to the proximal pole, is interrupted.[27]

The triquetral bone is the second most commonly fractured carpal bone in wrist injuries (about 18%–20%), caused by the avulsion of the radiotriquetral and ulnotriquetral ligaments. Triquetral fracture is more easily detected on lateral projections on the dorsal profile.

Fracture of the hamate and other carpal bones are less frequent, representing only 3% of carpal bone fractures. As these fractures are often challenging to recognize from standard radiographic projections, CT and MR imaging can be used as complementary examinations to confirm the diagnosis[28] (**Fig. 5**).

Pediatric bone injuries Pediatric bone injury patterns in wrist trauma are frequently different from fractures in adults and have a typical appearance. Because of the presence of unfused epiphyses, distal radius injury involves the epiphyseal growth plate preferentially, determining the

so-called *Salter-Harris fractures*. The most common fractures are those of type I and type II. The epiphysis is more frequently displaced dorsally[29] (**Fig. 6**).

Salter-Harris fractures can be challenging to detect on plain films with standard projections, especially if the physeal plate in not grossly widened or displaced. Attention should be paid to indirect signs, such as the presence of joint effusion or soft tissue swelling. In dubious cases or when there is clinical suspicion, MR imaging is indicated; the Salter-Harris injury is clearly evident on MR imaging as a physeal high-intensity line on T2 and fluid-sensitive sequences.[30]

Buckle (torus) fractures are pediatric fractures caused by compression forces, with disruption of the fibrous cortex but without disruption of the periosteal sleeve. In wrist injuries, buckle fractures can occur either at the distal or ulnar metaphysis. The radiographic appearance of the fracture is typical, with the crowning of the cortical profile. Sometimes, however, imaging signs appear days after the trauma when periosteal reaction or sclerosis begins to develop[31] (**Fig. 7**).

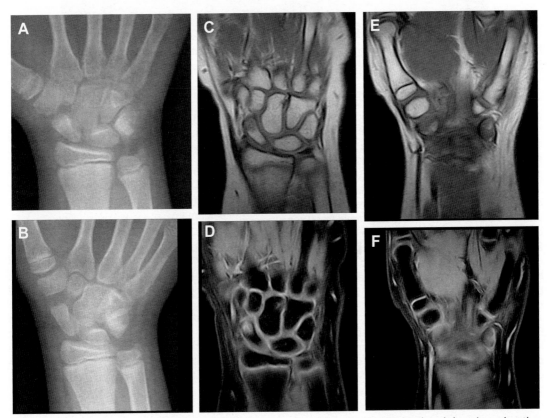

Fig. 5. Wrist AP (*A*) and dedicated AP projection for the scaphoid (*B*). Coronal T1 (*C, E*) and short inversion time inversion recovery (STIR). (*D, F*) MR imaging sequences in the same patient depict bone marrow edema and a fracture line at the proximal pole of the scaphoid. Note also the bone edema of the pisiform consistent with a bone contusion.

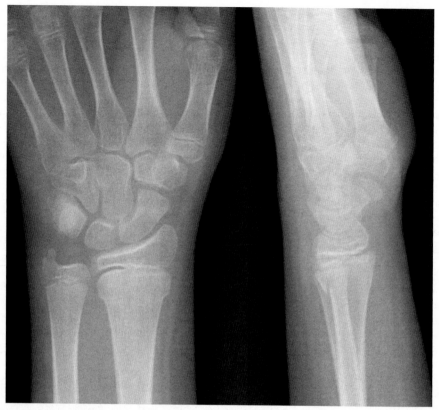

Fig. 6. Wrist AP and lateral view showing a Salter-Harris fracture of the distal radius. Note, in the lateral projection, the fracture line extending through the metaphysis (type II).

Greenstick fractures are characterized by cortical disruption on the tension side of the fracture, with an intact cortex on the contralateral compression side. Unlike buckle fractures, greenstick fractures are more unstable and may continue to displace after the first 2 weeks (**Fig. 8**).

Evaluating pediatric bone injuries, we should be aware and familiar with some normal variants of the pediatric skeleton that can mimic fractures or injury patterns. These include partial bone fusion (frequent at the level of lunate-triquetral), accessory ossicles (eg, os epilunatum, os hamulus) or developmental irregularities of bone profile (frequent at the level of the pisiform).[31]

Carpal instability Wrist injuries, especially those involving scaphoid fractures and disruption of carpal ligaments (mainly scapholunate and lunotriquetral ligament) are associated with a carpal dislocation, due to the break of bony and ligament linkage between the carpal rows. The proximal row of bones and the lunate are most commonly involved.[32] Imaging evaluation of suspected carpal instability requires accurate scrutiny of several direct and indirect signs (**Fig. 9**).

Mayfield[33] proposed a 4-part schematic progression of injury with extension, ulnar deviation, and carpal supination in wrist traumas, defined as progressive perilunar instability (PLI)[34] (**Fig. 10**).

- *Stage I: scapholunate dissociation.* There is a dorsal subluxation of the proximal pole of the scaphoid with disruption of the scapholunate ligament.
- *Stage II: perilunate dislocation.* Injury forces progress to the space of Poirier with further extension, ulnar deviation, and supination of the carpus. Carpal bones dislocate dorsally, and the lunate is still aligned with the distal radius.
- *Stage III: midcarpal dislocation.* Disruption of the lunotriquetral ligament, with displacement or fracture of the triquetrum. The capitolunate joint is also disrupted, and neither the capitate nor the lunate are aligned with the distal radius.
- *Stage IV: lunate dislocation.* Disruption of the dorsal radiocarpal ligament. This is more often an isolated finding, without associated fractures. The radiographic appearance of a lunate dislocation include: (i) intercarpal

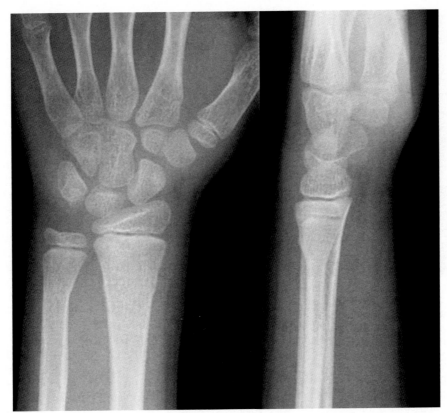

Fig. 7. Wrist AP and lateral view showing a buckle fracture of the distal radius.

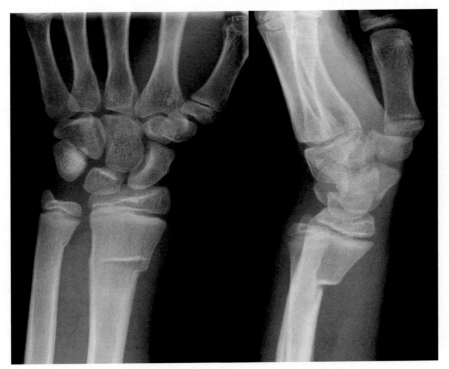

Fig. 8. Wrist AP and lateral view showing a greenstick fracture of the distal radius.

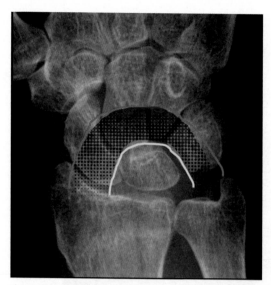

Fig. 9. The "zone of vulnerability" situated between the lesser arc (*yellow*) and the greater arc (*red*). Injuries along the lesser arc are consistent with *lunate dislocations*. Injuries along the greater arc are consistent with *preilunate dislocations*.

distance reduction and overlap of carpal bones on AP radiographic films and (ii) triangular appearance of the lunate, with volar displacement (look at the radio-luno-capitate alignment on lateral films)

Lesions of the *scapholunate ligament*, as described in PLI progression, determine the volar

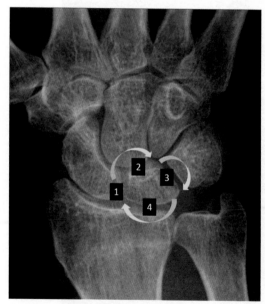

Fig. 10. Schematic representation of Mayfield perilunar instability (PLI) progression (Stages 1–4).

flexion of the scaphoid and dorsiflexion of the lunotriquetral block, with a resultant dorsal intercalated segmental instability pattern.[35] The main radiographic sign of scapholunate (SL) ligament injury is widening (>2–4 mm) of the SL distance ("Terry Thomas" sign) (**Fig. 11**). In doubtful cases or cases of dynamic instability, a clenched-fist projection, or views in ulnar and radial deviation, may be useful to load the capitate into the proximal carpal row and to produce increased widening. It is also essential to evaluate the contralateral wrist to exclude conditions of congenital SL ligament laxity. Another radiographic sign is the "signet-ring" sign, caused by the superimposition of the distal pole and the body of the scaphoid. Early recognizing of SL ligament injuries is of paramount importance, because a late severe complication of untreated scapholunate instability is scapholunate advanced collapse.[18,21]

As opposed to SL ligament injuries, *lunotriquetral ligament* disruption results from injuries in extension, radial deviation, and internal protonation, with consequent reverse PLI. In these injuries, the lunate remains attached to the scaphoid, and the triquetrum is dislocated dorsally, resulting in a volar intercalated segmental instability deformity.[36]

Even if carpal dislocations can be diagnosed with sufficient confidence using conventional radiography, MR imaging is the imaging modality of choice for the evaluation of the extrinsic ligaments of the wrist. MR imaging shows disruption or nonvisualization of incomplete tears of the ligament. Partial tears can be evident as fraying, thinning, elongation, or irregular course of the ligament, together with increased T2 signal intensity. The specificity of these MR signs is, however low, as there is a significant overlap with nontraumatic degenerative changes. The use of MR and CT arthrography with intra-articular contrast injection increases the diagnostic accuracy.[37]

SOFT TISSUE INJURIES
Triangular Fibrocartilage Complex Injuries

The triangular fibrocartilage complex (TFCC) is frequently injured during wrist traumas in protonation and extension, and anatomic factors such as a positive ulnar variance can increase the risk of a TFCC injury. Typical signs and symptoms of TFCC injuries include ulnar-sided swelling and pain with crepitus and instability during wrist movements.[38]

Because the treatment of TFCC injuries is strongly influenced by the pattern of injury, a precise and accurate diagnosis of the entity of the trauma is required for optimal treatment planning.

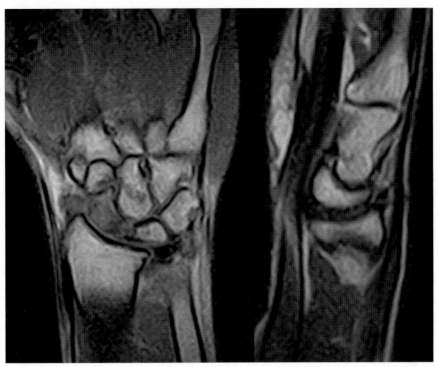

Fig. 11. Coronal and sagittal MR imaging of the wrist showing an SL ligament injury. In the coronal slice note the widening of the SL distance ("Terry Thomas" sign). In the sagittal cut, the dorsiflexion of the lunotriquetral block with dorsal intercalated segmental instability pattern is better appreciated.

TFCC tears can be divided into traumatic and degenerative according to the Palmer classification.[39]

Palmer class 1 tears include traumatic injuries and are subclassified according to the location as follows (**Fig. 12**):

- Class 1A tears, the most common subtype, involve the central fibrocartilage disk. Class 1A tears are most frequently localized at the radial side and frequently show a complex configuration.
- Class 1B tears are peripheral, near or at the insertion on the distal ulna. These tears may be associated with a fracture at the base of the ulnar styloid and DRUJ instability.
- Class 1C tears are distal avulsions, involving the volar ulnolunate or ulnotriquetral ligaments. Class 1C lesions are less common and can be associated with ulnar carpal instability due to palmar migration of the ulnar carpus.
- Class 1D tears are characterized by avulsion of the TFCC from its radial attachment at the sigmoid notch of the radius, and can be associated with an avulsion fracture of the sigmoid notch.

MR imaging is the modality of choice to assess TFCC injuries. MR imaging appearance of TFC tears is a linear high signal intensity defect on T2-weighted images. As reported for carpal ligaments, the sensitivity and specificity of standard MR imaging to detect peripheral tears is variable (reported sensitivity from 17% to 100%), as there are frequent cases of asymptomatic defects, especially in older patients.[2] The literature is mixed regarding the sensitivity and specificity of conventional MR imaging in detecting peripheral TFCC tears, ranging in sensitivity from 17% to 100%. Magnetic resonance arthrography visualization of contrast leakage through torn structures is the gold standard imaging examination, with sensitivity in detecting peripheral tears even higher than arthroscopy[40] (**Fig. 13**).

Distal Radioulnar Joint Instability

Injuries of the TFCC, especially when involving the dorsal and palmar radioulnar ligaments, and if associated with fracture of the distal radius or ulna, can result in instability of the DRUJ.[18] The mechanism of injury is a trauma in extension and extreme protonation. Typical fractures resulting in DRUJ instability are the Galeazzi

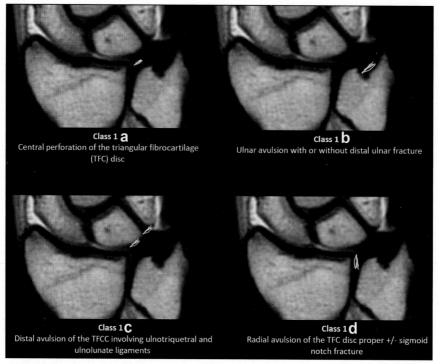

Fig. 12. TFCC injuries (palmer classification).

fracture-dislocation, in which there is a displaced radial fracture and an ulnar styloid fracture, and the Essex-Lopresti injury, a proximal radial head or neck fracture with interosseous ligament disruption. In DRUJ dislocation the ulna is dorsally dislocated in most cases.[4]

Isolated injuries of the DRUJ are less frequent, so detection of DRUJ dislocation should always raise suspicion for a more proximal radial fracture. The main clinical finding in these instabilities is the wrist locked in protonation with the patient unable to supinate. Diagnosis of DRUJ instability can be challenging on standard radiographic examination. The main imaging findings are an increased

distance (of 6 mm or more) between the distal radius and ulna on a true lateral projection, and an increased gap between the distal radius and ulna with dorsal dislocation or superimposition of the radius and ulna with volar dislocation on AP films.[29]

CT is frequently required to confirm the diagnosis. Several methods based on CT findings are described to evaluate DRUJ instability, namely the Mino method, the congruency method, and the epicenter method. The epicenter method is the most commonly used, being the most specific to detect radioulnar subluxation.[4] The epicenter method is evaluated determining the center of

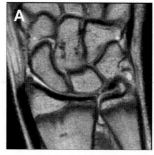
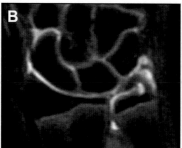
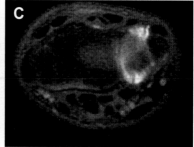

Fig. 13. Coronal T1 (A) and T2 fat-sat (B) and axial (C) magnetic resonance arthrography images of the wrist showing a TFCC tear near the radial side. There is also contrast medium leakage at the level of the distal radioulnar joint because of irregularity of the anterior ligamentous component of syndesmosis.

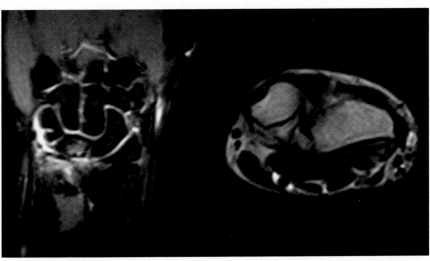

Fig. 14. Coronal STIR and axial T2 images of the wrist showing dorsal dislocation of the ulna. Note the bone marrow edema of the lunate, the distal ulna and radius fracture, and the high signal intensity at the level of the disrupted TFCC, findings consistent with severe DRUJ instability.

rotation of the DRUJ, halfway between the ulnar styloid and the center of the ulnar head. A perpendicular line is then drawn from the chord of the sigmoid notch to the center of rotation of the DRUJ. The DRUJ is considered normal if the line is in the middle half of the sigmoid notch[41] (Fig. 14).

Tendon Injuries

Wrist tendons are frequently involved in traumatic injuries. Even if the diagnosis of a tendon rupture is mainly based on the physical examination, imaging evaluation is essential to confirm the clinical diagnosis. For tendon injuries, MR imaging is the gold standard imaging examination, but US is a valuable imaging tool, capable of detecting traumatic changes and performing a dynamic functional examination of tendon function. Partial tendon tears can be detected on US as loss of fibrillar pattern, presence of hypoechoic/anechoic foci within the tendon, tendon swelling, and fluid in the tendon sheath. In complete tears, the tendon is discontinuous with a fluid gap at the rupture site. In some cases, injured tendons can retain morphologic integrity; in these cases, dynamic examination active-passive finger motion is helpful to detect reduced gliding of the tendon.[1,19,29]

Nerve Injuries

Wrist traumas can be frequently complicated also by nerve and vascular injuries, given the superficial location of these structures and the proximity to the bone. The most commonly damaged nerve in wrist injuries is the radial nerve, followed by the ulnar and median nerves.[1,18,42] Regarding tendon injuries, nerve involvement in wrist trauma is diagnosed clinically; however, there are several US and MR imaging findings to aid the diagnosis. On US, injured nerves show loss of the typical fascicular pattern, and swelling or thickening and decreased echogenicity of the nerve. Neuroma formation at the transected nerve end is a common late finding. At MR imaging, major signs of traumatic nerve injury include increased T2/short tau inversion recovery signal with enlargement of nerve fascicles.

SUMMARY

Instrumental imaging evaluation plays a fundamental role in the evaluation of the acutely injured wrist. Knowledge of different lesion patterns, diagnostic classifications, and indirect imaging signs is essential for an accurate diagnosis and to ensure the patient the best treatment strategy.

REFERENCES

1. Avery III DM, Rodner CM, Edgar CM. Sports-related wrist and hand injuries: a review. J Orthop Surg Res 2016;11(99):1–15.
2. Fotiadou A, Patel A, Morgan T, et al. Wrist injuries in young adults: the diagnostic impact of CT and MRI. Eur J Radiol 2011;77(2):235–9.
3. Obert L, Loisel F, Jardin E, et al. High-energy injuries of the wrist. Orthop Traumatol Surg Res 2015. https://doi.org/10.1016/j.otsr.2015.05.009.
4. Squires JH, England E, Mehta K, et al. The role of imaging in diagnosing diseases of the distal

radioulnar joint, triangular fibrocartilage complex, and distal ulna. AJR Am J Roentgenol 2014;203: 146–53.

5. Bruno F, Arrigoni F, Palumbo P, et al. New advances in MRI diagnosis of degenerative osteoarthropathy of the peripheral joints. Radiol Med 2019. https:// doi.org/10.1007/s11547-019-01003-1.

6. Bruno F, Barile A, Arrigoni F, et al. Weight-bearing MRI of the knee: a review of advantages and limits. Acta Biomed 2018;89. https://doi.org/10.23750/ abm.v89i1-S.7011.

7. Zappia M, Maggialetti N, Natella R, et al. Diagnostic imaging: pitfalls in rheumatology. Radiol Med 2019. https://doi.org/10.1007/s11547-019-01017-9.

8. Barile A, Bruno F, Arrigoni F, et al. Emergency and trauma of the ankle. Semin Musculoskelet Radiol 2017;21(3). https://doi.org/10.1055/s-0037-1602408.

9. Barile A, Bruno F, Mariani S, et al. What can be seen after rotator cuff repair: a brief review of diagnostic imaging findings. Musculoskelet Surg 2017;101. https://doi.org/10.1007/s12306-017-0455-2.

10. Salvati F, Rossi F, Limbucci N, et al. Mucoid metaplastic-degeneration of anterior cruciate ligament. J Sports Med Phys Fitness 2008;48(4): 483–7.

11. Barile A, Lanni G, Conti L, et al. Lesions of the biceps pulley as cause of anterosuperior impingement of the shoulder in the athlete: potentials and limits of MR arthrography compared with arthroscopy. Radiol Med 2013;118(1):112–22. https://doi.org/10.1007/ s11547-012-0838-2.

12. Barile A, Arrigoni F, Bruno F, et al. Computed tomography and MR imaging in rheumatoid arthritis. Radiol Clin North Am 2017. https://doi.org/10.1016/j. rcl.2017.04.006.

13. Reginelli A, Zappia M, Barile A, et al. Strategies of imaging after orthopedic surgery. Musculoskelet Surg 2017;101. https://doi.org/10.1007/s12306-017-0458-z.

14. Brink M, Steenbakkers A, Holla MI, et al. Single-shot CT after wrist trauma: impact on detection accuracy and treatment of fractures. Skeletal Radiol 2019; 48(6):949–57.

15. Rominger B, Bernreuter K, Kenney P, et al. MR imaging anatomy and of tears of wrist. Radiographics 1993;13:1233–46.

16. Mariani S, La Marra A, Arrigoni F, et al. Dynamic measurement of patello-femoral joint alignment using weight-bearing magnetic resonance imaging (WB-MRI). Eur J Radiol 2015. https://doi.org/10. 1016/j.ejrad.2015.09.017.

17. Starr HM, Sedgley MD, Means KR, et al. Ultrasonography for hand and wrist conditions. J Am Acad Orthop Surg 2016;24:544–54.

18. Davies AM, Grainger AJ, James SJ, et al. Imaging of the hand and wrist. Techniques and applications, Springer 2013.

19. Syed MA, Raj V, Jeyapalan K. Current role of multidetector computed tomography in imaging of wrist injuries. Curr Probl Diagn Radiol 2013; 42(1):13–25.

20. Ringler MD, Murthy NS. MR imaging of wrist ligaments. Magn Reson Imaging Clin N Am 2015; 23(3):367–91.

21. Sofka CM, Potter HG. Magnetic resonance imaging of the wrist. Semin Musculoskelet Radiol 2001;5(3): 217–26.

22. Little JT, Klionsky NB, Chaturvedi A, et al. Pediatric distal forearm and wrist injury: an imaging review. Radiographics 2014;34(2):472–91.

23. Goldfarb CA, Yin Y, Gilula LA, et al. Wrist fractures: what the clinician wants to know. Radiology 2013. https://doi.org/10.1148/radiology.219.1.r01ap1311.

24. Deroche AB, Dobson S. Wrist fractures. In: Anderson MR, Wilson SH, Rosenblatt MA, editors. Decision-making in orthopedic and regional anesthesiology: a case-based approach. Cambridge University Press; 2015. https://doi.org/10.1017/ CBO9781316145227.034.

25. Rettig AC. Athletic injuries of the wrist and hand. Part I: traumatic injuries of the wrist. Am J Sports Med 2003. https://doi.org/10.1177/03635465030310060801.

26. Doudoulakis KJ. Scaphoid fractures. In: Lasanianos NG, Kanakaris NK, Giannoudis PV, editors. Trauma and orthopaedic classifications: a comprehensive overview. Springer; 2015. https:// doi.org/10.1007/978-1-4471-6572-9_24.

27. Ring D, Jupiter JB, Herndon JH. Acute fractures of the scaphoid. J Am Acad Orthop Surg 2000. https://doi. org/10.5435/00124635-200007000-00003.

28. Mallee W, Doornberg JN, Ring D, et al. Comparison of CT and MRI for diagnosis of suspected scaphoid fractures. J Bone Joint Surg Am 2011. https://doi. org/10.2106/JBJS.I.01523.

29. Davis KW, Blankenbaker DG. Imaging the ligaments and tendons of the wrist. Semin Roentgenol 2010; 45(3):194–217.

30. Williams AA, Lochner HV. Pediatric hand and wrist injuries. Curr Rev Musculoskelet Med 2013. https:// doi.org/10.1007/s12178-012-9146-7.

31. Delgado J, Jaramillo D, Chauvin NA. Imaging the injured pediatric athlete: upper extremity. Radiographics 2016. https://doi.org/10.1148/rg.2016160036.

32. Miller RJ. Wrist MRI and carpal instability: what the surgeon needs to know, and the case for dynamic imaging. Semin Musculoskelet Radiol 2001;5(3):235–40.

33. Mayfield JK, Johnson RP, Kilcoyne RK. Carpal dislocations: pathomechanics and progressive perilunar instability. J Hand Surg Am 1980. https://doi.org/ 10.1016/S0363-5023(80)80007-4.

34. Caggiano N, Matullo KS. Carpal instability of the wrist. Orthop Clin North Am 2014;45(1):129–40.

35. Kuo CE, Wolfe SW. Scapholunate instability: current concepts in diagnosis and management. J Hand

Surg Am 2008. https://doi.org/10.1016/j.jhsa.2008.04.027.

36. Bednar JM, Osterman AL. Carpal instability: evaluation and treatment. J Am Acad Orthop Surg 2016. https://doi.org/10.5435/00124635-199309000-00002.

37. Kitay A, Wolfe SW. Scapholunate instability: current concepts in diagnosis and management. J Hand Surg Am 2012. https://doi.org/10.1016/j.jhsa.2012.07.035.

38. Skalski MR, White EA, Patel DB, et al. The traumatized TFCC: an illustrated review of the anatomy and injury patterns of the triangular fibrocartilage complex. Curr Probl Diagn Radiol 2015. https://doi.org/10.1067/j.cpradiol.2015.05.004.

39. Cody ME, Nakamura DT, Small KM, et al. MR imaging of the triangular fibrocartilage complex. Magn Reson Imaging Clin N Am 2015;23(3):393–403.

40. Moser T, Khoury MDV, Harris PG, et al. MDCT arthrography or MR arthrography for imaging the wrist joint? Semin Musculoskelet Radiol 2009;13(1):39–54.

41. Lo IKY, MacDermid JC, Bennett JD, et al. The radioulnar ratio: a new method of quantifying distal radioulnar joint subluxation. J Hand Surg Am 2001. https://doi.org/10.1053/jhsu.2001.22908.

42. Karabay N. US findings in traumatic wrist and hand injuries. Diagn Interv Radiol 2013;19:320–5.

Overuse Injuries of the Wrist

Eva Llopis, MD[a],*, Rodrigo Restrepo, MD[b], Ara Kassarjian, MD[c], Luis Cerezal, PhD[d]

KEYWORDS

• Overuse • Intersection • Impaction • Impingement • Tenosynovitis

KEY POINTS

- Anatomic variants and repetitive intense movement are the risk factors for developing wrist overuse injuries in sports and occupational environments.
- Tendon injuries occur secondary to friction, especially in areas where there is increase of pressure, such as crossing tendon regions or retinaculum thickening. Ultrasonography and magnetic resonance (MR) are excellent tools to assess the extent of the injury, allowing adequate treatment to be planned.
- Impaction syndromes of the wrist are degenerative disorders related to chronic compression of ulnar-sided structures with the carpal bones, and MR is essential to evaluate the spectrum of lesions.

MAGNETIC RESONANCE IMAGING OF ATHLETIC INJURIES OF THE WRIST: OVERUSE INJURIES

Introduction

Wrist and hand injuries are common in sports and represent between 3% and 9% of all athletic injuries.[1] With the ever-increasing rate of participation in sports by the general population, the number of wrist and hand injuries is also increasing. Work-related injuries are frequent, especially important acute finger open wounds that might lead to amputation[2,3]

However, up to 60% of work-related injuries are secondary to repetitive trauma and associated with long sick leave and therefore lost productivity.[3]

Wrist and hand injuries can be divided into acute traumatic injuries and chronic overuse-type injuries. Magnetic resonance (MR) imaging, in combination with physical examination and radiographs, is generally accepted as being one of the most important diagnostic tools in assessing the exact nature and extent of the injury. Such detailed assessment of the injury can aid in planning and executing the appropriate, and sometimes aggressive, therapy in order to get the patients back to competition or work as quickly as possible.[3]

This article reviews the mechanisms of injury, clinical signs and symptoms, usefulness of MR imaging, and therapeutic management of overuse wrist and hand injuries.

Epidemiology

Most acute injuries occur in the setting of contact sports or direct contact with mechanical or sharp-edged tools, and overuse injuries are secondary to repetitive hand intensive movements in combination with occupational and nonoccupational risk factors. Overuse wrist and hand injuries are more common in some specific sports, such as racquet sports, golf, and gymnastics; however, both types

Disclosure: The authors have nothing to disclosure.
[a] Department of Radiology, Hospital de la Ribera, Paseo Ciudadela 13, 15D, Valencia 46003, Spain; [b] Cedimed, Cll.7 N° 39-290 Piso 3, Medellin 050021, Colombia; [c] Elite Sports Imaging, SL, Calle Grecia 1, 28224 Pozuelo de Alarcón, Madrid, Spain; [d] Department of Radiology, Diagnostico Médico Cantabria, Calle Castilla, 6, Santander 39002, Spain
* Corresponding author.
E-mail address: evallopis@gmail.com

Radiol Clin N Am 57 (2019) 957–976
https://doi.org/10.1016/j.rcl.2019.05.001
0033-8389/19/© 2019 Elsevier Inc. All rights reserved.

of injuries can be seen in both contact and noncontact sports. In the context of work-related activities, the highest proportion are related to service industries, followed by manufacturing industries, assemblers, constructions laborers, supervisors in sales, carpenters, and cashiers, who are all prone to develop upper extremity work-related injuries.[3,4]

Athletic injuries have many consequences at all levels of competition. These consequences range from minor to significant loss of playing time, inability to return to preinjury performance levels, and the potential termination of a professional career. The often-used conservative wait-and-see approach for the general population is typically not appropriate with high-level athletes. In competitive athletes, a rapid and accurate diagnosis is crucial because it allows appropriate counseling regarding treatment options, rehabilitation programs, expected recuperation times, and prognosis regarding likelihood of return to the preinjury level of performance.[1,3,4]

Illness secondary to repetitive hand motion results in the longest absences from work, with a median of 18 to 20 days; carpal tunnel syndrome is associated with the highest median days away from work. Other causes are tendinitis or trigger fingers.[3]

The pathophysiology mechanism includes inflammation followed by repair with or without fibrotic scaring.

TENDONS

Overuse injuries involving the tendons of the wrist are common and typically take the form of tendinosis or tenosynovitis, although other lesions also occur.

Secondary to repetitive motion and load, progressive continuous pathophysiologic changes occur in the tendon and tendon sheath; a combination of early inflammatory signs is followed by fibrosis and proliferative response trying to repair the microscopic tissue injuries. If the mechanism continues, there is progressive functional impairment with degeneration and progressive fibrosis. Neurogenic changes associated with the adaptive mechanism to pain also play an important role in the lack of complete tissue repair.

Given the multiple tendons that traverse the dorsal aspect of the wrist, extensor tendons have been categorized into 6 compartments (**Fig. 1**).

De Quervain Syndrome

The most common tendinopathy about the wrist involves the first dorsal (extensor) compartment (abductor pollicis longus [APL] and extensor

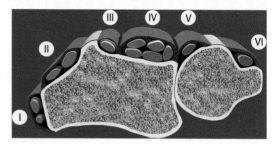

Fig. 1. Cross section of the 6 extensor tendon compartments of the wrist.

pollicis brevis [EPB]) and is referred to as de Quervain syndrome.[1–8] This tendinopathy (and stenosing tenosynovitis) results from shearing and microtrauma of the first dorsal compartment tendons during repetitive gliding over the radial styloid. This condition is most commonly seen in sports that require forceful grasping and ulnar deviation or repetitive use of the thumb and is thus encountered in golfers, rowers, certain racquet sport players, and fly fishers. Occupational related is more prevalent in women than in men (3:1), frequently seen in housekeeping tasks, typing, and knitting, and is particularly frequent in lactating woman secondary to lifting the baby under the axila with the webbing between the thumb and index finger under the baby.[1,5–10]

Comorbidities such as rheumatoid arthritis increase the risk of developing de Quervain syndrome.[11]

The classic clinical triad of de Quervain syndrome includes swelling at the level of the radial styloid, tenderness just proximal to the tip of the radial styloid, and a positive Finkelstein test. To perform the Finkelstein test, the patient is asked to make a fist with the thumb flexed and adducted under the fingers. The examiner then passively moves the wrist into ulnar deviation. If there is pain over the radial styloid during this passive ulnar deviation the test is said to be positive.[1,5–10]

The first step for imaging is to rule out anatomic variants that have been associated with increased risk for developing de Quervain disease (**Figs. 2–5**). Eighty-nine percent of the normal population have multiple APL tendon bundles ranging from 3 to 14 slips; less frequent is the presence of multiple EPBs (see **Figs. 3 and 5**). The presence of a septum dividing the first extensor compartment is important in the development of de Quervain but also for surgical planning. The septum can be complete or incomplete and its location can be distal or proximal to the radial styloid process. The septation is difficult to depict on MR imaging and only indirect signs, such as small indentation

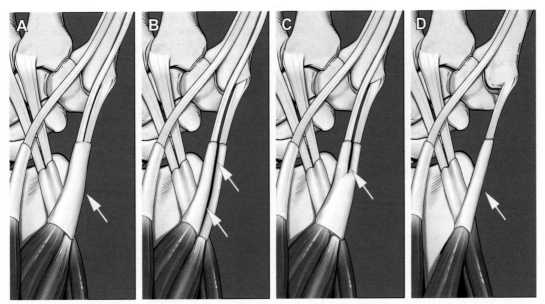

Fig. 2. The different anatomic variants of the first extensor compartment: (*A*) type I unique compartment (*white arrow*); (*B*) type II complete separation of the EPB and the APL sheaths (*white arrows*); (*C*) type III, incomplete septum limited to the distal part (they separate at the level of the radial styloid process) (*white arrow*); (*D*) type IV, absence of the EPB (*white arrow*).

on the lateral side of the radius, are usually seen on ultrasonography (US); however, it is much easier to detect the bony and fibrous or osseous ridge, the independent sheaths, and also the multiple bundles on 1 or both tendons. The patient is examined with the radial side of the forearm pointing up; the APL is more lateral and inserts onto the radial metacarpal base and the

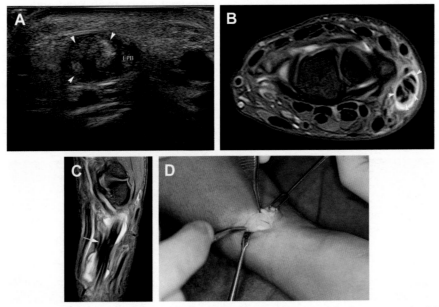

Fig. 3. De Quervain tenosynovitis in a 22-year-old male paddle tennis player. (*A*) Ultrasonography (US) axial image. (*B*) Axial fat-suppressed fast spin echo (FSE) T2-weighted image. (*C*) Sagittal fat-suppressed T2-weighted image shows multiple tendons of the APL (*arrowheads*) with tenosynovitis of the first extensor compartment; note a dumbbell shape of the tenosynovium secondary to thickening of the retinaculum (*arrow*). (*D*) Surgical release of the first compartment was performed because of the failing of the conservative treatments.

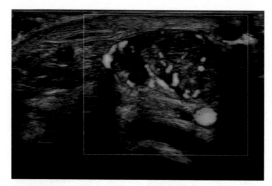

Fig. 4. De Quervain axial US with Doppler showing increased Doppler signal in the tenosynovial sheath and with the APL substance indicating tendinitis.

EPB is more medial. The septum is seen as an oblique linear structure from the extensor retinaculum dividing the 2 tendons. An osseous ridge can be also identified on US (see **Fig. 5**).

Four different variants have been defined. In type I, a there is a unique compartment where the tendons are difficult to separate at the level of the distal radius and can be individualized only at the level of the radial styloid process or radiocarpal joint. In type II, complete separation on US is easy to depict because they have a separated hypoechogenic halo with an oblique or vertical septumlike structure. Type III is incomplete and limited to the distal part; both tendons are within the same tendon sheath at the distal radius and at the level of the radial styloid process they separate and have their own hypoechogenic circular rim. In type IV, the EPB is absent[12] (see **Fig. 2**).

In cases of tenosynovitis, both US and MR show fluid within the tendon sheath of the first dorsal compartment (see **Figs. 3** and **4**). When there is a more advanced overuse injury and tendinosis is present, MR shows enlarged tendons with some increased signal intensity. If stenosing tenosynovitis is present, there will be a rim of T1 and T2 intermediate signal intensity surrounding the tendons[5,8,12] (see **Figs. 3–5**).

Management initially consists of a combination of steroid injections and oral nonsteroidal antiinflammatory drugs (NSAIDs). Nonoperative treatment is most effective in the early stages of the disease. In more chronic cases, there may be thickening of the retinacular roof of the first dorsal compartment, thereby leading to stenosis and poor gliding of the tendons. At this stage, surgical intervention may be necessary. Failure to recognize the subcompartment in the first extensor compartment may lead to inadequate decompression.[1,7]

Intersection Syndrome

The tendons of the second extensor compartment, extensor carpi radialis brevis (ECRB), and extensor carpi radialis longus (ECRL) cross twice in their path from the forearm to their metacarpal insertions. They cross first proximally by the first extensor compartment and 3 to 5 cm distally after the radiocarpal joint and the Lister tubercle. The fascia of the forearm covers the first crossing and the extensor retinaculum covers the second. These anatomic predisposing factors create a potential cause of mechanical friction with the motion of the thumb and hand and are named proximal or distal intersection syndromes[13,14] (**Fig. 6**).

Proximal Intersection Syndrome

Proximal intersection syndrome (also known as oarsmen's wrist, squeaker's wrist, or crossover syndrome) is a clinical entity characterized by repetitive friction approximately 4 to 6 cm proximal to the Lister tubercle at a point where the first dorsal myotendinous junction (APL and EPB) crosses over the second dorsal compartment unit (ECRL and ECRB). Pain, swelling, and occasionally

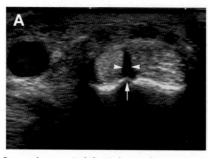
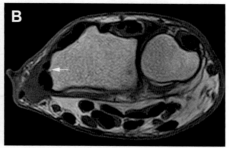

Fig. 5. De Quervain type II. (*A*) US shows the septum between the EPB and the APL as an oblique lineal structure separating the tendons (*arrow*), which are typically surrounded by a hypoechoic halo. The septum is associated with a small osseous crest (*arrowheads*) in the middle of the groove separating the 2 tendons of the first extensor compartment. (*B*) MR has difficulty depicting the septum; indirect signs, such as small crest in the lateral side of the radius, can help in the diagnosis (*arrow*). Note the multiple bundles of the APL.

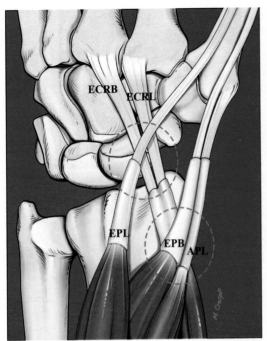

Fig. 6. The relation between the first, the second, and the third extensor compartments, showing the 2 crossing areas, which are vulnerable to friction and originate the proximal and distal intersection syndrome. Proximal intersection syndrome (squeaker's wrist). The inflammatory condition is caused by friction at the crossing points of the first dorsal compartment muscles (APL and EPB) and the radial wrist extensors (ECRL and ECRB). Distal to the radiocarpal joint the distal intersection syndrome secondary to the crossing between the extensor pollicis longus (EPL) over the second extensor compartment (ECRB and ECRL).

crepitus on palpation of this region are consistent with intersection syndrome. The crepitus may resemble a squeak and can be elicited either with wrist motion or direct palpation. This syndrome is secondary to repetitive wrist flexion and extension and is most commonly seen in oarsmen and other sports, such as racquet sports, rowing, and weight lifting. It also has been related to some occupational work, such as in secretaries, carpenters, and harvesters (see **Fig. 6**).[1,6,15]

The syndrome is thought to be caused by friction as the APL and the EPB muscle bellies cross over and rub along the surface of the radial wrist extensors, which can result in an inflammatory tenosynovitis and/or the development of an adventitial bursa. The extensor fascia of the forearm might play a role in the development of the intersection syndrome (see **Fig. 6**).[13,15]

The advantage of US is that allows a dynamic evaluation at the crossing point of the 2 compartments and shows tenosynovitis and soft tissue

edema. MR should be tailored if there is a clinical suspicion and should include the distal forearm in the field of view. MR imaging may show tendon thickening and peritendinous edema with fluid in the first and second dorsal extensor compartment tendon sheaths concentrated around the level where the first and second compartment tendons cross (**Fig. 7**). Peritendinous enhancement can be seen after contrast administration. They might also show loss of the normal ovoid appearance of the tendons and appear enlarged and rounded.[15]

Intersection syndrome is typically treated nonoperatively with oral NSAIDs, corticosteroid injections, and immobilization with the wrist in 20° of dorsiflexion. In refractory cases, surgical intervention may be necessary. In such cases, the crossing point of the first and second compartment tendons is explored, the overlying fascia is incised, and any existing adventitial bursa is excised.[1,13]

Distal Intersection Syndrome

Distal intersection syndrome is defined as tenosynovitis secondary to friction of the second extensor compartment as it is crossed by the extensor pollicis longus (EPL) distally to the Lister tubercle, and is less frequent than proximal intersection syndrome. Clinically it is difficult to differentiate from proximal intersection syndrome and de Quervain because they are close in the dorsolateral aspect of the wrist[14] (see **Fig. 6**).

The EPL runs from the forearm toward the thumb through the third extensor compartment lying within small groove of the dorsal radius, and the Lister tubercle serves as a pulley where its course is change to reach the base of the first metacarpal bone, crossing over the second extensor compartment. It is covered by the extensor retinaculum, which seals the groove and increases the pressure over the tendons. Moreover, there is a poorly vascularized area where the EPL enters the third extensor compartment. Anatomic configuration and the poor vascularization make it more vulnerable to friction and ruptures. Late EPL rupture is a well-known complication of nondisplaced radial fracture.[13,14]

Radiological diagnosis can be done with US and MR. Tendinosis and tenosynovitis of the EPL at the level of the Lister tubercle and usually of the second extensor compartment are the main findings that might be associated with increased signal on power Doppler hyperemia and bone marrow changes in the Lister tubercle area. EPL rupture has been reported as a complication[13,14] (**Fig. 8**).

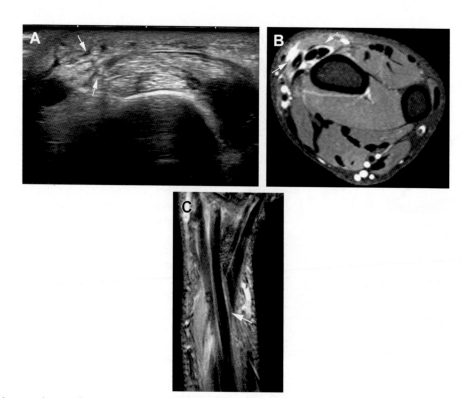

Fig. 7. Intersection syndrome in a 24-year-old male paddle player. (A) US axial plane proximal to the radiocarpal joint at the level of the crossing point of the first and second extensor compartments shows peritendinous edema (*arrows*). (B) Axial fat-suppressed T2-weighted image shows hyperintense fluid within the tendon sheaths and bursal distention at the intersection of the first and second extensor compartments (*arrows*). (C) Sagittal-oblique gradient echo T2-weighted image shows peritendinous edema and a small amount of fluid within the tendons sheaths of the first and second dorsal extensor compartments surrounding the area of intersection (*arrow*).

Extensor Carpi Ulnaris Tendinopathy

Extensor carpi ulnaris (ECU) tendinopathy (and associated tenosynovitis) is the second most common tendinopathy in athletes and is frequently seen in rowing, golf, and especially in racquet sports, particularly in the nondominant wrist of tennis players with 2-handed backhands.[1,5]

ECU tendinopathy manifests as pain and swelling just distal to the head of the ulna. This pain can be exacerbated with wrist extension, with the movements of pronosupination and ulnar deviation. ECU tendinopathy is typically seen in the setting of additional ulnar-sided wrist disorder, such as triangular fibrocartilage (TFC) complex tears, lunotriquetral ligament tears, anomalous tendon slips, nonunited ulnar styloid fractures, or a flat ECU tendon groove.[1,16,17] Isolated ECU tendon lesions, although possible, are less common.

The ECU extends through a longitudinal osseous groove in the dorsal aspect of the distal ulna and is stabilized by the extensor retinaculum and the linea jugata connecting the ulnar styloid

with the antebrachial fascia. A congenital variant with flat or convex ECU groove increases the risk of developing excessive friction and dislocation.

As with tendinopathy in other locations, MR imaging can show enlargement of the tendon with some increased intratendinous signal, peritendinous edema, and fluid within the tendon sheath[5] **(Fig. 9)**.

ECU tendinopathy is treated with rest, splinting, NSAIDs, and occasionally corticosteroid injections into the tendon sheath. If there is no response to these treatments, further investigation may be necessary to assess for an additional disorder that may be responsible for the symptoms.[16,17]

Subluxation of the Extensor Carpi Ulnaris

Subluxation (or dislocation) of the ECU tendon, although not strictly an overuse syndrome, should be considered as a possibility in athletes with ulnar-sided wrist pain.[1,5] The ECU has inherent instability with supination when the tendon shifts away from the osseous groove. Attenuation or rupture of the ECU tendon sheath, such as can

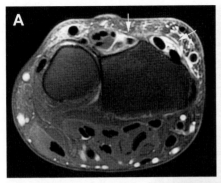
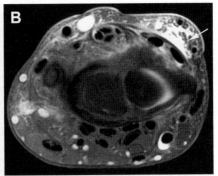
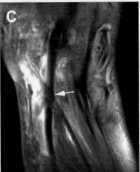

Fig. 8. Distal intersection syndrome. Axial fat-suppressed proton density (PD)–weighted consecutive images at the level of the Lister tubercle (*A*) and distal at the midcarpal level (*B*) show tenosynovitis of the second extensor compartment and of the EPL with dorsal soft tissue edema (*arrows*). (*C*) Coronal fat-suppressed PD-weighted image shows nicely soft tissue edema related to the crossing point (*arrow*).

be caused by sudden volar flexion and ulnar deviation, can allow subluxation of the ECU tendon out of the groove in the ulna. Such injuries have been reported in tennis, golf, baseball, and weightlifting.[1,5]

Patients with symptomatic ECU subluxation or dislocation complain of a painful snap along the dorsal ulnar aspect of the wrist during wrist supination and ulnar deviation. This subluxation may be visible and palpable.[16]

Dynamic MR imaging can show ECU tendon subluxation and dislocation during rotation of the forearm. In addition, MR can clearly show the morphology of the groove in the distal ulna as well as other associated lesions, if present[5,16] (**Fig. 10**).

Although some clinicians recommend casting of acute injuries for 6 weeks with the wrist in pronation and dorsiflexion, others recommend early open repair of acute injuries to ensure a more predictable outcome. In chronic cases, the subsheath may be surgically reconstructed.[16]

Wrist Flexor Tenosynovitis

Flexor carpi radialis (FCR) tenosynovitis is rare and may develop insidiously or be the result of direct

trauma. FCR tenosynovitis presents as pain over the FCR just proximal to the wrist flexor creases. It has been related to both occupational and sports activities, such as farming or industrial work and stick sports such as racquet sports or golf[1] (**Fig. 11**).

Flexor carpi ulnaris (FCU) tenosynovitis is more common than FCR tenosynovitis and can be seen in golf and racquet sports that involve excessive wrist motion, such as badminton and squash. Because the pisiform is a sesamoid within the substance of the FCU, pisotriquetral compression syndrome may accompany FCU tenosynovitis.[1] Patients with FCU tenosynovitis complain of pain over the pisiform or just proximal to the pisiform along the course of the FCU. This pain is exacerbated by resisted wrist flexion.

Again, ultrasonography and MR imaging show the typical features of tenosynovitis with fluid in the tendon sheath, thickening of the tendon sheath, and peritendinous inflammatory changes.[8]

Calcific tendinitis of the FCU can be secondary to local hypoxia caused by mechanical or vascular repetitive damage, or stress necrosis that leads to transformation of tendon into fibrocartilage. The chondrocyte activity produces calcifications. Calcifications are usually located close to the

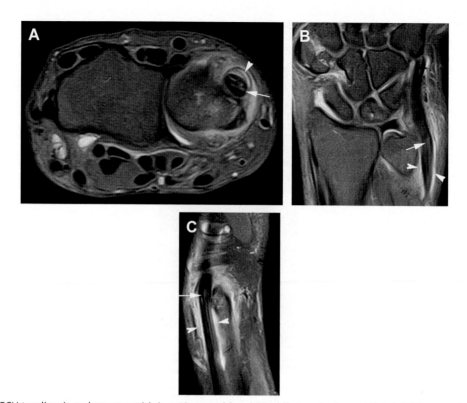

Fig. 9. ECU tendinosis and tenosynovitis in a 42-year-old male paddle tennis player. (*A*) Axial, (*B*) coronal, and (*C*) sagittal fat-suppressed FSE PD-weighted images reveal thickening and increased signal intensity of the ECU tendon (*arrows*) consistent with tendinosis; there is also increased fluid within the synovial sheath of the ECU (*arrowheads*) caused by tenosynovitis. Note the associated ill-defined bone marrow edema on the axial plane secondary to repetitive friction.

pisiform. Calcific tendinitis of FCU has been occupationally related to repetitive movement; although it is usually unilateral, bilateral cases have been reported.[18,19]

Flexor tendon tenosynovitis is typically treated with activity modification (if possible), NSAIDs, splint immobilization with the wrist slightly flexed, and corticosteroid injections. Refractory or chronic cases with tendinosis may require surgery

such as pisiform excision and lengthening of the FCU tendon with Z-plasty.[1]

BONES
Ulnar Impaction Syndrome

Ulnar impaction syndrome, also referred to as ulnocarpal impaction or ulnar abutment, is a chronic and degenerative condition resulting

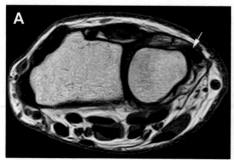
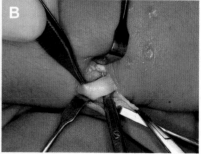

Fig. 10. ECU subluxation in a 36-year-old male paddle player. (*A*) Axial FSE T1-weighted image reveals complete rupture of the subsheath, ulnar dislocation of the ECU tendon (*arrow*), and soft tissue edema surrounding dorsal and lateral side of the wrist. (*B*) Intraoperative view confirmed the complete rupture of the ECU tendon subsheath.

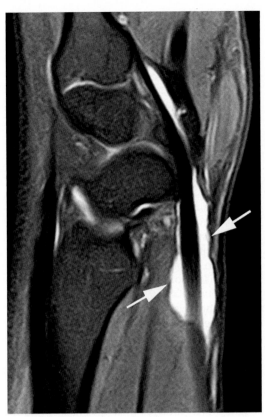

Fig. 11. FCR tenosynovitis. Sagittal fat-suppressed PD-weighted image shows fluid surrounding the FCR from its proximal side to its insertion on the base of the first metacarpal bone (*arrows*).

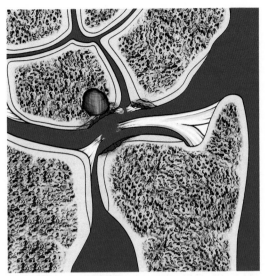

Fig. 12. The full spectrum of pathologic conditions in ulnar impaction syndrome, including chondromalacia of the ulnar head, and the ulnar side of the lunate bone; central perforation of the TFC; and lunotriquetral ligament tear.

On physical examination, there may be swelling and tenderness localized to the TFC complex and the lunotriquetral joint with limitation of forearm rotation and wrist motion.[20,22,23]

from repetitive impaction between the head of the ulna and the TFC complex and ulnar carpus. This repetitive impaction results in a continuum of pathologic changes with degenerative tearing of the TFC, chondromalacia of the lunate triquetrum and ulnar head, tear of the lunotriquetral ligament (with possible lunotriquetral instability), and eventually osteoarthritis of the distal radioulnar joint (DRUJ) and ulnocarpal joint (**Fig. 12**).[20–23]

Ulnar impaction syndrome most commonly occurs in the setting of positive ulnar variance, although it can also occasionally be seen with neutral or even negative ulnar variance.[20] Only 2.5 mm of ulnar positive variance increases the load to the ulnocarpal joint by 42%[24,25] (**Fig. 13**). The most common causes of positive ulnar variance are congenital, posttraumatic (eg, malunion of distal radial fracture or Essex-Lopresti fracture), postsurgical (eg, resection of radial head), and premature closure of the distal radial physis.[20,22,23] The end result is an elongated ulna (or shortened or dorsally tilted distal radius) with fixed increased loading of the distal ulna.

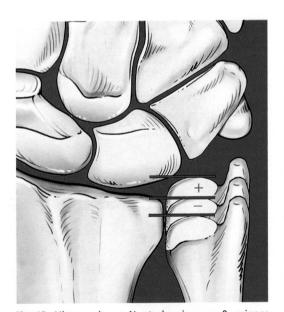

Fig. 13. Ulnar variance. Neutral variance or 0 variance is considered when the difference between the ulnar and the radial length is less than 1 mm, positive variance when the ulna abuts more distally than the radius (>1 mm), and negative variance when the ulnar is short compared with the radius (>1 mm).

The first step for imaging ulnar-sided pain is to obtain neutral radiological plain (0 rotation) posteroanterior and lateral films. This is the proper way to study ulnar variance, or the relation between the distal radius and the ulna; the fact that ulnar variance increases with pronation makes it more difficult to analyze on MR, where neutral position is more difficult to obtain. It is preferable to perform the MR imaging in the so-called superman position, taking care to support the patient's arm to make it as comfortable as possible so as to avoid movement. When MR imaging has to be performed with the wrist at the patient's side, the wrist coil should stand horizontal with the palm on the table to minimize the pronation.[11]

The role of MR imaging is to show the radiographically occult lesions (eg, TFC tear, cartilage defects) that can be present in the setting of ulnar impaction syndrome. In addition, MR imaging may reveal marrow edema in the cases in which the overlying cartilage is normal, even at arthroscopy, thereby suggesting that marrow edema may be a sensitive and early sign of ulnar impaction syndrome. As the disease progresses, more advanced changes can be seen, such as bone sclerosis (decreased signal on both T1-weighted and T2-weighted sequences) and subchondral cysts (well-circumscribed lesions that are hypointense on T1-weighted and hyperintense on T2-weighted imaging)[22,23,26] (see **Figs. 8** and **9**). In selected cases, MR arthrography may be used to better delineate the severity of the changes resulting from the ulnar impaction. MR arthrography is particularly useful in determining whether there is a perforation of the TFC (distinguish between Palmer IIB an IIC), whether the ulnocarpal ligaments are intact, and whether the lunotriquetral ligament is intact (distinguish between Palmer IIC and IID) (**Figs. 14–16**).[23,26] Computed tomography (CT) and MR arthrography are the methods of choice to distinguish between communicating and noncommunicating TFC tear, especially if there is suspicion of foveal detachment and to evaluate lunotriquetral ligament tears; its small size decreases the accuracy of MR without intra-articular contrast.[24,25,27,28]

Treatment strategies for ulnar impaction syndrome are complex and need to take into account multiple variables, including the amount of ulnar variance, the type of TFC lesion present, the shape of the sigmoid fossa and ulnar seat, and the presence or absence of associated lunotriquetral instability.[26] In cases without TFC perforation (Palmer class IIA and IIB), treatment may consist of an open wafer procedure, whereby the distal 2 to 3 mm of the dome of the ulnar head is resected, or formal ulnar shortening, whereby a section of the ulnar shaft 2 to 3 mm wide is resected, with subsequent rigid fixation of the shaft.[29] If there is perforation of the TFC (Palmer class IIC or IID), an arthroscopic wafer procedure may be performed with burring down of the head of the ulna (**Fig. 17**). The arthroscopic wafer procedure is minimally invasive, highly effective, and allows a rapid return to normal activities. In cases in which a Palmer class IIE lesion is present, a salvage procedure is often indicated. Options for a salvage procedure include partial or complete ulnar head resection (eg, Darrach procedure) or DRUJ arthrodesis with distal ulnar pseudoarthrosis (Sauvé Kapandji procedure)[29–32]

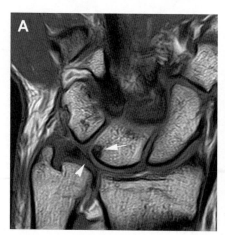
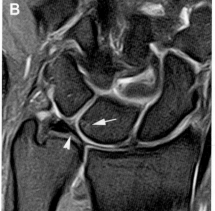

Fig. 14. Ulnar impaction syndrome in a 36-year-old male tennis player with insidious onset of ulnar-sided wrist pain. (*A, B*) Coronal T1-weighted and fat-suppressed T2-weighted images show positive ulnar variance with fraying of the ulnar side of the triangular fibrocartilage without central perforation of the TFC (*arrowheads*), and chondromalacia of the lunate bone with secondary subchondral changes (*arrows*) (Palmer class IIB lesion).

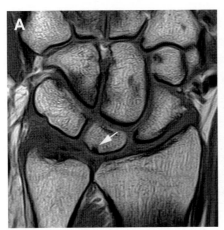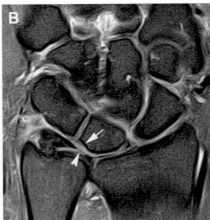

Fig. 15. Ulnar impaction syndrome in a 32-year-old male tennis player with ulnar-sided wrist pain. (*A, B*) Coronal FSE T1-weighted image and coronal fat-suppressed FSE PD-weighted image showing degenerative central perforation of the TFC (*arrowhead in B*) and small osteochondral lesion on the ulnar articular side of the lunate (*arrows*).

Ulnar Styloid Impaction Syndrome

Ulnar styloid impaction syndrome, as the name suggests, involves abnormal contact and impaction between the ulnar styloid and the triquetrum (and adjacent soft tissues)[23,26,33–36] (**Fig. 18**). An

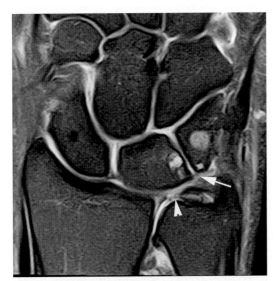

Fig. 16. Ulnar impaction syndrome in a 52-year-old male golf player with chronic ulnar-sided wrist pain. Coronal fat-suppressed T2-weighted image shows central perforation of the TFC (*arrowhead*), osteochondral lesions on the articular side of the lunate and triquetrum, and irregularity in the lunotriquetral ligament (*arrow*). Note also a lunotriquetral fibrocartilaginous coalition (Minaar type 1) with irregular narrowing of the proximal aspect of the lunotriquetral joint and marginal subchondral changes (associated with symptomatic lunotriquetral coalition).

elongated ulnar styloid is the most common cause for ulnar styloid impaction. This elongation may be congenital or may be the result of malunion of an avulsion fracture at the level of the ulnar fovea (type II fractures), which results in narrowing of the ulnocarpal distance and can result in repeated impaction between the ulnar styloid, the ulnar aspect of the lunate, and the radial aspect of the triquetrum.[12] Another congenital variant is a curved ulnar styloid with a parrot-beak configuration. The curvature is typically in a volar and radial direction, thereby resulting in narrowing of the distance between the styloid and the carpals. Dynamic ulnar styloid impact has also been described, based on ligamentous laxity instability or hyperloading activities, such as in racquet sports or golf.[26,36]

Normal styloid process measures between 3 and 6 mm, and greater than 7 mm is considered abnormal; however, it is preferable to calculate the ratio comparing the ulna head width and the styloid process length, with greater than 0.21 ± 0.07 being considered pathologic.[37]

MR imaging allows visualization of the integrity of the TFC complex and its ulnar attachments, presence of any nonunited bone fragments (and their relationship to TFC attachments), and any associated chondromalacia and subchondral changes in the adjacent carpal bones, especially at the tip of the styloid process and at the dorsal side of the triquetrum[23,26,33,38] (**Fig. 19**).

The treatment of choice for ulnar styloid impaction related to an elongated or curved styloid is resection of most of the ulnar styloid leaving the most proximal 2 mm intact so as not to affect the ulnar attachments of the TFC complex.[33,35,38]

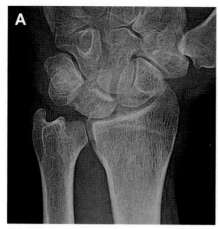
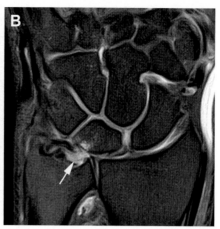

Fig. 17. Wafer procedure. (*A*, *B*) Posteroanterior radiograph and coronal fat-suppressed PD-weighted image after arthroscopic wafer procedure to shorten the ulnar head; note the central perforation of the TFC (*arrow in B*) and the osteochondral lesion on the articular side of the lunate.

The technique used to treat ulnar styloid impaction caused by styloid nonunion depends on the integrity and laxity of the TFC complex. If the TFC complex is lax, the ulnar styloid and the TFC complex are fixed into the ulnar fovea via a limited incision along the ulnar aspect of the wrist. If the TFC complex is not lax, the nonunited osseous fragment is resected.[26,33,35,38]

Hamatolunate Impaction Syndrome

In patients with a type II lunate bone, where there is an additional distal articular facet along the medial aspect of the lunate for articulation with the hamate, the biomechanics of the midcarpal row change and with ulnar deviation the hamate jumps over the extra lunate facet, increasing the loading over the proximal hamate. This extra facet measures approximately 4.5 mm with a variable depth. Chondromalacia at this hamatolunate articulation can result in ulnar-sided wrist pain. Repetitive abrasion and impingement at this articulation when the wrist is in full ulnar deviation may be the

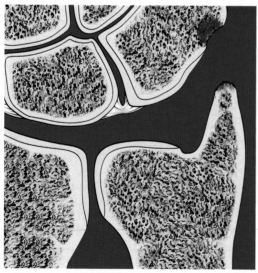

Fig. 18. The pathologic conditions that characterize ulnar styloid impaction syndrome, including elongated ulnar styloid process, and chondromalacia of the dorsal aspect of the triquetral bone and tip of the ulnar styloid.

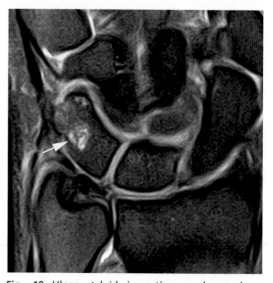

Fig. 19. Ulnar styloid impaction syndrome in a 24-year-old motorcyclist with chronic ulnar-sided pain without a history of trauma. Coronal fat-suppressed PD-weighted image reveals slightly elongated ulnar styloid with dorsal chondromalacia and bone marrow edema in the triquetrum (*arrow*).

A   **B**

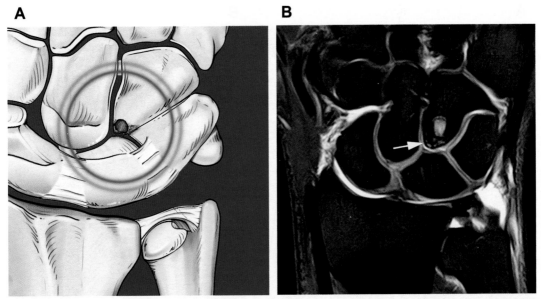

Fig. 20. (A) Diagram of hamatolunate impaction syndrome. Lunate type II of Viegas increases the risk of increasing the load on the proximal side of the hamate and early developing of osteochondral lesions. (B) Hamatolunate impaction syndrome in a 56-year-old man with ulnar sided wrist pain. Coronal T1 fat suppressed MR arthrography image demonstrates lunate type II with a deep extrafacet, chondral lesions on both articular surfaces and subchondral cyst on the hamate (*arrow*). Note the negative ulnar variance impinging on the lateral side of the radius.

cause of chondromalacia at this site (**Fig. 20**). Athletes with hamatolunate impaction complain of pain during full ulnar deviation of the wrist. Proximal chondral lesions of the hamate are the most frequent chondral lesions in the wrist.[22,23,39–42]

MR imaging shows the type II lunate with the extra articular facet and can show the articular cartilage defects, marrow edema, sclerosis, and subchondral cysts in the proximal pole of the hamate (see **Fig. 20**).[22,23,39–42]

Current treatment of hamatolunate impactions consists of arthroscopic burring of the apex of the hamate.

Ulnar Impingement

Negative ulnar variance causes abnormal contact between the ulna and the proximal ulnar side of the distal radius secondary to repetitive supination and pronation movements. Patients refer chronic proximal ulnar-side pain, that increase with forearm pronation and supination.[22,23] It can be congenital or secondary to early physis closure of the ulna but it is more frequently related to postsurgical procedures that shorten the ulna.[22,23] Plain films will show sclerosis and scalloping of the ulna impinging on the lateral side of the radius. MRI can also demonstrate bone marrow edema and synovitis (**Fig. 21**).[22,23]

Scaphoid Impaction Syndrome and Radial Styloid Impingement

Scaphoid impaction is secondary to chronic impaction of the dorsal rim of the scaphoid against the dorsal lip of the radius when the wrist is in forced hyperextension. Radiologically, a small ossicle or hypertrophic ridge at the dorsal scaphoid can be seen.

To differentiate this from radial styloid impingement, the patients indicate that pain is usually in the anatomic snuff box and produced by radial deviation with pressure exerted on the scaphoid tuberosity from the radial styloid.[43]

Dorsal Impingement Syndromes

Athletes that participate in sports that involve repetitive dorsiflexion, particularly with axial loading, as occurs in gymnastics, may have dorsal impingement syndromes.

The pathologic lesion is thought to be impingement of the dorsal capsule between the ECRB and the dorsal ridge of the scaphoid, and development of secondary redundant dorsal capsular thickening and synovitis. Underlying predynamic scapholunate instability or scaphoid rotatory subluxation should be ruled out.[44]

A

B

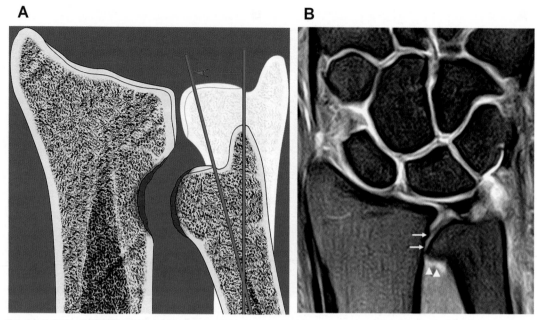

Fig. 21. (*A*) Diagram illustrating ulna impingement syndrome, with contraction of the extensor pollicis brevis, abductor pollicis longus and pronator quadratus muscle the ulna with negative variance converges over the lateral side of the radius. (*B*) Coronal PD fat suppressed MR showing negative ulnar variance, remodelation of the radius proximal to the sigmoid notch (*white arrow*) and synovitis (*arrowhead*).

It can also be related to the impingement of the rigid border of the strong fibrous extensor retinaculum with the extensor tendons of the fingers and thumb.[1,2]

The cause of the pain might be dorsal capsulitis or synovitis with subsequent capsular thickening. In more chronic cases, dorsal osteophytes may form along the rim of the distal radius, the scaphoid, and/or the lunate.[1] MR imaging can show such dorsal capsular thickening and associated osteophytes, although the major role of MR in dorsal impingement is to rule out other potential sources of dorsal pain, especially scapholunate tears.[45]

Although most cases resolve with splinting, rest, NSAIDs, and injections, refractory cases may require arthroscopic debridement of the synovitis and possibly any associated osteophytes. This debridement with posterior interosseous nerve excision may be curative.[1,44,45]

Dorsal Ganglion Cysts

An occult dorsal ganglion may be the result of athletic activity and can result in dorsal wrist pain.[1] Dorsal wrist ganglion can form part of the same spectrum of dorsal wrist impingement.[44]

The dorsal scapholunate region is composed of 3 distinct elements: the dorsal aspect of the scapholunate ligament, the dorsal intercarpal ligament, and the dorsal capsuloscapholunate septum contributing to the stabilization of the scapholunate interval. Dorsal ganglia are secondary to injury within these dorsal complex structures with mucoid degeneration and ganglia formation.[46]

The diagnosis can be suspected in athletes who complain of dorsal wrist pain with dorsiflexion, especially with loading.

MR imaging can show the exact location and size of the lesion as well as any associated injuries. A small percentage of dorsal ganglia are not detected by MR imaging, probably because of their small size. Is also important to rule out other causes of dorsal pain (**Fig. 22**).[1,46,47]

Cases that do not respond to rest and immobilization are preferably treated with arthroscopic or open excision.[1]

Gymnast's Wrist

The wrist is exposed in gymnastics to different types of stresses, including repetitive extreme wrist dorsiflexion motion, high-impact loading, axial compression, torsional forces, and distraction. Some exercises, such as floor routines and pommel horse, increase the load to the wrist up to 16 times body weight.[1,43,48,49]

Gymnasts with this condition complain of progressive dorsal wrist pain that is not associated

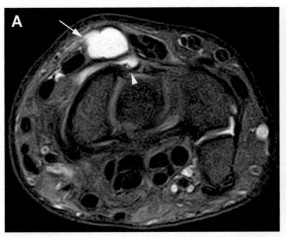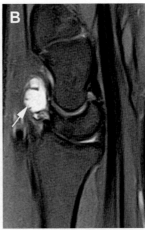

Fig. 22. Dorsal ganglion cyst. (*A, B*) Axial and sagittal PD and coronal fat-suppressed FSE PD-weighted image shows a dorsal ganglion cyst (*arrows*) depending on the dorsal aspect of the scapholunate ligament (*arrowhead in A*).

with an acute traumatic event. The pain is often worse immediately after training, particularly when performing exercises that require weight bearing on the hands.

Chronic overload to the growth plate might compromise its blood supply and lead to endo-chondral ossification and ultimately arrest of the distal radius physis. Children usually have negative ulnar variance and therefore the load to the wrist goes predominantly through the distal radius. Because older gymnasts have a higher prevalence of positive ulnar variance, this has been associated with chronic physis stress and earlier ossification.[43]

Although radiographs are typically normal, they might show widening of the growth plate, especially volarly and radially, cystic changes of the metaphyseal aspect of the growth plate, a beaked distal volar and radial physis, and haziness within the growth plate.

MR imaging can show widening of the distal radial physis and irregularity of the margin of the distal radial metaphysis. There may also be abnormally high signal along the distal radial metaphysis, possibly reflecting abnormal ossification of the physeal cartilage.[49]

Treatment consists of cessation of the offending activity. Growth arrest and acquired positive ulnar variance may result if the condition is not addressed[1,43,48,49] (**Fig. 23**).

Stress Reactions and Stress Fractures

Stress reactions and stress fractures of the distal ulna, scaphoid, hook of the hamate, and metacarpals are being increasingly recognized as causes of wrist and hand pain in athletes. These stress lesions most typically occur because of repetitive direct impaction or repetitive loading at tendon and ligament attachment sites.[50,51]

Of these stress injuries, the most commonly reported are those of the distal ulna from sports such as baseball, tennis, volleyball, and weight-lifting[52–54] (**Fig. 24**). Athletes with ulnar stress injuries present with pain and tenderness over the ulna during and after activity. Radiographs may be normal or may show mild periostitis or a small cortical lucency at the site of the stress fracture. MR imaging is very sensitive to these injuries and shows marrow edema

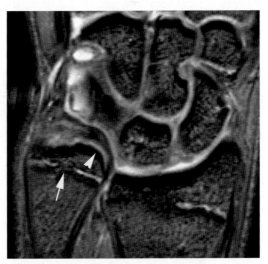

Fig. 23. Premature physeal arrest in a 16-year-old female gymnast (Gymnast's wrist). Coronal gradient echo T2-weighted image shows premature physeal arrest (*arrow*), with secondary marked positive ulnar variance and ulnocarpal impaction (*arrowhead*).

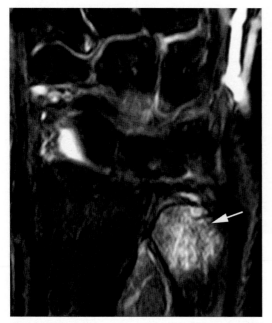

Fig. 24. Distal ulna stress reaction in a 34-year-old male tennis player. Coronal fat-suppressed T2-weighted image shows ill-defined bone marrow edema in the distal ulna (*arrow*).

(stress reaction) with a small hypointense fracture line (if a stress fracture is present). Stress fractures are treated with rest for 6 to 8 weeks.[51]

Kienböck Disease

Necrosis of the lunate (Kienböck disease, lunatomalacia) is most commonly seen in the dominant hand of men, particularly athletic men. This condition can be seen in athletes participating in sports that result in repetitive wrist loading, such as rowing, handball, football, and gymnastics.[55] Kienböck has also been associated with negative ulnar variance. Symptoms typically have an insidious onset with a dull ache along the mid-dorsal aspect of the affected wrist.

MR imaging is considered the gold standard for the early diagnosis of Kienböck disease. When radiographs are normal, MR imaging may show abnormal signal within the lunate. With contrast-enhanced MR imaging, the perfusion of the lunate can be assessed, thereby allowing determination of the size of the avascular (or necrotic) fragment of the bone[55] (**Fig. 25**). In more advanced stages, there may be collapse of the necrotic portion of the bone. Treatment strategies are variable but are typically prescribed based on the degree of necrosis, collapse, and associated osteoarthritis.

NERVES
Carpal Tunnel Syndrome

Carpal tunnel syndrome is the most common compressive peripheral neuropathy in athletes, occupational activities, and in the general population.[56,57] Carpal tunnel syndrome is caused by abnormal compression of the median nerve by the overlying flexor retinaculum. In athletes, the most common cause is flexor tenosynovitis, which is often related to repetitive motion. Chronic compression and increasing the pressure of the median nerve alters nerve function, blocks axonal conduction, reduces perfusion, and if the compression persists myelin degradation and neural fibrosis are induced. The condition can be related to bar work. Symptoms of carpal tunnel syndrome include pain and paresthesias in the

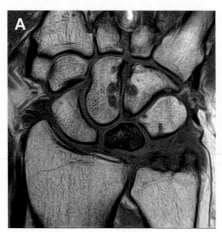
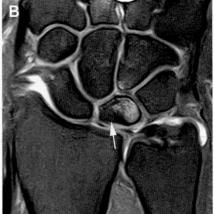

Fig. 25. Stage II Kienböck disease in a 34-year-old motorcyclist. (*A*) Coronal T1-weighted image shows uniform low-signal-intensity lunate marrow. (*B*) Coronal fat-suppressed T2-weighted image shows a partial necrotic lunate bone limited to the radial aspect (*arrow*). Note also an associated hamatolunate impaction syndrome.

distribution of the median nerve. Symptoms are often worse at night.[56,57]

At physical examination, median nerve distribution hyperesthesia, a positive Tinel sign (sensation of pins and needles provoked by tapping the median nerve), and a positive Phalen maneuver (reproduction of symptoms with forced wrist flexion) may be present. With more chronic disease, atrophy of the thenar eminence and weakness of median nerve distribution musculature may be seen.[56,57]

MR imaging's role is to rule out pathologic process within the carpal tunnel in the flexor compartment, such as flexor tenosynovitis, a ganglion, an anomalous muscle, or a neoplasm. Its role is limited in the evaluation of nerve compression and changes. The characteristic findings of carpal tunnel syndrome include enlargement and hyperintensity of the median nerve, and bowing of the flexor retinaculum (**Fig. 26**).

In athletes, when flexor tenosynovitis is the cause of carpal tunnel syndrome, rest, immobilization, NSAIDs, and occasionally steroid injections result in resolution of symptoms. Rarely, a short course of oral corticosteroids may be prescribed if initial treatment fails. Refractory cases may be treated with release of the flexor retinaculum (open or endoscopic).[57]

Guyon Canal Ulnar Neuropathy

Guyon tunnel ulnar neuropathy is typically seen in cyclists and is thus also referred to as cyclist's palsy.[57] This condition can also be presented in computer keyboard users as an occupational overuse syndrome[58]

This condition is typically caused by compression of the ulnar nerve within the Guyon canal, a space formed by the hook of the hamate, the pisiform, and the overlying volar carpal ligament. It is related to repetitive flexion and extension of the wrist and repeat pressure on the hypothenal eminence. Symptoms include numbness and paresthesias in the distribution of the ulnar nerve: the fifth finger and the ulnar side of the fourth finger. Weakness of the abductor digiti quinti, hypothenar atrophy, intrinsic hand muscle atrophy, and/or claw hand may also be seen.[57,58]

MR imaging may show enlargement and edema of the ulnar nerve and its branches, may show the site of compression, and can show a disorder that may be causing the compression, such as a hamate fracture, ganglion, ulnar artery aneurysm, or neoplasm[26] (see **Fig. 16**).

Treatment typically consists of modification of the handlebars, riding position, and grips. In rare cases, when conservative treatment is

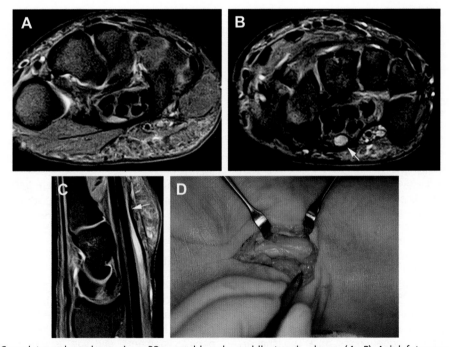

Fig. 26. Carpal tunnel syndrome in a 32-year-old male paddle tennis player. (*A, B*) Axial fat-suppressed T2-weighted consecutive images show median nerve compressive neuropathy manifested by proximal thickening and increased signal intensity of the median nerve (*arrow in B*). (*C*) Sagittal fat-suppressed T2-weighted image shows thickening of the flexor retinaculum (*arrow*). The median nerve is thickened proximally with increase signal intensity. (*D*) An open carpal tunnel release surgery was performed with complete relief of symptoms.

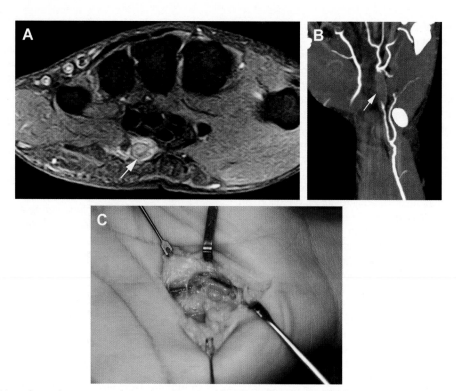

Fig. 27. Hypothenar hammer syndrome in a 30-year-old male cyclist. (*A*, *B*) Axial fat-suppressed T2-weighted and CT angiography images show a complete ulnar artery occlusion secondary to thrombosis (*arrows*). (*C*) Confirmation of ulnar artery thrombosis.

unsuccessful, or if there is an underlying focal lesion causing ulnar nerve compression, surgical release and/or excision of the offending lesion may be necessary.

Hypothenar Hammer Syndrome

Hypothenar hammer syndrome consists of vascular insufficiency caused by repetitive damage (or less frequently from a single blunt injury) to the unprotected ulnar artery that remains superficial when it exits the Guyon canal, resulting in damage to the arterial wall, decreased flow, thrombosis, and occasionally peripheral emboli. This condition can result in hand and finger ischemia and pain.[59] It was originally described in men using machinery, workers who use the ulnar palm as a tool to hammer objects, but hypothenar hammer syndrome can be seen in athletes, particularly those that use their hands for catching or striking (volleyball, baseball, football, karate, judo, handball) or those that grip a piece of equipment (baseball, racquet sports, golf). The ulnar artery is most prone to injury distally near the hook of the hamate because it is only covered by skin, subcutaneous fat, and the palmaris brevis muscle.[59]

MR angiography (and CT angiography) can show the injured segment of the ulnar artery and any associated stenosis or occlusion[5] (**Fig. 27**). With very-high-resolution imaging, distal embolic occlusions may also be seen.

Prevention is needed in the population that is inherently susceptible to developing hypothenar hammer syndrome by wearing proper protective equipment and changing grip techniques.[59]

Treatment can include activity modification, anticoagulants, oral vasodilators, thrombectomy, resection and anastomosis, and interpositional vein grafting.[60]

SUMMARY

Chronic wrist and hand pain is a common occupation-related complaint for both manual workers and athletes and may be caused by a variety of injuries involving the tendons, bones, nerves, ligaments, and soft tissues. US and MR imaging can accurately show the cause, location, severity, and associated lesions, thereby allowing accurate diagnosis and guiding appropriate therapy.

REFERENCES

1. Rettig AC. Athletic injuries of the wrist and hand: part II: overuse injuries of the wrist and traumatic injuries to the hand. Am J Sports Med 2004;32:262–73.

2. VanHeest AE, Luger NM, House JH, et al. Extensor retinaculum impingement in the athlete: a new diagnosis. Am J Sports Med 2007;35:2126–30.

3. Barr AE, Barbe MF, Clark BD. Work-related musculoskeletal disorders of the hand and wrist: epidemiology, pathophysiology, and sensorimotor changes. J Orthop Sports Phys Ther 2004;34:610–27.

4. Work related hand and wrist injuries in Australia (2008). ISBN 9780642327628.

5. Rosner JL, Zlatkin MB, Clifford P, et al. Imaging of athletic wrist and hand injuries. Semin Musculoskelet Radiol 2004;8:57–79.

6. McNally E, Wilson D, Seiler S. Rowing injuries. Semin Musculoskelet Radiol 2005;9:379–96.

7. Stern PJ. Tendinitis, overuse syndromes, and tendon injuries. Hand Clin 1990;6:467–76.

8. Clavero JA, Alomar X, Monill JM, et al. MR imaging of ligament and tendon injuries of the fingers. Radiographics 2002;22:237–56.

9. Ashraf MO, Devadoss VG. Systematic review and meta-analysis on steroid injection therapy for de Quervain's tenosynovitis in adults. Eur J Orthop Surg Traumatol 2014;24:149–57.

10. Stahl S, Vida D, Meisner C, et al. Systematic review and meta-analysis on the work-related cause of de Quervain tenosynovitis: a critical appraisal of its recognition as an occupational disease. Plast Reconstr Surg 2013;132:1479–91.

11. Stahl S, Vida D, Meisner C, et al. Work related etiology of de Quervain's tenosynovitis: a case-control study with prospectively collected data Pathophysiology of musculoskeletal disorders. BMC Musculoskelet Disord 2015;16:126.

12. Choi SJ, Ahn JH, Lee YL, et al. de Quervain disease: US identification of anatomic variants in the first extensor compartment with an emphasis on subcompartmentalization. Radiology 2011;260:480–6.

13. Parellada AJ, Gopez AG, Morrison WB, et al. Distal intersection tenosynovitis of the wrist: a lesser-known extensor tendinopathy with characteristic MR imaging features. Skeletal Radiol 2007;36:203–8.

14. Mattox R, Battaglia PJ, Scali F, et al. Distal intersection syndrome progressing to extensor pollicis longus tendon rupture: a case report with sonographic findings. J Ultrasound 2017;20:237–41.

15. de Lima JE, Kim HJ, Albertotti F, et al. Intersection syndrome: MR imaging with anatomic comparison of the distal forearm. Skeletal Radiol 2004;33:627–31.

16. Allende C, Le Viet D. Extensor carpi ulnaris problems at the wrist–classification, surgical treatment and results. J Hand Surg Br 2005;30:265–72.

17. Carneiro RS, Fontana R, Mazzer N. Ulnar wrist pain in athletes caused by erosion of the floor of the sixth dorsal compartment: a case series. Am J Sports Med 2005;33:1910–3.

18. Ryan WG. Calcific tendinitis of flexor carpi ulnaris: an easy misdiagnosis. Arch Emerg Med 1994;10:321–3.

19. Edmondson M, Skyrme A. Occupationally related bilateral calcific tendonitis of Flexor carpi ulnaris: case report. J Orthop Surg Res 2009;4:33.

20. Friedman SL, Palmer AK. The ulnar impaction syndrome. Hand Clin 1991;7:295–310.

21. Imaeda T, Nakamura R, Shionoya K, et al. Ulnar impaction syndrome: MR imaging findings. Radiology 1996;201:495–500.

22. Cerezal L, Del Pinal F, Abascal F, et al. Imaging findings in ulnar-sided wrist impaction syndromes. Radiographics 2002;22:105–21.

23. Cerezal L, Del Pinal F, Abascal F. MR imaging findings in ulnar-sided wrist impaction syndromes. Magn Reson Imaging Clin N Am 2004;12:281–99.

24. Schmitt R, Christopoulos G, Meier R, et al. Direct MR arthrography of the wrist in comparison with arthroscopy: a prospective study on 125 patients. Rofo 2003;175:911–9.

25. Braun H, Kenn W, Schneider S, et al. Direct MR arthrography of the wrist- value in detecting complete and partial defects of intrinsic ligaments and the TFCC in comparison with arthroscopy. Rofo 2003;175:1515–24.

26. Cerezal L, Abascal F, Del Pinal F. Wrist MR arthrography: how, why, when. Radiol Clin North Am 2005;43:709–31.

27. Haims AH, Schweitzer ME, Morrison WB, et al. Limitations of MR imaging in the diagnosis of peripheral tears of the triangular fibrocartilage of the wrist. AJR Am J Roentgenol 2002;178:419–22.

28. Cerezal L, de Dios Berná-Mestre J, Canga A, et al. MR and CT arthrography of the wrist. Semin Musculoskelet Radiol 2012;16(1):27–41.

29. Sachar K. Ulnar-sided wrist pain: evaluation and treatment of triangular fibrocartilage complex tears, ulnocarpal impaction syndrome, and lunotriquetral ligament tears. J Hand Surg Am 2012;37:1489–500.

30. Henderson CJ, Kobayashi KM. Minimally invasive approaches to ulnar-sided wrist disorders. Hand Clin 2014;30:77–89.

31. Minami A, Kato H. Ulnar shortening for triangular fibrocartilage complex tears associated with ulnar positive variance. J Hand Surg Am 1998;23:904–8.

32. Pirolo JM, Yao J. Minimally invasive approaches to ulnar-sided wrist disorders. Hand Clin 2014;30:77–89.

33. Topper SM, Wood MB, Ruby LK. Ulnar styloid impaction syndrome. J Hand Surg Am 1997;22:699–704.

34. Vezeridis PS, Yoshioka H, Han R, et al. Ulnar-sided wrist pain. Part I: anatomy and physical examination. Skeletal Radiol 2010;39:733–45.

35. Bell MJ, Hill RJ, McMurtry RY. Ulnar impingement syndrome. J Bone Joint Surg Br 1985;67:126–9.

36. Lees VC, Scheker LR. The radiological demonstration of dynamic ulnar impingement. J Hand Surg 1997;22:448–50.

37. Garcia-Elias M. Dorsal fractures of the triquetrum-avulsion or compression fractures? J Hand Surg Am 1987;12:266–8.

38. Tomaino MM, Gainer M, Towers JD. Carpal impaction with the ulnar styloid process: treatment with partial styloid resection. J Hand Surg Br 2001;26:252–5.

39. Thurston AJ, Stanley JK. Hamato-lunate impingement: an uncommon cause of ulnar-sided wrist pain. Arthroscopy 2000;16:540–4.

40. Viegas SF, Wagner K, Patterson R, et al. Medial (hamate) facet of the lunate. J Hand Surg Am 1990;15:564–71.

41. Malik AM, Schweitzer ME, Culp RW, et al. MR imaging of the type II lunate bone: frequency, extent, and associated findings. AJR Am J Roentgenol 1999; 173:335–8.

42. Pfirrmann CW, Theumann NH, Chung CB, et al. The hamatolunate facet: characterization and association with cartilage lesions–magnetic resonance arthrography and anatomic correlation in cadaveric wrists. Skeletal Radiol 2002;31:451–6.

43. Webb BG, Rettig LA. Gymnastic wrist injuries. Curr Sports Med Rep 2008;7:289–95.

44. Henry M. Arthroscopic management of dorsal wrist impingement. J Hand Surg 2008;33:1201–4.

45. Matson A, Dekker T, Lampley A, et al. Diagnosis and arthroscopic management of dorsal wrist capsular impingement. J Hand Surg Am 2017;42:e167–74.

46. Mathoulin C, Gras M. Arthroscopic management of dorsal and volar wrist ganglion. Hand Clin 2017; 33:769–77.

47. Borisch N. Arthroscopic resection of occult dorsal wrist ganglia. Arch Orthop Trauma Surg 2016;136:1473–80.

48. Morgan WJ, Slowman LS. Acute hand and wrist injuries in athletes: evaluation and management. J Am Acad Orthop Surg 2001;9:389–400.

49. Dobyns JH, Gabel GT. Gymnast's wrist. Hand Clin 1990;6:493–505.

50. Pepper M, Akuthota V, McCarty EC. The pathophysiology of stress fractures. Clin Sports Med 2006;25: 1–16.

51. Jones GL. Upper extremity stress fractures. Clin Sports Med 2006;25:159–74.

52. Fragniere B, Landry M, Siegrist O. Stress fracture of the ulna in a professional tennis player using a double-handed backhand stroke. Knee Surg Sports Traumatol Arthrosc 2001;9:239–41.

53. Guha AR, Marynissen H. Stress fracture of the hook of the hamate. Br J Sports Med 2002;36:224–5.

54. Parsons EM, Goldblatt JP, Richmond JC. Metacarpal stress fracture in an intercollegiate rower: case report. Am J Sports Med 2005;33:293–4.

55. Trumble TE, Katolik LI. Treatment of Kienböck disease in athletes. Atlas Hand Clin 2006;11:45–65.

56. Akuthota V, Plastaras C, Lindberg K, et al. The effect of long-distance bicycling on ulnar and median nerves: an electrophysiologic evaluation of cyclist palsy. Am J Sports Med 2005;33:1224–30.

57. Aulicino PL. Neurovascular injuries in the hands of athletes. Hand Clin 1990;6:455–66.

58. Chan JC, Tiong WH, Hennessy MJ, et al. A Guyon's canal ganglion presenting as occupational overuse syndrome: a case report. J Brachial Plex Peripher Nerve Inj 2008;3:4.

59. Henderson CJ, Kobayashi KM. Ulnar-sided wrist pain in the athlete. Orthop Clin N Am 2016;47(4):787–98.

60. Mueller LP, Rudig L, Kreiter KF, et al. Hypothenar hammer syndrome in sports. Knee Surg Sports Traumatol Arthrosc 1996;4(3):167–70.

Imaging the Postsurgical Upper Limb
The Radiologist Perspective

Alberto Bazzocchi, MD, PhD[a],*,
Maria Pilar Aparisi Gómez, MBChB, FRANZCR[b,c,d],
Paolo Spinnato, MD[a], Alessandro Marinelli, MD[e],
Alessandro Napoli, MD, PhD[f], Roberto Rotini, MD[e],
Carlo Catalano, MD[f], Giuseppe Guglielmi, MD[g]

KEYWORDS

• Shoulder • Elbow • Wrist • Joints • Upper extremity • Postoperative period • Radiology
• MR imaging

KEY POINTS

- All imaging modalities play important roles in postsurgical assessment.
- Good knowledge and understanding of the different surgical procedures help in providing as much information as possible to guarantee a favorable outcome of treatment, therefore improving levels of care and prognosis.
- Familiarity with expected postsurgical appearances is mandatory, to be able to discern these from complications.

INTRODUCTION

Imaging plays a fundamental role in postsurgical assessment. As much as knowledge on processes and mechanisms causing disorder, radiologists need to be familiar with the different options of treatment, especially surgical procedures, to be able to reassure about expected postsurgical appearances and detect potential complications.

This article reviews the surgical procedures that are most frequently used in the shoulder, elbow, and wrist, with a focus on the indications, normal postsurgical appearances, and imaging features of potential complications. Emphasis is made on points that should not be overlooked in the surgical planning.

Disclosure: The authors confirm that this article has not been published elsewhere and is not under consideration by another publisher. All authors have approved the article and agree with submission for your consideration. The authors have no conflicts of interest or funding information to disclose.
[a] Diagnostic and Interventional Radiology, IRCCS Istituto Ortopedico Rizzoli, Via G. C. Pupilli 1, Bologna 40136, Italy; [b] Department of Radiology, National Women's Hospital, Auckland City Hospital, Greenlane Clinical Center, Auckland District Health Board, 2 Park Road, Grafton, Auckland 1023, New Zealand; [c] Department of Ultrasound, National Women's Hospital, Auckland City Hospital, Greenlane Clinical Center, Auckland District Health Board, 2 Park Road, Grafton, Auckland 1023, New Zealand; [d] Department of Radiology, Hospital Nisa Nueve de Octubre, Calle Valle de la Ballestera, 59, Valencia 46015, Spain; [e] Shoulder and Elbow Surgery, IRCCS Istituto Ortopedico Rizzoli, Via G. C. Pupilli 1, Bologna 40136, Italy; [f] Department of Radiologic, Oncologic and Pathologic Sciences, La Sapienza University of Rome, V.le Regina Elena 324, Rome 00180, Italy; [g] Department of Radiology, University of Foggia, Viale Luigi Pinto 1, Foggia 71100, Italy
* Corresponding author.
E-mail address: abazzo@inwind.it

Table 1
Positive and negative features for the different types of approach for surgical procedures in the shoulder

Open Surgery

Positives	Negatives
• Better long-term results, given the visualization of the cuff and subacromial space is more clear and the handling easier	• Higher morbidity and involves detaching the origin of the anterior and/or middle heads of the deltoid in the acromion, with the chance of potential long-term complications

Arthroscopy

Positives	Negatives
• Fewer complications during and after surgery • Allows good intraarticular visualization	• Requires a reasonable amount of experience

MIni-open Procedures

Helpful in certain procedures that cannot be completed with arthroscopy alone
The deltoid is only split and not detached

SHOULDER
Surgical Options

Shoulder surgery can be performed through an open approach or via arthroscopy. MIni-open procedures are a combination of both. Pros and cons are summarized in **Table 1**.

The detachment of the deltoid is an unusual (8%) delayed complication (1–5 months) after open procedures (much less frequent in mini-open). Recent studies have shown no difference in clinical outcomes among the 3 approaches.[1,2]

Subacromial decompression

Subacromial decompression consists of the resection of the anteroinferior aspect of the acromion. The role of subacromial descompression alone has decreased through the years.

Resection of the coracoacromial ligament can also be performed,[3] if this is thickened, but many surgeons opt for debriding, especially in young patients, to prevent superior migration of the humeral head with time.

If there is associated acromioclavicular (AC) joint degeneration, the joint is resected, along with up to 1 cm of the distal clavicle (Mumford procedure).

Indications Indications are summarized in **Box 1**.

Things to assess beforehand Impingement tests can be performed. Patients may have undergone diagnostic/therapeutic injections. Significant relief of pain or symptoms after injection can pinpoint impingement as the cause and help select patients for subacromial decompression.[4]

Patients with advanced age, with a minimal activity level, with medical conditions, or with expectations out of proportion may not be good candidates.

It is important to mention that if there is the suspicion of instability as the origin of symptoms, this should be investigated thoroughly before proceeding with decompressive surgery. Eccentric loading of the cuff or internal glenoid impingement leads to further damage of shoulder structures later in life, and symptoms of impingement in these cases can be a consequence, not an causal factor. Acromioplasty does not represent a treatment of the original problem in these cases, and on some occasions worsens the condition. Acromioplasty can only be useful in these cases as a complementary technique if the bursa is involved, and after addressing the origin of the problem.[5]

Normal postsurgical appearances It is always important to compare with presurgical imaging,

Box 1
Indications for subacromial decompression

- Symptoms: painful shoulder with signs of impingement
- Failure of conservative management/rehabilitation
- Coexisting cuff disease (combination with cuff repair). Impingement signs, and lesion on bursal side > lesion on articular side
- Young, active patients
- Preoperative findings consistent with impingement on MR imaging (severe AC joint degenerative disease, type 3 acromion, thick coracoacromial ligament)

Data from Dzirkale A, Paruchuri NB, Zlatkin MB. Postoperative shoulder. In: Pope TL, Bloem HL, Beltran J, Morrison WB, Wilson DJ, eds. Imaging of the Musculoskeletal System, 2nd edition. Philadelphia: Saunders Elsevier; 2015. p. 1123-1135.

to be able to assess the change in anatomy in the osseous outlet. Direct postsurgical assessment can be performed with magnetic resonance (MR) or computed tomography (CT). Ultrasonography (US) is useful in the assessment of associated cuff disorder.

Expected postsurgical appearances are summarized in **Box 2**.

On MR imaging, there can be artifact caused by residual microscopic metal fragments (**Fig. 1**). In the cases in which an open or mini-open approach has been used, sutures will be visible on the middle or proximal part of the deltoid (foci of artifact on MR imaging or small hyperechoic foci with no shadowing on US). Fibrosis in relation to the site of acromioplasty can also be detected on MR imaging (with low T1 and low T2).

In some cases, there is an improvement in the radiological appearances of the rotator cuff, but this is not consistent, and abnormal signal may persist.

Abnormal postsurgical appearances/complications Abnormal postsurgical appearances and complications are summarized in **Table 2** and **Fig. 2**.

How is possible rotator cuff disorder assessed after acromioplasty? In some cases, persistent abnormal signal of the rotator cuff tendons is a confounding factor in assessing potential

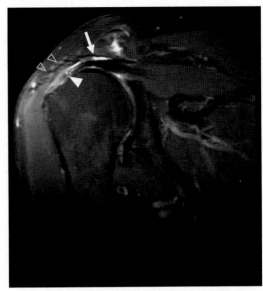

Fig. 1. Postacromioplasty change. Coronal proton density-weighted spectral attenuated inversion recovery shows metallic susceptibility artifact (PDW SPAIR) (*arrowheads*). Note that the AC joint appears mildly hypertrophic, with effusion. A band of fluid is present between the tendon and the undersurface of the acromion (*white arrow*); this does not represent the bursa, because it has been resected. The tendon is thin and attenuated, in keeping with rotator cuff tendinosis, with incomplete rupture (*white arrowhead*).

Box 2
Expected postsurgical appearances after subacromial acromioplasty decompression

- Acromion: may show an inferior flat surface (compared with previous morphology). The anterior one-third of the acromion should not be present because this is the resected portion.

- Resection of the AC joint: there may be absence of the distal clavicle with widening of the joint.

- Resection of the bursa: there will be scar tissue in this location, and it is also possible to see a band of fluid, which is important given that the presence of fluid in this location will not be a useful indicator of cuff injury in subsequent assessment.

- Resection-debridement of the coracoacromial ligament: absence of it or increased signal intensity in water-sensitive sequences (normally at the acromion end).

Data from Mohana-Borges AV, Chung CB, Resnick D. MR imaging and MR arthrography of the postoperative shoulder: spectrum of normal and abnormal findings. Radiographics 2004;24(1):69–85.

---

progression of disorder of the rotator cuff after acromioplasty. MR imaging remains sensitive but is not as specific for rotator cuff tendon abnormalities. It remains fairly sensitive (84%) and specific (87%) for residual impingement, though.[6] Arthrography may be useful to detect tears.

Rotator cuff repair or debridement
The normal steps for repair are subacromial decompression, rotator cuff mobilization, and repair of the tendon (depending on degree and type of lesion). In some cases, a bursal release/resection may also be performed.[7]

The aim of cuff repair is to reestablish continuity of the tendon without generating tension (**Fig. 3**).

Indications Indications are summarized in **Box 3**.

Things to assess beforehand As preparation, thorough cuff assessment is necessary, with US or MR imaging. US has the same accuracy as MR in expert hands.[8]

It is paramount to accurately characterize the tear, as well as to detect associated findings, which may represent potential causes (impingement). This characterization guides the type of treatment[9] (summarized in **Table 3**).

Table 2
Abnormal postsurgical appearances/ complications of subacromial decompression

General postsurgical complications	Adhesive capsulitis, synovitis, infection (arthritis, osteomyelitis), chondrolysis, potential retention of foreign bodies, and bleeding
Inadequate resection	In these cases, the presence of factors that could lead to recurrent impingement will be seen, such as spurs or acromion fragments
Residual AC joint degeneration	Hypertrophy
Excessive scarring and fibrosis	Stiffness, pain
Persistence of an os acromiale	Reproduce symptoms during deltoid contraction
Detachment or atrophy of the deltoid	Unusual (8%) delayed complication (1–5 mo) after open procedures (much less frequent in miniopen)
Presence of an undiagnosed instability	Original symptoms persist or worsen

Data from Magee TH, Gaenslen ES, Seitz R, et al. MR imaging of the shoulder after surgery. AJR Am J Roentgenol 1997;168(4):925-928.

In massive or chronic tears, mobilization of other muscles may be needed and therefore an open approach is adequate, although arthroscopy has also been advocated.[10]

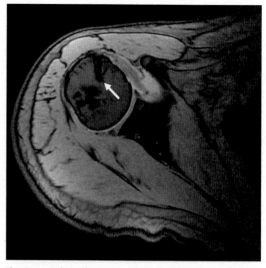

Fig. 3. Axial gradient-recalled echo (GRE) T2* shows a repair with a tunnel for anchor in the lesser tuberosity (*white arrow*).

Severe muscle atrophy or severe retractions are likely to result in failure of the procedure, so it is important to assess muscle belly characteristics:
Degree of atrophy (edema in the muscle is the most reliable sign).
Fat infiltration: Goutallier classification (0–4).
Advanced age, poor activity level, and comorbidities are factors to consider because they may be relative contraindications to surgery.

Normal postsurgical appearances Comparison with previous imaging is useful, as well as gathering information on the type of surgery performed. Expected postsurgical appearances are summarized in **Box 4**.
US and MR imaging have been shown to offer the same accuracy in postoperative assessment

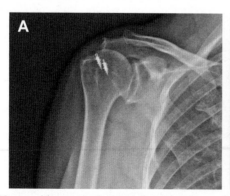
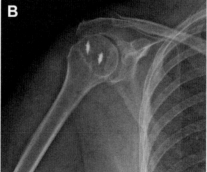

Fig. 2. A 58-year-old woman submitted after extensive acromial resection and rotator cuff repair. There was instability and persistent pain. (*A*) Anteroposterior (AP) radiograph shows superior subluxation of the humeral head, and signs of osteoarthritis, with marginal osteophytes and subtle subchondral sclerosis in the humeral head. Note the rotator cuff repair anchors, in their expected locations. The acromial segment removed was too large, and superior instability developed as a result. (*B*) Abducted and externally rotated view shows the extent of acromial resection.

Box 3
Indications for rotator cuff repair or debridement

- Physical signs and symptoms of cuff disease: impingement, pain, weakness
- Consideration of degree of tear and patient activity level
- Full-thickness tears are surgically managed unless symptoms are minimal and strength and range of motion are preserved
- Tears increasing in size
- Subacromial decompression and bursal release are often added (especially in bursal tears)

Data from Dzirkale A, Paruchuri NB, Zlatkin MB. Postoperative shoulder. In: Pope TL, Bloem HL, Beltran J, Morrison WB, Wilson DJ, eds. Imaging of the Musculoskeletal System, 2nd edition. Philadelphia: Saunders Elsevier; 2015. p. 1123-1135.

---

of the rotator cuff, with lower sensitivity for partial-thickness tears.[11]

It is important to mention that if a retracted torn tendon is reinserted, the location will be in a more medial part of the greater tuberosity, which means that a region of bare bone in the lateral part of the tuberosity does not mean recurrent tear.[12]

After repairs of high-grade or large full-thickness tears the tendon can be medialized (**Fig. 4**).

On MR arthrography the presence of contrast through the tendon is normal (this is no longer watertight) and does not indicate a tear long as there are no defined tendon defects.[13] Today metatallic, peek and all-suture anchors can be used, with different implications for imaging.

Abnormal postsurgical appearances/complications Abnormal postsurgical appearances and complications are summarized in **Table 4** and **Fig. 5**.

Sensitivity and specificity of MR imaging to detect recurrent tears is high (84% and 91% for full thickness, and 83% and 83% for partial thickness, respectively) (**Figs. 6** and **7**).[6]

MR arthrography is indicated in cases of presence of granulation tissue and when there is important interfering artifact.[13]

Repairs of glenohumeral instability
May be unidirectional, bidirectional, multidirectional, and anterior, posterior, inferior, or superior. Unidirectional tends to be the result of a single traumatic event (generally anterior dislocation) and is associated with damage to labrum, ligaments, and capsule (Bankart lesion and variants). Multidirectional instability tends to be atraumatic.[14]

Surgical techniques are direct or indirect, although today indirect techniques are rarely indicated (**Box 5**).

Indications Indications are summarized in **Box 6**.

Things to assess beforehand Characterization of the type of injury causing instability with adequate

---

Table 3
Types of treatment of rotator cuff tears

Type of Tear	Treatment	Approach
Low grade (<50% depth)	Simple debridement	Arthroscopy
Intermediate	Debridement with suturing of the defect created by debridement	Arthroscopy
High grade (>50% depth)	Excised and treated as full thickness	Arthroscopy/open
Full Thickness		
Small	Side-to-side suturing	Arthroscopy/open
Large	Reattachment tendon to bone Transosseous fixation with a direct tendon-to-bone attachment	Open, mini-open, arthroscopy
Massive	Mobilization of other tendons (long head of biceps, subscapularis)	Open/Arthroscopy
Irreparable tears	Tendon transfer (latissimus) Subacromial decompression Use of grafts/meshes	Open/Arthroscopy

Data from Morag Y, Jacobson JA, Miller B, et al. MR imaging of rotator cuff injury: what the clinician needs to know. Radiographics 2006;26(4): 1045-1065.

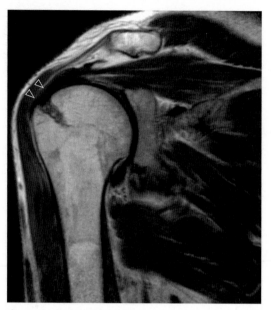

Fig. 4. Coronal PDW image shows a tunnel for anchor in the greater tuberosity. Note slight thinning of the reinserted tendon (*arrowheads*).

information on the status of glenoid, cartilage, labrum, ligaments, capsule, and tendons is necessary to plan surgery.

The goal of surgery is to repair structures to achieve a degree of stability as close as possible to the anatomic.

In cases of traumatic instability, patients may originally be treated with closed reduction and immobilization and then a rehabilitation program, to strengthen the dynamic stabilizers of the shoulder.

In young patients, surgery is performed to repair the labrum (placing suture anchors, absorbable tacks, or knotless fixation) and/or the capsule (capsulorrhaphy, reinforcement with sutures, capsular shifts) (**Fig. 8**). If there are bony defects, reduction of the fragment or grafting is performed.

Bony defects on the glenoid may lead to reversal of the normal pear shape of the glenoid, with recurrent dislocation. Defects representing greater than 6 or 8 mm or greater than 20% to 25% of the inferior glenoid diameter need surgery (fixation, coracoid transfer, bone grafting).[15] Assessment of the glenoid can be done with multidetector CT (MDCT), using oblique sagittal reformatted images (or three-dimensional [3D] imaging with digital subtraction of the humeral head),[16] but MR imaging has also been validated[17] to accurately quantify the amount of bone loss. Each 1.5 to 1.7 mm of glenoid bone loss approximately corresponds to a 5% increase in loss of glenoid bone stock.[18]

A glenoid defect of more than 25% with instability is definitely an indication for open surgery[19] and bone grafting. The most relevant treatment when there is a large glenoid fracture, glenoid wear caused by multiple dislocations, or a Bankart repair has failed is the transfer of the coracoid with its attached tendons (modified Bristow-Latarjet).[14]

In patients with glenoid bone loss, a concurrent Hill-Sachs lesion can have different

Table 4
**Abnormal postsurgical appearances/
complications of rotator cuff repair or
debridement**

General postsurgical complications	Adhesive capsulitis, synovitis, infection (arthritis, osteomyelitis), chondrolysis, potential retention of foreign bodies, and bleeding
Recurrent Tear	
US	Reliable indicators of a tear are nonvisualization of the tendon, focal defects, retraction from anchors or fixation, and demonstration of loose sutures
MR imaging	Reliable indicator of a tear is absence or retraction of the tendon, and then the presence of fluid signal within a tendon defect
MR arthrography	Identification of partial tears in cases of presence of granulation tissue and when there is important artifact
Axillary or suprascapular nerve injury	Atrophy of the teres minor and supraspinatus and infraspinatus
Inadequate acromioplasty	Failure to address osteoarthritis of the AC joint: recurrence of symptoms
Chondral defects of the glenoid	Mimic the symptoms of subacromial impingement
Aggressive debridement	Iatrogenic tears
Detachment or atrophy of the deltoid	Unusual (8%) delayed complication (1–5 mo) after open procedures much less frequent in miniopen

Data from Refs.[6,13,14]

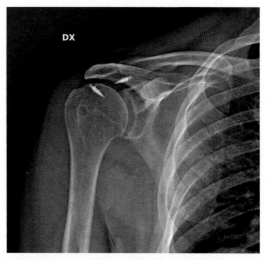

Fig. 5. A 71-year-old man with recurring pain symptoms after rotator cuff repair. AP radiograph shows migration of a rotator cuff anchor into the subacromial space, in keeping with repair detachment.

consequences, as Burkhart and DeBeer[15] described with the concept of significant bone loss. Depending on the orientation and position of the Hill-Sachs defect, the abnormal glenoid may be engaged with much less force and anterior translation in the athletic position (90° abduction and 90° of external rotation), and dislocation then occurs.[20] According to this, Hill-Sachs lesions could be engaging or nonengaging, or, as has

more recently been coined, to differentiate the true engaging lesions after Bankart repair (and not merely caused by ligament laxity or injury) off-track or on-track depending of the risk of recurrence of dislocation.[21]

- Medial margin of Hill-Sachs lesion is within the glenoid track (on-track): bone support.
- Medial margin of Hill-Sachs lesion is more medial than the glenoid track (off-track): no bone support.

Accurate description of the size, and of the size, depth, and orientation of the bone loss, in the glenoid and the humerus respectively allows clinicians to describe the bipolar model (bone loss glenoid–humeral head defect) and the risk of recurrent dislocation, and therefore helps with the planning of surgical options. The surgical aim to achieve stability is to convert off-track lesions into on-track lesions.[22]

Assessment is performed with MDCT (3D reconstructions)[22] or arthroscopy (normally both shoulders are scanned and anatomic measurements obtained from the healthy one) (**Box 7**).

Engaging Hill-Sachs lesions may be treated with bone graft augmentation, to restore sphericity of the humeral head, or increasingly the use of the remplissage technique (filling the defect with capsule and rotator cuff tendon).[16] If the loss is greater than 40%, replacement of the humeral head is necessary.[23]

Isolated labral (superior labrum anteroposterior) tears with no instability can be treated with debridement.[24]

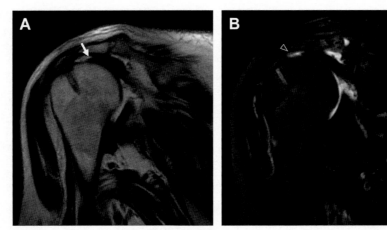

Fig. 6. A 57-year-old woman with impaired abduction, 2 years after rotator cuff repair. (*A*) Coronal PDW shows the bony anchor, with the groove for reattachment slightly higher in the humeral head than the anatomic attachment in the greater tuberosity. There is complete discontinuity of the supraspinatus tendon, which shows retraction (*white arrow*). (*B*) Coronal T2 fat saturation also shows interposed fluid (*arrowhead*).

Posterior instability is normally treated similarly to anterior, with repair of the labrum and capsular reinforcement or shift. Bone defects are treated with bone grafts, or osteotomies if there is glenoid dysplasia, which is commonly associated with posterior labral tears and multidirectional instability.[25]

Multidirectional instability is normally treated conservatively, and is associated with ligament laxity or, as mentioned, glenoid dysplasia. In cases in which the conservative treatment fails, surgical repair is performed with an inferior capsular shift.[25]

Paralabral cysts can be decompressed/removed arthroscopically, but if these are large they may need open surgery and deroofing.[24]

In general, the larger the extent of the injury causing instability, the more likely an open approach will be needed.

Volitional dislocators are not candidates for surgery to reestablish stability.

Normal postsurgical appearances Normal postsurgical appearances are summarized in **Box 8** (see **Fig. 8**).

MR arthrography is preferred to noncontrast MR imaging to study the labrum and capsule. Residual tear or recurrent tear is identified with up to 92% accuracy.[26]

On US, suture materials and anchors may be visible (especially if anchors are displaced).[27]

Abnormal postsurgical appearances/complications Abnormal postsurgical appearances and complications are summarized in **Table 5** and **Fig. 9**.

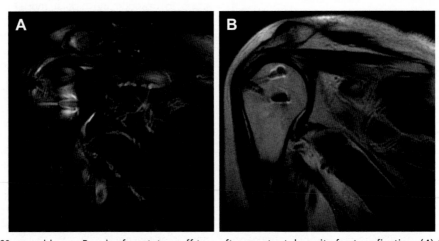

Fig. 7. A 60-year-old man. Repair of a rotator cuff tear after greater tuberosity fracture fixation. (*A*) Coronal T2 fat saturation shows artifact from fixation screws in the humeral head, and an anchor tunnel in the region of the greater tuberosity. Note the band of fluid overlying the tendon. (*B*) Coronal PDW shows less artifact. The rotator cuff shows normal postsurgical appearances, with slightly heterogeneous signal.

Box 5
Types of surgery to address glenohumeral instability

Direct	Indirect
Labral, ligamentous, or capsular injury is directly repaired More often performed (either arthroscopic or open approach)	Alteration of anatomy to aid without addressing the problem per se (eg, capsular tightening) Less frequently performed now (Putti-Platt procedure, Magnuson-Stack, Bristow)

Data from Jacobson JA, Miller B, Bedi A, et al. Imaging of the postoperative shoulder. Semin Musculoskelet Radiol 2011 Sep;15(4):320-39.

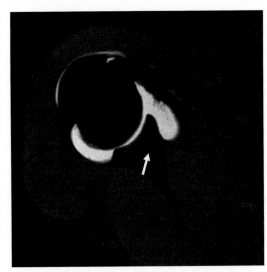

Fig. 8. MR arthrogram shows a glenoid anchor for anterior labrum repair (*white arrow*). These appearances are expected, with no fluid signal interposed between the labrum and glenoid, which would indicate detachment.

Rapid-onset chondrolysis is a severe complication that has been reported in young patients. The exact cause remains uncertain. It was first hypothesized as a response to thermal energy in capsulorrhaphy, but this has not been proved.[28] Some investigators suggest an immune response. Symptoms are pain and loss of range of motion during the first 3 to 12 months. MR imaging shows complete loss of the cartilage, with no reactive osteophyte formation and no synovitis (differential with osteoarthritis and infection respectively).

Shoulder arthroplasty

Shoulder arthroplasty is the technique of choice for patients with articular damage and pain who do not respond to other conservative or surgical measures.

It is also useful in cases of shoulder dysfunction and loss of motion that have become unacceptable to the patient as a result of osteonecrosis, osteoarthritis, trauma, or inflammatory arthritis.

Components are generally metal alloys and ultrahigh-molecular-weight polyethylene, with or without cement and screw fixation.

Indications Indications are summarized in **Table 6**.

Box 6
Indications for glenohumeral instability repair

- Anterior instability in young patients
- Repair of posterior or multidirectional instability tends to be performed after failure of rehabilitation program, with an inferior capsular shift
- If there are paralabral cysts causing nerve compression and denervation symptoms, surgery is indicated

Box 7
Steps of assessment of off-track and on-track lesions (computed tomography)

1	Measure, D, either by arthroscopy or from 3D CT scan
2	Determine, d
3	Calculate GT: GT = 0.83D − d
4	Calculate the width of the HSI, which is the width of the HS plus the width of the BB between the rotator cuff attachments and the lateral aspect of the HS HSI = HS + BB
5	HSI>GT, the HS is off-track or engaging HSI<GT, the HS is on-track or nonengaging

Abbreviations: BB, bone bridge; d, width of the anterior glenoid bone loss; D, diameter of the inferior glenoid; GT, width of the glenoid track; HS, Hill-Sachs lesion; HSI, Hill-Sachs interval.

Data from Di Giacomo G, Itoi E, Burkhart SS. Evolving concept of bipolar bone loss and the Hill-Sachs lesion: from "engaging/non-engaging" lesion to "on-track/off-track" lesion. Arthroscopy 2014;30(1):90-8.

Things to assess beforehand The selection of the optimal technique depends on the type of damage and the extent.

Integrity of the rotator cuff in cases in which total arthroplasty is considered determines whether a conventional (intact rotator cuff) or reverse (tear or deficiency of the cuff)[29] procedure is indicated.

Unsatisfactory postoperative performance is often caused by muscle deficit, so careful assessment of periscapular muscles, mainly the deltoid, is mandatory.

Reverse arthroplasties have a higher complication rate and are reserved for cases in which functional demands are lower.[19] The typical complication is anterior dislocation, seen in up to 20%.[30]

The only contraindication is active infection.

Normal postsurgical appearances Initial basic assessment is performed with radiographs.

- Anatomic alignment
- Presence of a fracture
- Hardware failure

A distance of less than 2 mm between the hardware and the bone is considered normal. If this is increased, assessment for stability is recommended.[31] There could be loosening, infection, or particle disease.

The prosthetic head should sit proud, at about 5 mm from the greater tuberosity. The prosthetic head base should parallel the humeral neck's cut surface with 35° or 45° of articular retroversion (arm in neutral at side or 90° elbow flexion).[31]

Alignment has to be carefully correlated clinically. Alignment is initially assessed with radiographs. MR imaging and MDCT with artifact reduction can assess abnormal alignment and version alteration, and give information on the status of articular surfaces or bone stock. Minor humeral head replacement migration relative to the glenoid may be normal, mainly caused by preoperative loss of other stabilizers.[31]

If there is concern after a rotator cuff tear, US is indicated, given the prosthetic material generates artifact on MR imaging. Immediately after surgery, the rotator cuff tendons may appear heterogeneous. The subscapularis tendon assessment may be challenging, and dynamic assessment is useful.[14]

Abnormal postsurgical appearances/complications Abnormal postsurgical appearances and complications are summarized in **Table 7** and **Fig. 10**.

CT or MR imaging assessment is recommended in the first instance if there is the suspicion of infection or particle disease. Aspiration may be necessary to further elucidate this.[14]

ELBOW
Surgical Options

Most surgical procedures in the elbow have the purpose of repairing bone and soft tissues. In cases of catastrophic trauma with extensive damage to bone structures or important osteoarthritis, elbow arthroplasty is considered.

Typical complications include malunion, nonunion, displacement, and infection.

Fixation of most common fractures
The main tool for assessment is radiographs, followed by CT. Whenever injury to vascular structures is suspected, techniques such as MR angiography, Doppler US, and arthrography are needed. In cases of suspicion of nerve injury, MR or US are useful.

Table 5
Abnormal postsurgical appearances/complications in glenohumeral instability repair

General postsurgical complications	Adhesive capsulitis, synovitis, infection (arthritis, osteomyelitis), chondrolysis, potential retention of foreign bodies, and bleeding
Recurrent labral tear	MRA preferred method of diagnosis, because of the presence of artifact, granulation tissue, and scarring
Capsular detachment	MR imaging/magnetic resonance: capsular attachment is more medial than a type 3
Loosening of the anchors	Better seen on radiographs or CT, but can also be picked on MR imaging, as abnormal signal surrounding the anchor If displaced, it can be found with any modality in the joint recesses
Nonunion, displacement, or infection of bone graft	Radiographs and CT (also MR imaging)
Inadequate paralabral cyst resection	Nerve compression: evident as atrophy and fatty infiltration of the muscle
Suprascapular nerve injury	Atrophy and fatty infiltration of the muscle
Failure to address occult instability in a different direction	Exacerbation of symptoms of the unmasked instability
Overtight repair	Degenerative change, or in instability in the opposite direction; possible in multidirectional instability
Detached staples, tacks, sutures	Early osteoarthritis
Rapid-onset chondrolysis	Young patients. The exact cause remains uncertain. Symptoms are pain and loss of range of motion during the first 3–12 mo MR imaging shows complete loss of the cartilage, with no reactive osteophyte formation and no synovitis (differential with OA and infection respectively)
Screw or other surgical devices protruding into the joint	Early osteoarthritis

Abbreviations: MRA, MR angiography; OA, osteoarthritis.

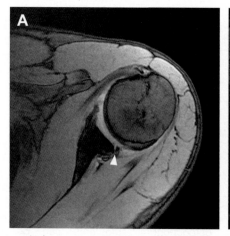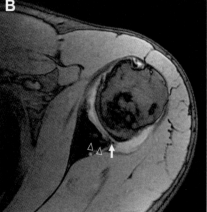

Fig. 9. Postsurgical assessment in a 49-year-old patient with recurrent symptoms after labral repair. Axial GRE T2* at 2 different levels. (*A*) At a more cranial level, a tear of the posterior labrum is evident as a hyperintense line (*white arrowhead*). (*B*) More caudally there is labral loss and marginal glenoid irregularity (*white arrow*). Note the anchors present in the glenoid (*arrowheads*); this was a repair of an extensive labral tear involving the labrum from 3 to 9 o'clock. There is joint effusion and narrowing of the articular space, with loss of cartilage thickness in both aspects. The posterior capsule appears distended, suggesting the possibility of a component of multidirectional instability, possibly resulting in labral retear/early osteoarthritis.

Table 6
Indications for arthroplasty

Arthroplasty		Indications	Potential Typical Complications
Total arthroplasty Disorder involves both articular aspects	Conventional Cemented humeral head or resurfacing component Cemented glenoid	Intact rotator cuff	Loosening
	Reverse Glenoid ball: humeral socket	Tear or deficiency of the rotator cuff	Loosening Anterior dislocation Acromion fracture
Hemiarthroplasty Disorder involves the humeral head	Replacement Stemless or Stemmed (cemented or press fit)	Rotator cuff arthropathy fractures Osteoarthritis Avascular necrosis	Glenohumeral osteoarthrosis (progressive joint space narrowing)
	Resurfacing Anatomy minimally distorted. Maintains soft tissue balancing.	Mild osteoarthritis avascular necrosis	Glenohumeral osteoarthrosis (progressive joint space narrowing)

Data from Refs.[29–31]

Indications Indications are summarized in **Table 8**.

Things to assess beforehand Displaced, comminuted, or open fractures or situations of nerve entrapment or vascular injury require open reduction and internal fixation.

Loose bodies and fragments should be described in number and location.

Radial head fractures can become displaced after reduction.[32]

When a radial head prosthesis is planned, it is important to assess for uniformity in width of the adjacent ulnohumeral joint, which is done through carefully selecting the size of the head so that there is no asymmetry between the medial and lateral aspects of the ulnohumeral joint, which could lead to osteoarthritis and ligament injury.[33]

Abnormal postsurgical appearances/complications Abnormal postsurgical appearances and complications are summarized in **Table 8**.

Normal postsurgical appearances
Distal humerus Near-anatomic alignment. A line drawn following the anterior aspect of the humerus should ideally intersect the capitellum at the junction of the anterior and middle thirds; however, slight displacement may be present.[34]

The elbow should maintain a slight valgus.

Radius The radial head should line up with the capitellum on anteroposterior (AP) and lateral views.[34]

If there is replacement, alignment of the prosthetic head has to be similar (**Fig. 11**).

Repair of osteochondral fractures
Valgus stress can result in osteochondral injury to the capitellum.

Nondisplaced, stable fragments are treated conservatively or with arthroscopic drilling.

Loose fragments can be removed or reattached. If the fragment is reattached to the bone, anatomic alignment is expected in imaging analysis.

Other techniques are also used, such as mosaicplasty, chondrocyte transplant, and allograft reconstruction.[35]

Osteochondral plugs and chondrocyte transplant need to be assessed with MR imaging. If satisfactory, the signal of the cartilage becomes normal over time. If there has been grafting, the fragment has to be incorporated into the normal contour of the subchondral bone. Loosening of osteochondral fragments can be seen as increased lucency with the parent bone on radiographs, but evaluation should be performed with MR imaging or MR/CT arthrogram. It may appear as a cleft on MR imaging or as a cleft filled with intraarticular contrast on MR angiography or CT arthrogram.

Table 7 Abnormal postsurgical appearances/ complications of shoulder arthroplasty	
General postsurgical complications	Adhesive capsulitis, synovitis, infection (arthritis, osteomyelitis), potential retention of foreign bodies, and bleeding
Loosening	Distance of more than 2 mm between hardware and bone (radiographs, CT, MR imaging)
Osteoarthrosis	More frequent in hemiarthroplasty
Dislocation	Generally traumatic Reverse total arthroplasty
Instability	
Superior	Rotator cuff dysfunction (most frequent)
Inferior	Improper humeral length restoration
Anterior	Anteversion of either component Deltoid laxity or deltoid temporary hypotonia
Posterior	Retroversion of either component
Infection	Radiographs are always performed but CT or MR assessment is recommended in the first instance Aspiration
Particle disease	CT or MR assessment is recommended in the first instance Aspiration

Total arthroplasty

Total arthroplasty is indicated in the case of nonunion, advanced osteoarthritis, or severely comminuted fractures.

There are 3 types of elbow arthroplasty, depending on the rigidity of fixation of the humeral component to the ulnar component[36] (**Table 9**).

Plain radiographs are the preferred method for the evaluation of arthroplasties.

The stem of the humeral and ulnar components has to be in the middle of the shafts. For semiconstrained arthroplasties, a line drawn through the anterior humeral cortex should bisect the area between the anterior flange and the posterior humeral cortex. On the lateral view, the ulnar component should start in line with the olecranon tip.

A potential complication with arthroplasty, as in other locations, is the possibility of periprosthetic fracture (**Fig. 12**).

Ligament reconstruction

Medial collateral ligament The medial collateral ligament MCL is the most important stabilizer against varus stress, especially the anterior bundle.

The most frequent type of injury, as previously mentioned, results from repetitive microtrauma with valgus stress, which is typical of overhead throwing athletes.

The first MCL reconstruction was performed in 1974, based on a figure-of-eight repair with a graft. Since then many modifications on the technique have been developed, most of them based on muscle splitting.[34]

After surgery the ligament appears hyperintense because of granulation tissue and suture material. Approximately 6 months postsurgery, signal

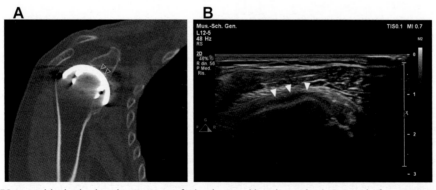

Fig. 10. A 56-year-old who had undergone resurfacing humeral head prosthesis 6 years before presents with pain and decreased range of movements. (*A*) CT coronal plane reconstruction shows marked narrowing of joint space (*arrowheads*) with advanced degenerative change in the glenoid, which is a typical complication of this type of repair. (*B*) On US, a complete tear of the supraspinatus tendon with a sliver of interposed fluid was noted (*white arrowheads*).

Table 8
Types of surgical treatment and complications

	Fractures for Surgery		Treatment	Complications
Distal humerus	Supracondylar		Percutaneous pins in children, plates and screws in adults	• Varus deformity. Cubitus varus may result in lateral fracture with throwing sports, and needs to be corrected with an osteotomy • Nerve injuries can occur in the context of reduction or placement of pins • Posterolateral displacement can result in medial nerve and brachial artery injury • Posteromedial displacement is associated with radial nerve injury • Volkmann ischemic contracture can happen if the brachial artery has been injured
Radius	Type II or III		ORIF Resection fragments	• General • Injury to the radial or ulnar nerve and their branches • Radial head may migrate proximally, and subluxate asymptomatically, with subsequent development of osteoarthritis
	Type III or IV		Radial head prosthesis	• Loosening • Proximal migration • Subluxation • Dislocation • Fracture • Osteoarthritis and capitellar erosion
Ulna	Coronoid	Type II or III	ORIF (compression screw)	• General
	Olecranon	Displaced	Tension band and Kirschner wires ORIF and dorsal plate and screws	• General • Olecranon bursitis

General complications include malunion, nonunion, displacement, and infection.
Abbreviation: ORIF, open reduction and internal fixation.
Data from Bazzocchi A, Aparisi Gómez MP, Bartoloni A, et al. Emergency and Trauma of the Elbow. Semin Musculoskelet Radiol. 2017 Jul;21(3):257–81.

intensity decreases on all sequences, with possible thickening of the ligament. In some cases, mild hyperintensity remains in the proximal aspect of the ligament, but this is not pathologic. Tunneling defects can be seen in the humerus and ulna.

Sometimes in the ulna the tunnel is distal to the sublime tubercle.

Techniques such as US, MR imaging, and MR arthrography are the best ones to assess the reconstructed ligament.

The presence of discontinuity, laxity, thinning, and irregularity in any of the mentioned techniques indicates injury to the reconstructed ligament. Avulsion fractures of the medial epicondyle are rare complications.[37]

Stress radiographs and CT arthrography can also be used, but they may be normal in the presence of a rupture unless there is abnormal valgus angulation of dislodgement of the metal anchors and screws, if they are present.

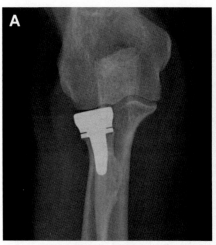 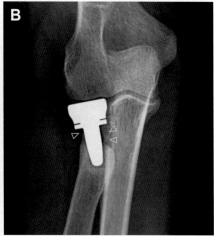

Fig. 11. A 58-year-old woman with radial arthroplasty. (*A*) Early radiograph shows expected appearance of the radial head prosthesis, correctly aligned with the radius. There is no lucency around the stem. (*B*) Eighteen months later, radiograph shows marked resorption of radial neck around the prosthetic stem (*arrowheads*).

Table 9
Types of elbow arthroplasty

Type of Arthroplasty	Characteristics
Fully constrained (performed in the past)	• Cemented • Metal-to-metal hinge type • Not frequently used because of high rate of complication with loosening and periprosthetic fracture
Unconstrained (unlinked)	• 2 parts, consisting of metal to high-density polyethylene resurfacing components, with the parts unlocked (replicate normal surfaces) • Require intact ligaments • Have the lowest incidence of loosening but can dislocate
Semiconstrained (linked)	• 2 or 3 parts, consisting of metal to high-density polyethylene connected by a locking pin • Have the advantage of a certain valgus and varus laxity, which helps to dissipate forces • Lowest rate of complications (only 10%) compared with the other types • Most commonly used

Data from Bertolini M, Giacalone F, Pontini I. Elbow Arthroplasty. In: Albanese CV, Faletti C, eds. Imaging of the Prosthetic Joints: A Combined radiological and Clinical Perspective. Milano: Springer Milan; 2014: 135–48.

The ulnar nerve may have been surgically transposed from the cubital tunnel into a subcutaneous or submuscular location. It is important to assess for signs of neuropathy.

Other possible postoperative potential complications are excessive scarring or fibrosis, heterotopic bone formation, and infection.

Lateral collateral ligament The presence of symptomatic posterolateral rotatory instability is an indication for surgical repair of the lateral collateral ligament (LCL).

Acute ligament repair is only recommended when there is marked instability after reduction of the elbow or in open reduction after fracture dislocations, especially when there has been internal fixation of the radial head or the coronoid process.[38]

The LCL can be primarily reconstructed or grafted (**Fig. 13**).

The presence of discontinuity, laxity, thinning, and irregularity may indicate injury to the reconstructed ligament. Recurrent dislocation can occur.

Other possible postoperative potential complications are excessive scarring or fibrosis, heterotopic ossification, and infection[38] (**Fig. 14**).

Epicondylitis

Most cases are treated conservatively (physical therapy, antiinflamatories, icing, bracing) with a 90% success rate. Percutaneous treatment with corticosteroid injection can be indicated if pain persists for 3 months. Other techniques, such as prolotherapy, dry needling, and platelet-rich plasma injection, can also be attempted. If symptoms do not improve after 6 months, surgery is considered.

On the lateral aspect, the usual technique is debridement of the extensor carpi radialis brevis (ECRB), with decortication of the lateral

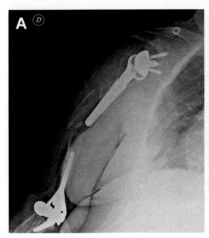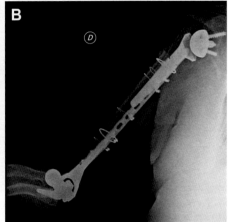

Fig. 12. A 74-year-old woman with reverse shoulder arthroplasty and total elbow arthroplasty, for severe post-traumatic osteoarthritis. The patient had a fall. (*A*) Comminuted humeral-periprosthetic fracture of the humerus is evident. The distal humeral component of the elbow total arthroplasty shows no signs of loosening. (*B*) The fracture was repaired with bone grafting and a plate.

epicondyle, performed through an open approach (Nirschl procedure) or arthroscopically, with comparable results.[39] In some cases, reinforcement with an anconeus flap is also performed, improving outcomes.[40] Percutaneous tenotomy is performed under US guidance, with very good results at follow-up.[41]

On the medial aspect, the use of surgery is much less common, and less successful in general, given the association with ulnar nerve disorder. Patients generally respond to conservative treatment and injection. Most surgical techniques consist of the release of the flexor origin and excision of diseased tissue. A new technique consists of fascial elevation and tendon origin resection, with an 80% rate of success.[42]

Things to assess beforehand The most commonly involved tendons are the ECRB, in the lateral aspect, and the flexor carpi radialis and pronator teres medially. Lateral epicondylitis may be associated with underlying ligament disorder and instability, and posterior interosseous nerve compression.

Medial epicondylitis is frequently associated with ulnar neuropathy (up to 50% of cases).[43]

Normal postsurgical appearances Postoperative assessment is better performed with MR imaging. The signal intensity of the tendon may remain altered for some time after surgery, with progressive evolution to low signal and thickening.[44]

It is important to mention that recently injected tendons show increased signal intensity.

Abnormal postsurgical appearances/complications Lateral epicondylitis may be associated with underlying ligament disorder, and this has to be

carefully looked for in cases of persistent pain after surgery.

Potential complications of medial epicondylitis surgery are persistent nerve symptoms. US shows a thickened, hypoechoic ulnar nerve. MR imaging shows abnormal signal intensity and thickening.

Incomplete resection of the pathologic tissue has an appearance similar to tendinosis or a tendon tear. Fibrosis or excessive scarring, and formation of an adventitious bursa, can occur.

Distal biceps repair
Surgery is the preferred treatment in the case of rupture of the biceps tendon. Full-thickness tears of single or bifid tendons are more commonly treated surgically than partial tears.[45]

Normally, the tendon is reattached to the radial tuberosity with suture anchors. In chronic cases attachment to the brachialis muscle can be performed. In some cases of delayed diagnosis and scarring of the muscle, an allograft can be placed.

Postsurgical evaluation is performed with MR imaging (ABER [abduction and external rotation] position), although US can also be useful. The tendon usually shows intermediate signal intensity and appears thickened.[46]

Complications include rerupture and suture or anchor rupture.

There is the possibility of nerve damage, involving median, radial, and posterior interosseus nerves and heterotopic ossification, which is best seen on radiographs or CT.

Triceps repair
Partial tears can be treated conservatively. Full-thickness tears are treated with reattachment to

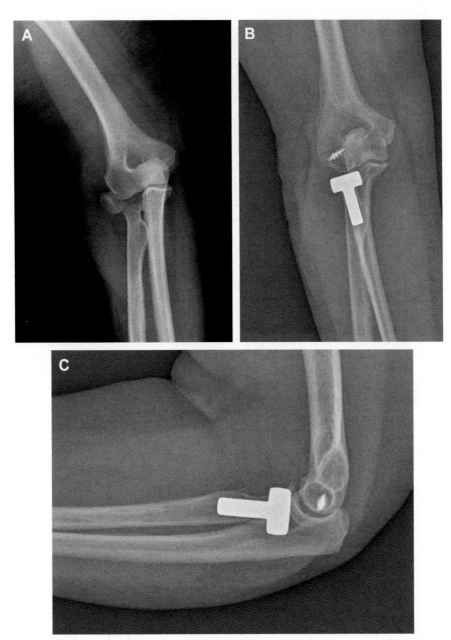

Fig. 13. A 64-year-old woman. (*A*) AP radiograph shows a displaced fracture of the radial head. The fracture was treated with a radial head arthroplasty and LCL repair. (*B*) AP and (*C*) lateral radiographs show normal expected postsurgical appearances of the humeral head prosthesis and lateral humeral anchor of the repaired LCL.

the ulna with drill holes, and on some occasions (chronic cases) grafts are used. If there is a large avulsion fragment, this is reattached with a screw.

Postsurgical evaluation is performed with MR imaging or US. The tendon usually shows intermediate signal intensity and appears thick in immediate postsurgical status. Signal intensity decreases progressively within a year.[33]

Complications include rerupture and olecranon bursitis.

There is the possibility of ulnar nerve damage and heterotopic ossification.

Olecranon bursa resection

Most bursitis is treated with aspiration and corticosteroid injections.

Bursectomy is performed if this treatment fails, through an open or endoscopic approach. The endoscopic approach has good outcomes with minimal complications.[47]

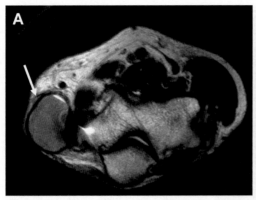
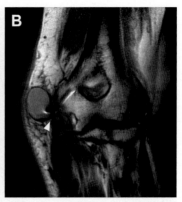

Fig. 14. A 68-year-old man. LCL repair 10 years ago. Progressive pain with swelling in the lateral aspect of the elbow. (A) Axial T2-weighted image shows susceptibility artifact from anchor in the region of the lateral epicondyle. Associated with this, there is a fluid-filled structure within the lateral soft tissues, with thick walls (*white arrow*). (B) Coronal T1-weighted image shows fluid content to be high in signal, and a small tail connecting the fluid-filled structure with the location of the anchor (*white arrowhead*). Surgical drainage/excision showed inflammatory changes with development of particle disease.

Focal scarring and absence of fluid are normal in postoperative imaging.

Poor wound healing, excessive deep scarring, synoviocutaneous fistula, and tears of the biceps are described complications.

WRIST
Surgical Options

This article focuses on distal forearm fractures, carpal tunnel intervention, and fractures of the scaphoid and trapezometacarpal joint.

Fixation of most common forearm fractures at the wrist

Fixation of most common forearm fractures at the wrist are summarized in **Table 10**.

Normal postsurgical appearances Radiographs are the first tool for assessment.

Anatomic alignment must be achieved, with no significant displacement.

On lateral view, the radius has a neutral or volar tilt. On posteroanterior view, the radius may have an ulnar inclination of approximately 15°. Articular surfaces must be regular, and if there are step-offs these must not surpass 2 mm. Ulnar variance should be neutral.

Bone grafting is sometimes used and this should not be mistaken for fragments. Ulnar styloid fractures may require treatment depending on the type of fracture - involved structures.[48]

Abnormal postsurgical appearances/complications Evaluation is normally performed with radiographs and CT. Eventually MR imaging will be

useful for the study of soft tissues. MR arthrograms are useful for the study of triangular fibrocartilage complex and carpal ligaments (see **Table 10**).

The wrist is the most common site in the body for fracture malunion (up to 5%).[48]

Carpal tunnel syndrome

Carpal tunnel syndrome (CTS) is the most common nerve entrapment syndrome in the upper limb. Causes are repetitive or acute trauma, infection, variants, infiltrative disorder, mass lesions, or a combination of these.

Treatments of some causes are splinting, medication, injections, and avoidance of activities.

Masses (ganglia, tumors) need resection.

Patients that do not improve with conservative management or meet electrophysiologic test criteria for severity go to surgery.[49]

Surgery can be performed through an open approach or endoscopically, and consists of decompression with section of the carpal transverse ligament, release of the flexor retinaculum with division on the ulnar side, and occasionally epineurotomy.

Normal postsurgical appearances Assessment is performed with US and MR imaging. Normal postsurgical appearances are sometimes difficult to discern from persistent pathologic changes.

Volume is usually increased, with volar convexity and displacement of contents. The transverse ligament shows a discontinuity where a segment has been resected.[50]

The fat plane at the floor of the carpal tunnel, dorsal to the flexor digitorum profundus, is another usual finding.

Table 10
Indications for fixation of wrist fractures

Indication for Surgical Fixation in Distal Forearm Fractures		Complications
• Unstable lesion	Closed reduction external fixation	• Malunion: most common site in the body (up to 5%)
• Severe comminution	ORIF	• Nonunion
• Intraarticular fractures with more than 2 mm of articular surface step-off (risk of osteoarthritis)		• Nerve retraction
		• Unstable internal fixation
		• Extension of screws into articular surface
• Barton (dorsal lip of the radius with carpal subluxation)		• Loss of reduction or fixation
• Reverse Barton (volar lip of the radius with carpal subluxation)		• Infection
		• Peritendinous adhesions
• Radial styloid fractures (buttress plate fixation)		• Ulnocarpal impaction syndrome: resulting from nonsatisfactory reduction of radial fracture with shortening and positive ulnar variance
• Compression fractures of the radial articular surface		• TFCC injury: resulting from nonsatisfactory reduction of radial fracture with shortening and positive ulnar variance
• Rotated fragments		
• Significantly displaced fragments		• Other ligamentous injuries (proximal row intrinsic ligaments, extrinsic carpal ligaments)

Abbreviation: TFCC, triangular fibrocartilage complex.
Data from Steinbach L, Chung C. Postoperative elbow, wrist and hand. In: Pope TL, Bloem HL, Beltran J, Morrison WB, Wilson DJ, eds. Imaging of the Musculoskeletal System, 2nd edition. Philadelphia: Saunders Elsevier; 2015: 1136–1161.

Normally there is improvement in signal and size of the median nerve (not complete). On US, significant increase in volume at the level of pisiform-hamate, as well as increase in volume of the carpal tunnel at this level, has been reported.[51]

On MR imaging, the signal and volume of the medial nerve normalizes. A study found that the best predictor of recurrence of CTS was enlargement of the median nerve at the level of the pisiform, with persistent tenosynovitis also a good indicator.[52]

Abnormal postsurgical appearances/complications Abnormal postsurgical appearances and complications are summarized in **Box 9**.

Scaphoid fracture

Scaphoid fractures are the most common carpal bone fractures and result from falling onto an outstretched hand. They may easily be missed in the early imaging assessment.

The waist is the most common location, followed by the proximal and distal poles.

Vascular supply to the scaphoid runs from proximal to distal, and this makes proximal fracture fragments more prone to necrosis.

Indications for surgery are summarized in **Box 10**.

Surgery can be performed through open procedures or arthroscopy. Surgical procedures include closed reduction with percutaneous pinning or compression screw and open reduction

---

Box 9
Abnormal postsurgical appearances/complications after carpal tunnel release

- Incomplete release: more frequent with endoscopic procedure (MR imaging/US: transverse ligament remains continuous between the pisiform and hook of the hamate)

- Reconstitution with inflammation and scarring (MR imaging/US: scarring, fibrosis, granulation tissue)

- Laceration of the nerve (potentially with formation of a neuroma)

- Ulnar artery laceration

- Fracture of the hook of the hamate.

Data from Beck JD, Jones RB, Malone WJ, et al. Magnetic resonance imaging after endoscopic carpal tunnel release. J Hand Surg Am 2013;38(2):331–5.

Box 10
Indications for fixation of scaphoid fracture

- Fracture of the proximal pole
- Comminution
- Displacement of more than 1 mm
- Scapholunate angle of more than 60° (normal, 30°–60°)
- Radiolunate or capitolunate angle of more than 15° (normal, −15° to +15°)
- Delayed presentation
- Evidence of nonunion or necrosis
- Occupational requirement (use of long casting not possible)

---

with Kirschner wires or compression screw[53] or staple[54] (**Fig. 15**). Comminution and nonunion may require bone grafting.

Other salvage procedures for nonunions are radial styloidectomy, excision of the proximal fragment, carpectomy of the proximal row, and total or partial arthrodesis of the wrist.

Normal postsurgical appearances Assessment begins with radiographs. Fragments should be reduced, and normally aligned. Hardware traverses the fracture line. Fractures should be consolidated in 20 weeks.

CT is optimal for spatial resolution, and useful to assess potential malunion and other complications. At present, MR imaging is used as a screening tool in most situations of negative radiographs and clinical suspicion, given its sensitivity to detect bone contusion and soft tissue–related causes for pain.[55]

US has also been proved useful in expert hands.

Abnormal postsurgical appearances/complications Abnormal postsurgical appearances and complications are summarized in **Table 11** and **Fig. 16**.

Recent studies have shown that dynamic contrast-enhanced MR imaging does not add additional predictive value to standard delayed contrast-enhanced MR imaging for the assessment of viability of the proximal fragment.[56,57]

Surgical treatment of trapezometacarpal joint osteoarthritis

Trapezometacarpal joint osteoarthritis can be treated with partial trapeziectomy, with resection arthroplasty, ligament reconstruction, and tendon interposition with flexor carpi radialis tendon.

The techniques provide pain relief (**Fig. 17**). Complications are typical of surgical procedures, with none specifically associated with the use of the tendon.[58]

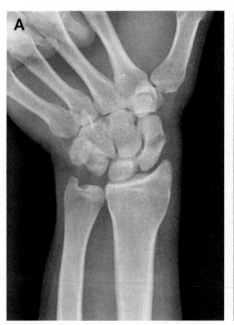
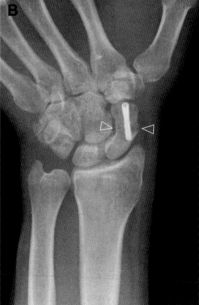

Fig. 15. A 44-year-old man, delayed presentation after fall on outstretched hand 3.5 weeks before. (*A*) Scaphoid view shows a fracture of the waist of the scaphoid, with a region of lucency around the fracture line. (*B*) The fracture was repaired with a screw. Postsurgical radiograph shows correct placement of a screw, with satisfactory progressive fracture healing (*arrowheads*).

Table 11
Abnormal postsurgical appearances/complications in fixation of scaphoid fracture

Complications of Scaphoid Fracture Treatment	Imaging	Treatment
Nonunion: • Complication of conservative or postsurgical repair • Potential evolution to scaphoid nonunion advanced collapse	X-Ray/CT • Sclerosis • Bone cysts	Grafting Styloidectomy Excision of the proximal fragment Carpectomy of the proximal row Total or partial arthrodesis of the wrist
Malunion: • Dorsal angulation (humpback deformity) • Dorsal intercalated segment instability	X-Ray/CT • Deformity	Osteotomy
Avascular necrosis: Can result with or without nonunion Usually proximal	CT • Sclerosis is not specific MR imaging • Low T1 and T2 likely MR imaging + Gd • Enhancement is not specific for viability	Grafting Salvage proximal fragment: Styloidectomy Excision of the proximal fragment Carpectomy of the proximal row Total or partial arthrodesis of the wrist

Abbreviations: Gd, gadolinium; TFCC, triangular fibrocartilage complex.

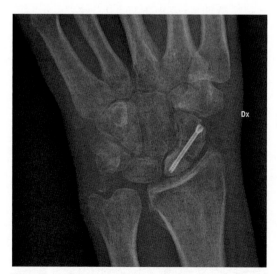

Fig. 16. A 27-year-old man. Follow-up dedicated scaphoid view radiograph shows persistence of a lucent line in the waist of the scaphoid, months after fixation. Note the generalized osteopenia caused by prolonged immobilization, and the presence of an os styloideum.

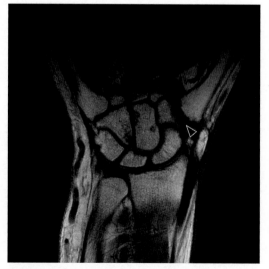

Fig. 17. A 57-year-old woman, treated with trapeziectomy because of severe osteoarthritis and pain. Coronal T1-weighted MR image shows the expected appearance after trapezium bone resection. The base of the metacarpal now articulates with the trapezoid (*arrowhead*). Results were satisfactory for pain palliation.

SUMMARY

This article reviews the most common surgical procedures performed in the shoulder, elbow, and wrist, with their expected postsurgical appearances and potential complications. The correct understanding of the different types of surgical management helps to identify normal postsurgical appearances and recognize potential complications.

ACKNOWLEDGMENTS

The authors would like to kindly thank Dr Francisco Aparisi from Valencia for his help in preparing the figures.

REFERENCES

1. Morse K, Davis AD, Afra R, et al. Arthroscopic versus mini-open rotator cuff repair: a comprehensive review and meta-analysis. Am J Sports Med 2008;36(9):1824–8.
2. Mohtadi NG, Hollinshead RM, Sasyniuk TM, et al. A randomized clinical trial comparing open to arthroscopic acromioplasty with mini-open rotator cuff repair for full-thickness rotator cuff tears: disease-specific quality of life outcome at an average 2-year follow-up. Am J Sports Med 2008;36(6): 1043–51.
3. Mohana-Borges AV, Chung CB, Resnick D. MR imaging and MR arthrography of the postoperative shoulder: spectrum of normal and abnormal findings. Radiographics 2004;24(1):69–85.
4. Cameron BD, Iannotti JP. Clinical evaluation of the painful shoulder. In: Zhatkin MB, editor. MRI of the shoulder. Philadelphia: Lippincott Williams & Wilkins; 2003. p. 47–84.
5. Kvitne RS, Jobe FW, Jobe CM. Shoulder instability in the overhand or throwing athlete. Clin Sports Med 1995;14(4):917–35.
6. Magee TH, Gaenslen ES, Seitz R, et al. MR imaging of the shoulder after surgery. AJR Am J Roentgenol 1997;168(4):925–8.
7. Woertler K. Multimodality imaging of the postoperative shoulder. Eur Radiol 2007;17(12):3038–55.
8. Corazza A, Orlandi D, Fabbro E, et al. Dynamic high-resolution ultrasound of the shoulder: how we do it. Eur J Radiol 2015;84(2):266–77.
9. Morag Y, Jacobson JA, Miller B, et al. MR imaging of rotator cuff injury: what the clinician needs to know. Radiographics 2006;26(4):1045–65.
10. Burkhart SS. Shoulder arthroscopy. New concepts. Clin Sports Med 1996;15(4):635–53.
11. Gilat R, Atoun E, Cohen O, et al. Recurrent rotator cuff tear: is ultrasound imaging reliable? J Shoulder Elbow Surg 2018;27(7):1263–7.
12. Bianchi S, Martinoli C. Shoulder. In: Bianchi S, Martinoli C, editors. Ultrasound of the musculoskeletal system. Berlin: Springer; 2007. p. 189–333.
13. Duc SR, Mengiardi B, Pfirrmann CW, et al. Diagnostic performance of MR arthrography after rotator cuff repair. AJR Am J Roentgenol 2006;186(1): 237–41.
14. Jacobson JA, Miller B, Bedi A, et al. Imaging of the postoperative shoulder. Semin Musculoskelet Radiol 2011;15(4):320–39.
15. Burkhart SS, De Beer JF. Traumatic glenohumeral bone defects and their relationship to failure of arthroscopic Bankart repairs: significance of the inverted-pear glenoid and the humeral engaging Hill-Sachs lesion. Arthroscopy 2000;16(7):677–94.
16. Larribe M, Laurent PE, Acid S, et al. Anterior shoulder instability: the role of advanced shoulder imaging in preoperative planning. Semin Musculoskelet Radiol 2014;18(4):398–403.
17. Gyftopoulos S, Hasan S, Bencardino J, et al. Diagnostic accuracy of MRI in the measurement of glenoid bone loss. AJR Am J Roentgenol 2012;199: 873–8.
18. Huysmans PE, Haen PS, Kidd M, et al. The shape of the inferior part of the glenoid: a cadaveric study. J Shoulder Elbow Surg 2006;15(6):759–63.
19. Dzirkale A, Paruchuri NB, Zlatkin MB. Postoperative shoulder. In: Pope TL, Bloem HL, Beltran J, et al, editors. Imaging of the musculoskeletal system. 2nd edition. Philadelphia: Saunders Elsevier; 2015. p. 1123–35.
20. Gyftopoulos S, Yemin A, Beltran L, et al. Engaging Hill-Sachs lesion: is there an association between this lesion and findings on MRI? AJR Am J Roentgenol 2013;201(4):W633–8.
21. Yamamoto N, Itoi E, Abe H, et al. Contact between the glenoid and the humeral head in abduction, external rotation, and horizontal extension: a new concept of glenoid track. J Shoulder Elbow Surg 2007;16(5):649–56.
22. Di Giacomo G, Itoi E, Burkhart SS. Evolving concept of bipolar bone loss and the Hill-Sachs lesion: from "engaging/non-engaging" lesion to "on-track/off-track" lesion. Arthroscopy 2014;30(1):90–8.
23. Lynch JR, Clinton JM, Dewing CB, et al. Treatment of osseous defects associated with anterior shoulder instability. J Shoulder Elbow Surg 2009;18(2): 317–28.
24. Keener JD, Brophy RH. Superior labral tears of the shoulder: pathogenesis, evaluation, and treatment. J Am Acad Orthop Surg 2009;17(10):627–37.
25. Harper KW, Helms CA, Haystead CM, et al. Glenoid dysplasia: incidence and association with posterior labral tears as evaluated on MRI. AJR Am J Roentgenol 2005;184(3):984–8.
26. Probyn LJ, White LM, Salonen DC, et al. Recurrent symptoms after shoulder instability repair: direct

MR arthrographic assessment-correlation with second-look surgical evaluation. Radiology 2007; 245(3):814–23.

27. Major NM, Banks MC. MR imaging of complications of loose surgical tacks in the shoulder. AJR Am J Roentgenol 2003;180(2):377–80.

28. Levine WN, Clark AM Jr, D'Alessandro DF, et al. Chondrolysis following arthroscopic thermal capsulorrhaphy to treat shoulder instability. A report of two cases. J Bone Joint Surg Am 2005;87(3): 616–21.

29. Ricchetti ET, Abboud JA, Kuntz AF, et al. Total shoulder arthroplasty in older patients: increased perioperative morbidity? Clin Orthop Relat Res 2011; 469(4):1042–9.

30. Roberts CC, Ekelund AL, Renfree KJ, et al. Radiologic assessment of reverse shoulder arthroplasty. Radiographics 2007;27(1):223–35.

31. Feldman F. Radiology of shoulder prostheses. Semin Musculoskelet Radiol 2006;10(1):5–21.

32. Rosas HG, Lee KS. Imaging acute trauma of the elbow. Semin Musculoskelet Radiol 2010;14: 394–411.

33. Bazzocchi A, Aparisi Gómez MP, Bartoloni A, et al. Emergency and trauma of the elbow. Semin Musculoskelet Radiol 2017;21(3):257–81.

34. Crosby NE, Greenberg JA. Radiographic evaluation of the elbow. J Hand Surg Am 2014;39(7):1408–14.

35. Iwasaki N, Kato H, Ishikawa J, et al. Autologous osteochondral mosaicplasty for osteochondritis dissecans of the elbow in teenage athletes: surgical technique. J Bone Joint Surg Am 2010;92(Suppl 1 Pt 2):208–16.

36. Bertolini M, Giacalone F, Pontini I. Elbow Arthroplasty. In: Albanese CV, Faletti C, editors. Imaging of the prosthetic joints: a combined radiological and clinical perspective. Milano (Italy): Springer Milan; 2014. p. 135–48.

37. Kaplan LJ, Potter HG. MR imaging of ligament injuries to the elbow. Magn Reson Imaging Clin N Am 2004;12(2):221–32. v-vi.

38. Olsen BS, Søjbjerg JO. The treatment of recurrent posterolateral instability of the elbow. J Bone Joint Surg Br 2003;85(3):342–6.

39. Kwon BC, Kim JY, Park KT. The Nirschl procedure versus arthroscopic extensor carpi radialis brevis débridement for lateral epicondylitis. J Shoulder Elbow Surg 2017;26(1):118–24.

40. Ruch DS, Orr SB, Richard MJ, et al. A comparison of débridement with and without anconeus muscle flap for treatment of refractory lateral epicondylitis. J Shoulder Elbow Surg 2015;24(2):236–41.

41. Seng C, Mohan PC, Koh SB, et al. Ultrasonic percutaneous tenotomy for recalcitrant lateral elbow tendinopathy: sustainability and sonographic progression at 3 years. Am J Sports Med 2016;44(2): 504–10.

42. Kwon BC, Kwon YS, Bae KJ. The fascial elevation and tendon origin resection technique for the treatment of chronic recalcitrant medial epicondylitis. Am J Sports Med 2014;42(7):1731–7.

43. Gabel GT, Morrey BF. Operative treatment of medial epicondylitis. Influence of concomitant ulnar neuropathy at the elbow. J Bone Joint Surg Am 1995;77(7): 1065–9.

44. Steinbach L, Chung C. Postoperative elbow, wrist and hand. In: Pope TL, editor. Imaging of the musculoskeletal system. 2nd edition. Philadelphia: Saunders Elsevier; 2015. p. 1136–61.

45. Hayter CL, Giuffre BM. Overuse and traumatic injuries of the elbow. Magn Reson Imaging Clin N Am 2009;17:617–38.

46. Giuffrè BM, Moss MJ. Optimal positioning for MRI of the distal biceps brachii tendon: flexed abducted supinated view. AJR Am J Roentgenol 2004; 182(4):944–6.

47. Rhyou IH, Park KJ, Kim KC, et al. Endoscopic olecranon bursal resection for olecranon bursitis: a comparative study for septic and aseptic olecranon bursitis. J Hand Surg Asian Pac Vol 2016;21(2): 167–72.

48. Herrera M, Chapman CB, Roh M, et al. Treatment of unstable distal radius fractures with cancellous allograft and external fixation. J Hand Surg Am 1999; 24(6):1269–78.

49. Fernández-de-Las-Peñas C, Cleland J, Palacios-Ceña M, et al. The effectiveness of manual therapy versus surgery on self-reported function, cervical range of motion, and pinch grip force in carpal tunnel syndrome: a randomized clinical trial. J Orthop Sports Phys Ther 2017;47(3):151–61.

50. Beck JD, Jones RB, Malone WJ, et al. Magnetic resonance imaging after endoscopic carpal tunnel release. J Hand Surg Am 2013;38(2):331–5.

51. Lee CH, Kim TK, Yoon ES, et al. Postoperative morphologic analysis of carpal tunnel syndrome using high-resolution ultrasonography. Ann Plast Surg 2005;54(2):143–6.

52. Wu HT, Schweitzer ME, Culp RW. Potential MR signs of recurrent carpal tunnel syndrome: initial experience. J Comput Assist Tomogr 2004;28(6): 860–4.

53. Dias JJ, Dhukaram V, Abhinav A, et al. Clinical and radiological outcome of cast immobilisation versus surgical treatment of acute scaphoid fractures at a mean follow-up of 93 months. J Bone Joint Surg Br 2008;90(7):899–905.

54. Dunn J, Kusnezov N, Fares A, et al. The scaphoid staple: a systematic review. Hand (N Y) 2017; 12(3):236–41.

55. Bergh TH, Lindau T, Soldal LA, et al. Clinical scaphoid score (CSS) to identify scaphoid fracture with MRI in patients with normal x-ray after a wrist trauma. Emerg Med J 2014;31(8):659–64.

56. Cerezal L, Abascal F, Canga A, et al. Usefulness of gadolinium-enhanced MR imaging in the evaluation of the vascularity of scaphoid nonunions. AJR Am J Roentgenol 2000;174(1):141–9.

57. Larribe M, Gay A, Freire V, et al. Usefulness of dynamic contrast-enhanced MRI in the evaluation of the viability of acute scaphoid fracture. Skeletal Radiol 2014;43(12):1697–703.

58. Varitimidis SE, Fox RJ, King JA, et al. Trapeziometacarpal arthroplasty using the entire flexor carpi radialis tendon. Clin Orthop Relat Res 2000;(370): 164–70.

Imaging of Common Rheumatic Joint Diseases Affecting the Upper Limbs

Mikael Boesen, MD, PhD[a,b,c], Frank W. Roemer, MD, PhD[d,e],
Mikkel Østergaard, MD, PhD, DMSc[c,f], Mario Maas, MD, PhD[g],
Lene Terslev, MD, PhD[f], Ali Guermazi, MD, PhD[d,*]

KEYWORDS

- Imaging • Rheumatology • Conventional radiography • CT • MR imaging • Ultrasound
- Osteoarthritis • Rheumatoid arthritis

KEY POINTS

- Imaging plays an important role in diagnosis and monitoring of rheumatic diseases of the upper limb.
- Many rheumatic diseases present with similar clinical pictures, especially in the early stages.
- Imaging findings in inflammatory and degenerative joint diseases often are nonspecific, especially in the early stages.
- Imaging findings should be interpreted in light of the clinical context—clinical and paraclinical findings.
- Good referrals with short clinical history, main clinical findings, disease-involved joint(s), pain distribution, and relevant blood tests increase the likelihood of a correct diagnosis.

INTRODUCTION

Imaging plays an important role in diagnosis and monitoring of rheumatic diseases affecting the upper limb and can be used to distinguish normal tissue from disease changes. Many rheumatic diseases show upper limb involvement. This article focuses on the most common arthritic conditions: osteoarthritis (OA), rheumatoid arthritis (RA), psoriatic arthritis (PsA), gout (arthritis urica), calcium pyrophosphate deposition disease (CPPD), and hydroxyapatite deposition disease (HADD) affecting the hand, elbow, and shoulder.

Uniform for all rheumatic joint conditions is the presence of 1 or more painful and swollen joints leading eventually and, if untreated, to disability and decreased function. Because many conditions may present with a similar clinical picture, the differential diagnosis based on clinical and imaging findings may be challenging. The anatomic joint distribution of the disease and some specific imaging features as observed on conventional radiography (CR), MR imaging, CT, or ultrasound (US), together with clinical and serologic findings, may help establish a definite diagnosis and inform disease severity (**Table 1**). Nuclear medicine

Disclosures: See last page of article.
[a] Department of Radiology, Bispebjerg and Frederiksberg Hospital, Copenhagen University, Bispebjerg Bakke 23, 2400 Copenhagen N, Denmark; [b] Parker Institute, Bispebjerg and Frederiksberg Hospital, Copenhagen University, Bispebjerg Bakke 23, 2400 Copenhagen N, Denmark; [c] Department of Clinical Medicine, University of Copenhagen, Bispebjerg Bakke 23, 2400 Copenhagen N, Denmark; [d] Department of Radiology, Boston University School of Medicine, 820 Harrison Avenue, FGH Building, 3rd Floor, Boston, MA 02118, USA; [e] Department of Radiology, Friedrich-Alexander University Erlangen-Nürnberg (FAU) and Universitätsklinikum Erlangen, Maximiliansplatz 3, 91054 Erlangen, Germany; [f] Department of Rheumatology, Rigshospitalet Glostrup, Copenhagen University, Nordre Ringvej 57, 2600 Glostrup, Denmark; [g] Department of Radiology, AMC Hospital, Meibergdreef 9, 1105 AZ Amsterdam, the Netherlands
* Corresponding author.
E-mail address: Ali.Guermazi@bmc.org

Radiol Clin N Am 57 (2019) 1001–1034
https://doi.org/10.1016/j.rcl.2019.03.007

Table 1
Imaging features and distribution of various joint arthritides of the upper extremity

	Osteoarthritis	Rheumatoid Arthritis	Psoriatic Arthritis	Gout	Calcium Pyrophosphate Deposition Disease	Hydroxyapatite Deposition Disease
Joint affections	Asymmetric affections of DIP, PIP, CMC1, and STT joints Primary OA in the elbow and shoulder is rare and usually a consequence of underlying arthritis or trauma.	Symmetric affection of MCP and wrist joints Less frequently the shoulder, even less in the elbow	Asymmetric DIP and PIP joints Less frequently the wrist, shoulder, elbow, in decreasing order. Enthesitis and tenosynovitis are frequent. Can precede skin psoriasis	Asymmetric affection of various finger and wrist joints, extra-articular tophi, and erosions Less frequently the elbow and shoulder	Asymmetric affection of MCP and first RC row in the wrist Less frequent elbow and shoulder; associated with hyperparathyroidism	Asymmetric affection of single joints. More often extraarticular affection of soft tissue and tendons in the shoulder elbow and hand, in decreasing frequency
CR/CT	Normal mineralization Asymmetric JSN Central erosions giving a seagull appearance Subchondral sclerosis Osteophytes Cysts Radial or ulnar subluxations	Decreased mineralization Periarticular soft tissue swelling Uniform JSN Juxta-articular and generalized halisteresis Marginal erosions starting in bare areas Ulnar and volar subluxations Ankylosis especially in wrist bones	Normal mineralization Bone proliferation Rapid JSN that occasionally can look widened Marginal erosions—mimicking mouse ears Pencil in cup Telescoping digits Ankylosis of finger and wrist joints Acro-osteolysis	Normal mineralization Tophi Relatively preserved joint space Punch-out erosions with sclerotic borders and overhanging edges can occur intra-articularly, periarticularly, or extra-articularly	Normal mineralization Uniform JSN Subchondral sclerosis Osteophytes with hook-like configuration in the MCP joints Pronounced cystic bone changes	Heterogeneous presentation with normal mineralization but periarticular calcification primarily in tendons and ligaments with linear dense depositions that develop to homogeneous well delineated circular appearance around shoulder, elbow and wrist

MR imaging	Osteophytes Cysts Synovitis BME Effusion Asymmetric JSN Capsulitis Tendinosis Ligament lesions	Erosions Synovitis BME Effusion Symmetric JSN Tenosynovitis Soft tissue edema Subluxations Ankylosis	Bone proliferation Erosions Enthesitis Effusion Capsulitis Synovitis BME Tenosynovitis Soft tissue edema Ankylosis	Distribution of soft tissue masses (tophi) Erosions BME Effusion Soft tissue edema	Osteophytes Cysts Synovitis BME Effusion Asymmetric JSN capsulitis Tendinosis Ligament lesions	Soft tissue masses with heterogeneous signal in the involved tendons Bursitis If joints are affected: Erosions Synovitis BME
US	Osteophytes Synovitis Effusion Capsulitis Enthesitis Tendinosis	Synovitis Effusion Erosions Tenosynovitis Capsulitis Enthesitis Subluxations	Bone proliferation Erosions Enthesitis Effusion Capsulitis Synovitis Tenosynovitis Soft tissue edema	Soft tissue masses (tophi) Erosions Effusion Synovitis Soft tissue edema	Osteophytes Erosions Synovitis Effusion Capsulitis Tendinosis Calcifications in the cartilage and TFCDC	Soft tissue masses with hyperechoic signal in the involved tendons Bursitis If joints are affected: Erosions Synovitis Effusion

Abbreviation: JSN, joint space narrowing.

currently is not widely used in the clinical context, mainly due to the use of a substantial radiation and nonspecificity of most nuclear medicine examinations. Hybrid imaging techniques, however, like PET-CT, single-photon emission CT (SPECT)-CT, and, recently, PET–MR imaging, are increasingly applied in the research setting to understand metabolic changes of soft tissue and bone in rheumatic diseases.[1]

OSTEOARTHRITIS

OA is the most frequent form of arthritis and a leading cause of physical disability, affecting millions worldwide, with huge social economic costs.[2] OA is considered a degenerative disease with pain, fatigue, and physical constraints that have a negative impact on the ability to perform common daily activities and is the main cause of reduced or lost ability to work. The Food and Drug Administration recognized OA as a serious disease with an unmet need for therapies that modify the underlying pathophysiology of the disease and can potentially change its natural course to prevent long-term disability (https://www.fda.gov/downloads/drugs/guidancecompliance regulatoryinformation/guidances/ucm071577.pdf).

Even though OA affects primarily the joints of the spine and the lower limb, that is, knee and hip joints, it is the most frequent form of arthritis of the upper limb inpatients over 45 years old.[3] It also is important to emphasize that OA may coexist with other joint diseases, including inflammatory joint diseases. Trauma and inflammatory joint diseases ultimately may progress to OA, which can give differential diagnostic challenges.

In the upper extremity, the hand is often affected by OA with a typical clinical picture of asymmetric stiff and painful distal finger joints and or pain at the radial side of the wrist (base of thumb) with or without swelling and tenderness. Over time, development of Heberden nodes in the distal interphalangeal (DIP) finger joints or Bouchard nodes in the proximal interphalangeal (PIP) joints can be seen. The disease is more predominant in women and on CR the disease typically is distributed asymmetrically in the DIP and PIP joints as well as the first carpometacarpal joint (CMC1) and scaphotrapeziotrapezoidal (STT) joint of the wrist (**Fig. 1**), with relative sparing of the metacarpophalangeal (MCP) joints. In the affected joints and similar to any OA affected joints, there are normal mineralization, asymmetric joint space narrowing, osteophytes, subchondral sclerosis, and subcortical central cysts (**Fig. 2**) that can lead to radial or ulnar subluxation when the disease progresses.

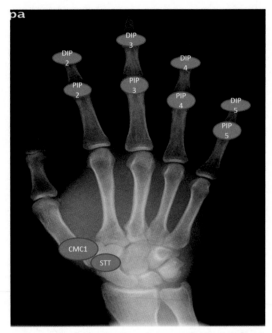

Fig. 1. Typical distribution pattern of hand OA primarily affecting the PIP and DIP joints as well as CMC1 and STT joint of the wrist with relative sparing of the MCP joints.

Volar subluxation of the fingers, as seen in advanced cases of RA, is seldom seen in hand OA.

Erosive OA (EOA) has been viewed as a subset of hand OA, with demonstrable joint erosions, and also is referred to as an inflammatory OA.[4] It classically affects the interphalangeal joints of the hands symmetrically, typically in postmenopausal women with an estimated female-to-male ratio of 12:1.[5] Large joints, such as the shoulder, knee, and hip, are rarely involved.[6] There is moderate to severe synovitis, but the precise etiology is yet to be determined.[7] Clinical symptoms of EOA include pain, swelling, and tenderness of the small joints of the hands as well as throbbing paresthesia of the fingertips and morning stiffness.[5] EOA starts from the DIP joints and later involves the PIP joints and also may affect the first CMC, STT, and other intercarpal joints.[8] The affected articulations commonly are characterized by deformities, which can include subluxations, flexion contractions, Heberden and Bouchard nodes, ankylosis of DIP and PIP joints, and opera-glass deformity.[9]

Characteristic radiographic changes of EOA include a combination of osseous proliferation and erosions. Although the presence of erosions is an essential hallmark for the diagnosis of EOA, osteophytes that are characteristic of nonerosive OA sometimes may be absent. The precise

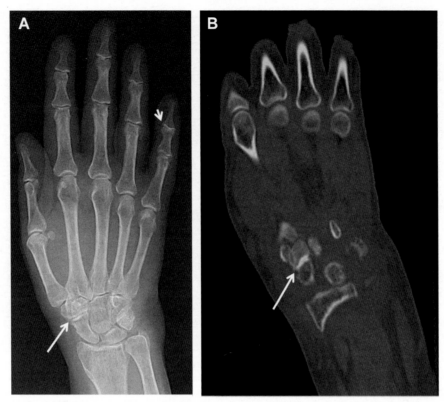

Fig. 2. A 66-year-old woman with right radial wrist pain and remitting-relapsing pain in the DIP joints of the right hand. (*A*) Posterior anterior radiograph of the right hand shows osteoarthritic changes in the radial side of the wrist, especially in the STT joint with joint space narrowing, subchondral sclerosis, and osteophytes (*arrow*). Note the mild osteoarthritic changes with marginal osteophytes and asymmetric joint space narrowing in several DIP joints, especially in the fifth DIP joint (*arrowhead*). (*B*) Long-axis coronal CT reformat of the same hand shows more detailed bony changes compared with the radiograph, such as osteophytes, joint space narrowing, and sclerosis (*arrow*).

diagnostic criteria of EOA are not well reported, including the type, number, and locations of the affected joints.[7] A recent systematic review of the literature revealed there is little agreement about even a radiographic definition of this disease, despite a heavy reliance on radiographic findings.[10]

Erosions affecting small joints of the hand have been illustrated in the revised atlas by Altman and Gold.[11] Typically, lesions begin at the central portion of the joint as a sharply marginated defect, usually preceded by joint space narrowing.[7] This may be associated with a crumbling erosion of the central bony surface.[12] Progression of the disease process leads to the characteristic gull-wing deformity due to marginal sclerosis and osteophytes of the distal side of the joints, while the proximal side is centrally eroded and thinned[7] (**Fig. 3**). Another characteristic erosion, found particularly at PIP joints, is the sawtooth erosion (see **Fig. 3**A; **Fig. 4**), which may later lead to ankylosis. The crumbling erosions affecting PIP joints

are seen less commonly. Joint space narrowing and erosions may be seen in the early stage of EOA, whereas marginal osteophytes leading to Heberden and Bouchard nodes are seen at a later stage of the disease.[7] The population-based Framingham Osteoarthritis Study showed that radiography-detected hand EOA is associated with MR imaging–detected subchondral bone attrition in the knee joint—an association likely explained by a heightened burden of disease.[13]

The use of bone scintigraphy has been described in the imaging of hand EOA, and its possible role in predicting clinical and radiographic progression of the disease was explored.[14] A more recent study comparing bone scintigraphy and high-resolution multi-pinhole SPECT, however, demonstrated that multi-pinhole SPECT was able to differentiate between early RA and EOA based on the pattern of tracer uptake, whereas bone scintigraphy could not.[15] The role of nuclear medicine imaging specifically for hand EOA is not well established to date.

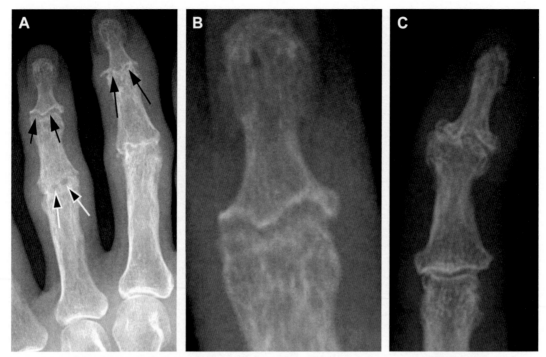

Fig. 3. (*A*) Anteroposterior radiograph shows gull-wing features (*black arrows*) in the DIP joints. In addition, PIP joint of digit 4 shows a so-called sawtooth erosion (*white arrows*). (*B, C*) Anteroposterior radiograph shows other examples of gull-wing appearance in EOA. In PsA, erosions more typically have a mouse-ear configuration characterized by a periosteal apposition in the marginal aspects of distal phalanges of the DIP joints. Erosions are marginally located and there is frequent involvement of other sites in the body, in particular the sacroiliac joints. Acro-osteolysis, pencil-like deformities, and arthritis mutilans are seen in PsA but not in EOA.

For imaging of the hand and the wrist using the standard 1.5T or 3T closed-bore MR imaging system, patients typically are placed prone with the hand to be imaged extended above the head (Superman position)[16] or along the side of the body in the newly developed wide-bore magnets. Alternatively, a dedicated extremity MR imaging system can be used if a patient is claustrophobic or too obese to fit in the magnet, but extremity MR imaging systems usually are limited to a lower strength magnet (1.5T or less).[17] Erosions typically are evaluated on axial and coronal planes using a T1-weighted non–fat-suppressed spin-echo sequence, and associated synovitis can be assessed using T1-weighted fat-suppressed sequences with or without contrast enhancement[18] (**Fig. 5**). Dynamic contrast-enhanced (DCE)–MR imaging also has been shown to enable differentiation between EOA and PsA, with different degrees of late enhancement at 15 minutes post–intravenous (IV) gadolinium administration[19] (**Fig. 6**). Studies have shown that thanks to its multiplanar capabilities MR imaging is significantly more sensitive to the detection of erosions than radiography,[16,20] and a semiquantitative MR imaging scoring system called the Outcome Measures in Rheumatoid Arthritis Clinical Trials (OMERACT) Hand Osteoarthritis Magnetic Resonance Imaging Scoring System has been developed and shown good reliability and responsiveness for erosion assessment.[21]

US has been shown more sensitive than CR for detection of erosion and osteophytes.[22,23] Additionally, US can detect the presence of active inflammatory changes in and around the synovial joint by means of gray-scale and color Doppler imaging (**Fig. 7**). In the context of hand EOA, it has been shown that synovial tissues lining the surface cavity of bone erosions potentially are subjected to an inflammatory process.[24] US thus can detect the presence of synovitis that is closely related to erosive changes in hand EOA. Several recently published studies showed US-detected inflammatory signs in hand EOA[22,25,26] that also seem to predict erosive progression.[27]

CT is the reference method for imaging bony changes and shows osteophytes, subcortical sclerosis, cysts and erosions in 3-D (see **Fig. 2**), but CT remains less frequently used compared with MR imaging because CT uses radiation and cannot detect bone marrow edema (BME) and soft tissue changes like MR imaging can (**Table 2**).

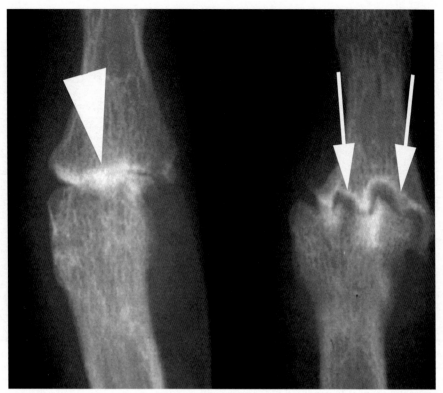

Fig. 4. Magnification of an anteroposterior radiograph depicts a classical sawtooth erosion in the fourth PIP joint (*right, arrows*) whereas the third PIP joint exhibits a nonerosive appearance of advanced OA with joint space narrowing and subchondral sclerosis (*left, arrowhead*). The main difference between the 2 subtypes of OA is the presence or absence of radiographic erosions. Clinical aspects sometimes may be indistinguishable, although EOA is characterized by more frequent inflammatory episodes, which may involve several joints simultaneously and may persist for years.

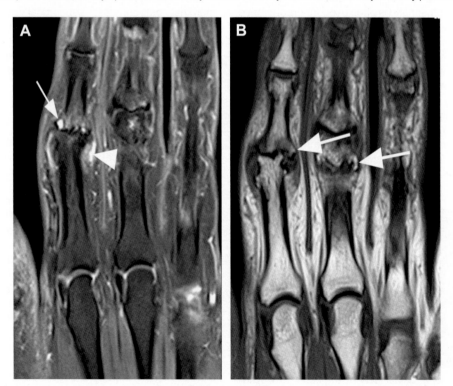

Fig. 5. (*A*) Coronal T1-weighted fat-suppressed contrast-enhanced MR imaging shows synovial inflammation (*arrowhead*) and subchondral cystic changes (*arrow*). (*B*) The corresponding coronal T1-weighted MR imaging more distinctly shows marginal osteophytes (*arrows*) characteristic of OA.

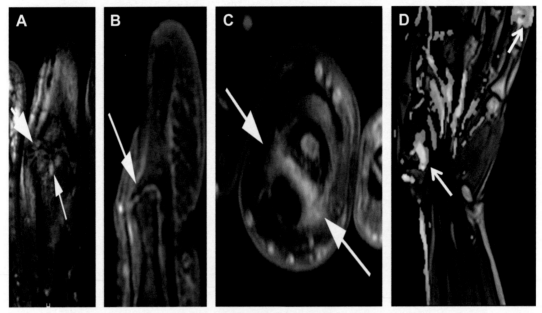

Fig. 6. EOA on MR imaging. (*A*) Coronal fat-suppressed proton density–weighted MR imaging shows a subchondral cystic lesion (*arrow*) and a classic marginal osteophyte (*arrowhead*). (*B*) Osteophytes commonly are observed dorsally at the joint margin as depicted in this sagittal fat-suppressed proton density–weighted MR imaging (*arrow*). (*C*) Corresponding axial T1-weighted MR imaging with contrast-enhanced fat-suppression at the level of the joint line shows marked synovitis reflected as hyperintense contrast enhancement (*arrows*). (*D*) DCE–MR imaging in a different patient with inflammatory hand OA shows marked enhancement, which appears as brighter yellow in the first carpometacarpal and fifth DIP joints (*arrows*).

CT on the other hand is often used for preoperative planning and in research settings. Micro-CT provides near histologic images of bony changes widely used to study the trabecular pattern changes after various arthritis conditions, especially in animal models.[28,29]

Primary OA of the elbow and shoulder is rare and usually secondary to trauma or another underlying arthritis. Similar to other joints, the typical appearance on CR is normal bone mineralization with asymmetric joint space narrowing, joint effusion with extension of the capsule along with

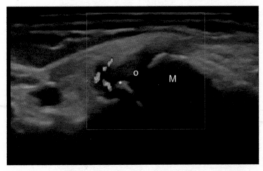

Fig. 7. US longitudinal view of the CMC1 with synovial hypertrophy (o) and Doppler activity and osteophyte (*). M, metacarpal bone.

marginal osteophytes, subcortical cysts, and subcortical sclerosis. CT, MR imaging, and US can be used to support the diagnosis similar to that seen in the hand, where MR imaging and US in particular are used to study potential ligament and tendon disease and damage.

RHEUMATOID ARTHRITIS

RA is a chronic inflammatory joint disease with an unpredictable clinical course.[30] In two-thirds of cases it presents as symmetric arthralgia and arthritis in the small joint of the hands and feet and may lead to severe skeletal changes and destruction of the affected joints.[31] RA has a great impact on all aspects of life due to joint-related symptoms, including pain and impaired physical function as well as general malaise and fatigue. RA affects approximately 1% of the adult population in the Western World with a female-to-male ratio of 2:1. In the hand, the typical clinical picture is symmetric, painful, swollen joints affecting the wrist and MCP and PIP joints but never the DIP joints (**Fig. 8**). Symptoms often are accompanied with elevated C-reactive protein or sedimentation ratio as well as positive rheumatic factor and/or elevated anticyclic citrulinated peptides.

Table 2
Sensitivity of the different imaging methods for detection of typical pathologic changes seen in inflammatory joint arthritis in the upper extremity

	Conventional Radiography	CT	MR Imaging	Ultrasound
Synovitis	NA	+	+++(+)	+++
BME	NA	+(#)	+++	NA
Capsulitis	NA	+	+++(+)	++
Enthesitis	NA	+	+++(+)	+++
Erosions	++	++++	+++	++
Bony sclerosis	++	++++	+	NA
Soft tissue calcifications	++	++++	+	+++
Joint space narrowing	++	+++	++	+
Subluxations	++	+++	+++	+
Tenosynovitis	NA	+	+++(+)	+++
Ligaments	NA	+	+++	+++
Effusion	NA	+	+++(+)	++

(+) Increased detection if IV gadolinium contrast is used; (#) increased detection using DECT and virtual noncalcium images.

In the early disease stages, CR of the hands is normal with a possible soft tissue swelling, which is followed by periarticular halisteresis (osteopenia) and later by uniform narrowing of joint spaces

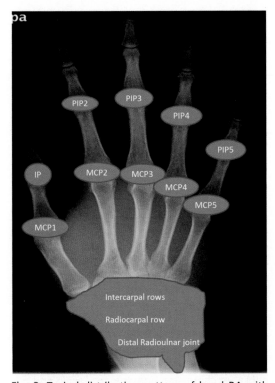

Fig. 8. Typical distribution pattern of hand RA with symmetric painful and swollen joints that can affect the 3 compartments of the wrist, and the MCP and PIP joints but never the DIP joints.

and development of erosions (**Fig. 9**A). Erosions can be seen within the first 3 months to 6 months of the disease, with a predilection for the bare areas of the bone and vascular channels penetrating the bone,[32] and is present in up to approximately 50% of all newly diagnosed RA patients.[33,34] As erosions become more pronounced, generalized halisteresis and volar subluxation at the MCP joints may be followed by subsequent ulnar deviation of the fingers, potential swan neck deformity, and in the end stages ankylosis, especially in the wrist, if the disease is not adequately treated (**Fig. 9**B, C). These end-stage CR changes fortunately are rare today due to more effective treat-to-target algorithms using standardized fast escalation of treatment with synthetic disease-modifying antirheumatic drugs (DMARDs) alone or in combination with glucocorticoids (often injected) and, in cases of insufficient response, biological DMARDs.[35]

Even though it is well known that CR shows only late RA bone changes, CR is still the only imaging modality accepted by the Food and Drug Administration to allow pharmaceutical companies to claim structural damage inhibition for new drugs. This is despite that MR imaging has been shown much more sensitive for detection and monitoring of early bone damage in several studies,[36–38] using the validated OMERACT RA MRI scoring system (RAMRIS).[39] Furthermore, MR imaging can show early signs of arthritis, such as synovitis, BME, and tenosynovitis—especially after IV gadolinium contrast administration (**Fig. 10**). After IV gadolinium contrast administration, the sensitivity and

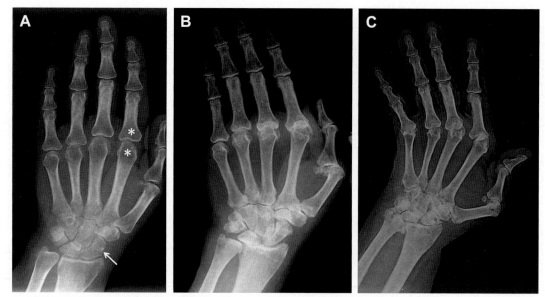

Fig. 9. A 35-year-old woman with early RA. (*A*) Anteroposterior radiograph shows periarticular osteopenia in the all MCP joints (*), soft tissue swelling around the wrist, and a small erosion in the scaphoid bone (*arrow*). (*B*) Same patient 9 years later; radiograph shows severe progressive erosive disease and joint space narrowing of the first carpal row and MCP joints as well as subluxations of first to third MCP joints and evolving ulnar deviation. Also, note the progressive osteopenia seen as thinning of the cortex of the MCP bones and the relative sparing of PIP joints. (*C*) A 48-year-old woman with 11-year history of RA. Anteroposterior radiograph of the left hand shows joint space narrowing, multiple erosions in wrist and MCP joints, osteopenia, ulnar subluxations of MCP joints, and soft tissue swelling. (*Courtesy of* Dr. Guillermo Valenzuela, Plantation, FL, US.)

specificity for synovitis[40] and tenosynovitis[41] detection improve and it is also possible to differentiate joint fluid from synovial pannus (**Fig. 11**). Contrast-enhanced MR imaging also allows differentiation between active inflammation and fibrotic inactive pannus, especially when a DCE–MR imaging sequence is performed. DCE–MR imaging can differentiate inactive from active disease and shows very fast treatment response after therapy in clinical trials and research studies similar to US Doppler[42] (**Fig. 12**). DCE–MR imaging thus may become a clinical tool to monitor early treatment response similar to its use in oncology that is, prostate, breast, and brain cancer imaging.[43–45] Furthermore, with MR imaging, bone erosion in patients with RA can be seen a mean of 2 years before they are evident on CR (see **Fig. 10**; **Fig. 13**),[46] and 20% to 30% of the metacarpal bone can be eroded on MR imaging and still not be apparent on CR[47,48] (see **Fig. 10**D). In addition, MR imaging can show ligament, cartilage, and tendon damage. MR imaging also is the only accepted modality currently for detection of BME, which has been shown to predict future bone erosions[49–51] (**Fig. 14**). Perioperative biopsy samples taken from patients with severe RA have shown that BME reflects true bone marrow inflammation[52] and erosions can

develop from the bone marrow through an inflammatory release of cytokines that stimulate osteoclasts to resorb the bone.[49]

US allows bedside assessment of inflammatory and structural changes in both early and late stages of RA, such as synovitis, tenosynovitis, and bone erosions, using both gray-scale and color Doppler (**Figs. 15–17**). US is more sensitive than clinical examination for the detection of tenosynovitis and synovitis in both symptomatic and asymptomatic joints,[53–55] and with a sensitivity comparable to MR imaging.[56] This has resulted in both US and MR imaging signs of synovitis included in the new classification criteria for RA for detection of subclinical synovitis.[57,58] Furthermore, the presence of synovial hypertrophy in the MCP and wrist joints in patients with very early disease is an independent predictor for developing RA.[59] The higher the grade of the synovial hypertrophy, the better the specificity (from 79.4% to 93.4%) at the expense of sensitivity (78%–56.1%).[60] US is, however, not fully implemented in the diagnostic setup for RA patients. A consensus-based scoring system recently was published that takes both the gray-scale and color Doppler findings into account when monitoring treatment response; however, data suggest that routine US monitoring is not necessary if applying

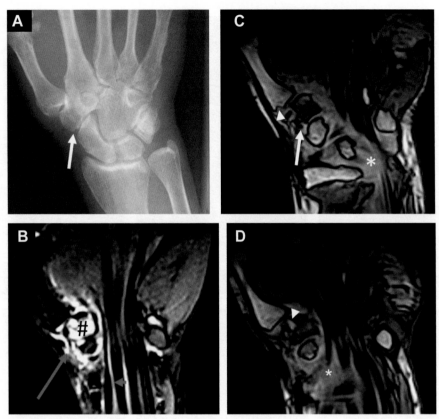

Fig. 10. A 42-year-old woman with RA for 7 years and clinical signs of activity in the right wrist. (*A*) Anteroposterior radiograph shows a small erosion in trapezium bone (*arrow*). (*B–D*) Low-field 0.2T images taken 2 years before A. (*B*) Coronal short TI inversion recovery MR imaging with severe BME of the trapezium bone (#), surrounding synovitis (*red arrow*) and tenosynovitis (*red arrowhead*). Coronal contrast-enhanced gradient-echo T1-weighted MR imaging consecutive slices without fat suppression show severe synovitis in the wrist (*C, D, asterisks*) and the same erosion in the trapezium bone (*C, arrow*) as seen on the radiograph as well as several erosions in both the trapezium and base of the first metacarpal bone that cannot be seen on the radiograph (*C, D, arrowheads*).

a tight clinical control.[61] Tenosynovitis of the extensor carpi ulnaris is frequently involved in early RA (see **Fig. 16**)[62] and also has been shown to predict erosive disease after 1 year. Similarly, a high Doppler score in joints also is associated with erosive progression after 1 year in patients with active disease as well as in patients in clinical remission (see **Fig. 12**A, B).[63–65] For structural changes, US is more sensitive than CR in detecting bone erosions in MCP, PIP, and MTP joints,[66,67] but US is inferior to MR imaging in the ability to follow erosive changes over time in the wrist and hand.[68] The reason for the lower sensitivity is explained partly by the fact that some areas of the joints are inaccessible to US. When evaluating only the areas that are accessible by US in MCP joints, however, the sensitivity, specificity, and accuracy were 71%, 95% and 90%, respectively,[69] with CT as the reference indicating that bone erosions found on US are true erosions.

The clinical relevance of MR imaging and US findings in RA is emphasized by the fact that 20% to 30% patients in clinical and biochemical remission have radiographic progression after 1 year,[70] as defined by both the American College of Rheumatology (ACR) and the European League Against Rheumatism (EULAR) guidelines. Many of these patients might have had subclinical inflammatory synovitis and BME on MR imaging (**Fig. 18**) and increased Doppler activity on US which are known to predict erosive disease progression on CR[71] but it has yet to be shown that treating subclinical US or MR imaging symptoms is better than the usual standard care for preventing future joint damage.[61,72]

CT is the technology of reference for detecting erosion and calcifications but due to radiation issues it is not often used in assessment of hand RA, even though it has been shown to detect more erosions in the wrist and MCP bones than

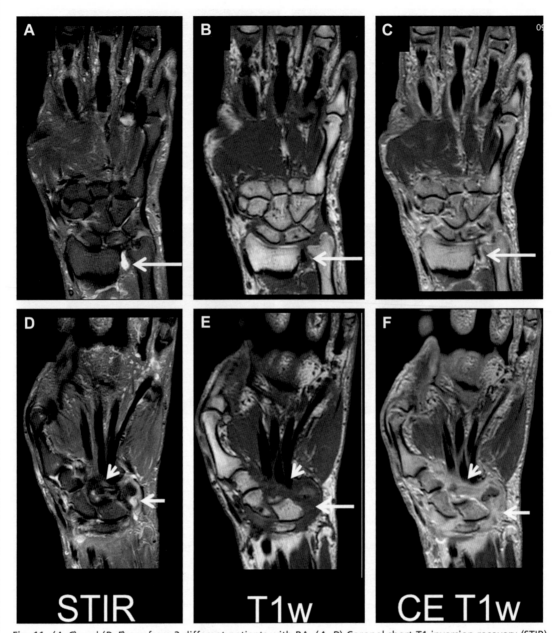

Fig. 11. (*A–C*) and (*D–F*) are from 2 different patients with RA. (*A, D*) Coronal short T1 inversion recovery (STIR) MR imaging, (*B, E*) coronal T1-weighted MR imaging without fat suppression, and (*C, F*) coronal contrast-enhanced T1-weighted MR imaging without fat-suppression. Approximately 50% of the increased signal intensity in the radioulnar joints on the (*A*) STIR image corresponds to joint effusion, only visible as the (*C*) hypointense area within the enhancing synovium (*arrows*). (*F*) The severe enhancement of synovium is barely visible on the (*D*) STIR image (*arrows and arrowheads*). This means that STIR MR imaging can both overestimate and underestimate the amount of synovitis compared with the contrast-enhanced T1-weighted images. CE, contrast-enhanced; T1w, T1-weighted.

MR imaging, US, or CR.[68,73] CT often is used for preoperative planning, but newer CT scanners that can obtain 3-D CT images with dual-energy CT (DECT) technology and low radiation dose have made it possible to study BME by using virtual noncalcium images that enable quantification of the water content in a bone with fatty marrow. This is feasible even in small wrist and hand bones[74] but the technique still has challenges and lacks standardized acquisition and post-processing protocols.[75] Nevertheless, it seems entirely possible that in the near future acquiring DECT images with a very low radiation dose in less than 1 minute that can detect and

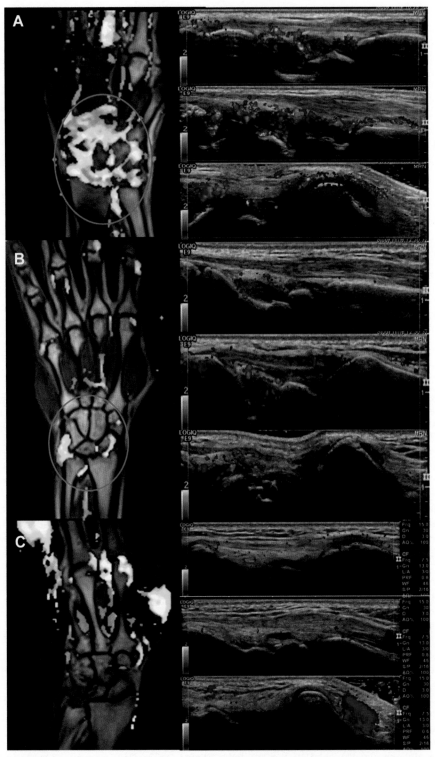

Fig. 12. DCE–MR imaging and corresponding color Doppler longitudinal US examination in the central and dorsal synovium of the wrist in patients with (*A*) severe inflammation, (*B*) low to moderate inflammation, and (*C*) no inflammation in the wrist (*red circles*). Note that DCE–MR imaging also depicts inflammation in several MCP and PIP joints (*A–C*).

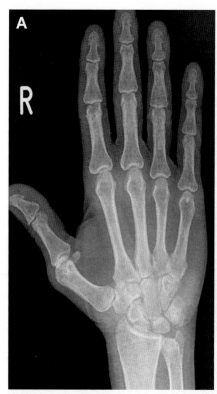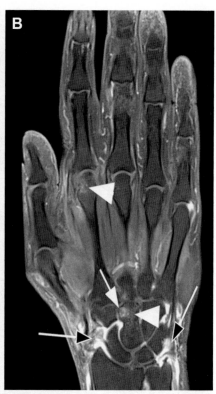

Fig. 13. A 48-year-old woman with pain primarily in the wrist. No established diagnosis of an inflammatory disorder. (*A*) Anteroposterior radiograph does not show any pathology suggestive of RA. There are no erosive changes, no focal periarticular osteopenia, and no soft tissue swelling. (*B*) The corresponding coronal contrast-enhanced fat-suppressed T1-weighted MR imaging shows several features characteristic of active RA, including osteitis (*arrowheads*), a bony erosion (*small white arrow*), and marked carpal synovitis (*long black arrows*). This example emphasizes the role of MRI in detecting early disease and characterizing disease activity.

monitor erosions in 3-D and simultaneously provide an estimate of potential BME in the bone may be possible.

RA also affects the elbow in approximately 30% and the shoulder in approximately 60% of the patients presenting clinically with pain and limited range of motion. In the elbow, an extension of the capsule and elevated fat pad are seen on the lateral CR followed by generalized halisteresis, uniform joint space narrowing, and cystic/erosive changes without new bone formation and osteophytes (**Fig. 19**). In the shoulder, there can be uniform joint space narrowing of all joint compartments without the presence of osteophytes along with generalized halisteresis and migration of the humeral head toward the inferior surface of the acromion. Erosions are late manifestations usually seen at the rotator cuff insertion sites (bare area) and the acromio-clavicular joint (**Fig. 20**). Later in the disease, large cystic changes can occur in the humeral head due to invasive synovium creating a differential diagnostic challenge to a bony tumor (ie,

chondroblastoma). CT can show all bony features in 3-D with much higher sensitivity than CR whereas MR imaging can show BME, synovitis, cystic and erosive changes, capsulitis, and ligament and tendon damage as well as nerve and muscle involvement in both the elbow and shoulder.

PSORIATIC ARTHRITIS

Between 5% and 40% of people with cutaneous psoriasis develop PsA that typically presents in the upper extremity as oligoarthritis with asymmetric joint affection of the DIP and PIP joints, wrist, MCP, shoulder, and elbow joints in decreasing frequency[76] (**Fig. 21**). In the early disease stages, CR of the hand and fingers in patients with PsA shows normal bones with potential soft tissue swelling. Relatively specific signs of PsA are nail changes and the clinical entity of a swollen inflamed digit, that is, dactylitis (often referred to as sausage finger), even though it also can be seen in other spondylarthritides.[77]

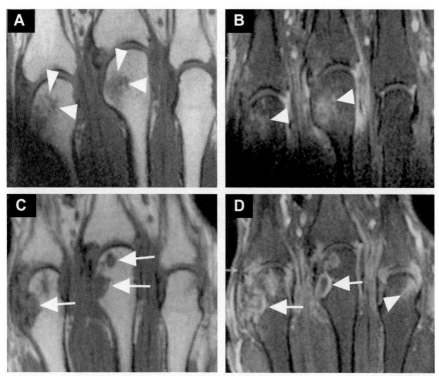

Fig. 14. Example of disease progression prior the era of biologic therapy. (*A*) T1-weighted MR imaging shows areas of bone marrow edema (osteitis) in the metacarpal heads but no erosive disease (*arrowheads*). These are characterized by diffuse ill-defined hypointensity on (*A*) T1-weighted images and hyperintensity (*arrowheads*) on (*B*) contrast-enhanced fat-suppressed T1-weighted MR imaging. (*C*) Follow-up T1-weighted MR imaging 17 months later shows marked bony destructions at the metacarpal heads with erosions that have developed in areas of prior osteitis (*C* [*arrows*]). BME is one of the strongest predictors of subsequent erosive disease. (*D*) The corresponding T1-weighted fat-suppressed contrast-enhanced MR imaging shows the erosions (*arrows*) and an area of newly developed osteitis in the fourth metacarpal head that was not present at baseline (*arrowhead*).

Over time, periostitis with irregular thickening of the cortex or periosteal layers of new bone along the long bones of the fingers will be seen on CR as clouded fluffy densities (**Fig. 22**). The bones in typical cases have preserved bone mineralization even though transient periarticular halisteresis can occur. Bone proliferation is also a relatively specific sign of PsA that happens along

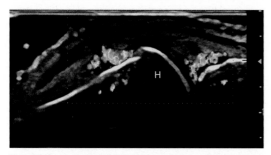

Fig. 15. Longitudinal US view of the second metacarpal joint in RA with synovitis (synovial hypertrophy and Doppler activity). H, metacarpal head.

shafts of the long bones, adjacent to erosions, at ligament, capsular, and tendon insertions.[78,79] Later marginal erosions become apparent in the DIP joints on CR and CT scans in conjunction with bone proliferation that looks like mouse ears (**Fig. 23**). If the disease is not treated development of so-called pencil-in-cup configuration can be seen before potential ankylosis of finger joints occurs.[78,79] At this stage, some patients exhibit generalized halisteresis (see **Fig. 22**C). In approximately 5% of PsA patients, arthritis mutilans, is seen[80] with rapidly progressing disease changes associated with nail changes and telescoping digits. In these patients, a resorption of the distal phalanges called acro-osteolysis occasionally occurs.

MR imaging can show both the inflammatory and structural lesions after PsA in the hand, elbow, and shoulder, such as synovitis, enthesitis, tenosynovitis, BME, bone erosion, periarticular inflammation, and to a lesser extent bone proliferation (**Fig. 24**).[81–83] Synovitis, enthesitis, tenosynovitis,

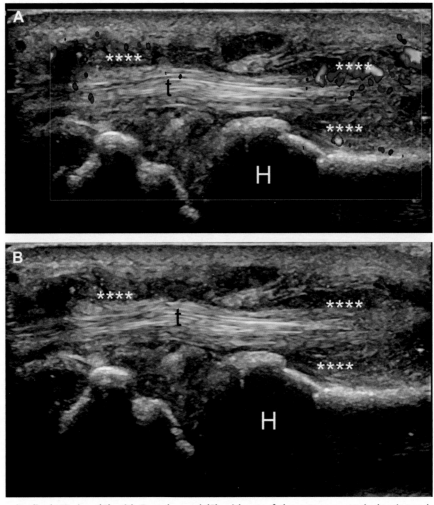

Fig. 16. Longitudinal US view (*A*) with Doppler and (*B*) without of the extensor carpi ulnaris tendon (t) in RA showing tenosynovitis (****). H, head of ulna.

and periarticular inflammation are better visualized when IV gadolinium contrast is used. Dactylitis on MR imaging seems to be caused by a combination of tenosynovitis, synovitis, capsulitis, and periarticular inflammation (**Fig. 25**).[84,85] DCE–MR imaging may add additional information about inflammation (**Fig. 26**) but needs further study. Consensus-based MR imaging definitions of important pathologies in the PsA hand, and a corresponding semiquantitative scoring system has been developed and validated for monitoring disease activity and joint damage in PsA clinical trials.[86,87] More recently, consensus-based definitions and a scoring system for enthesitis have been developed and currently are in press. Whole-body MR imaging allows simultaneous assessment of peripheral and axial joints and entheses[88] but requires more validation before use in clinical practice.

US in PsA is characterized by inflammation of both intra-articular (synovitis and erosions) and extra-articular (enthesitis, tendinitis, and tenosynovitis) structures. US has a higher sensitivity than clinical examination[89–94] for detecting these features (**Figs. 27** and **28**). The appearance of synovitis on US is nonspecific. Hence, for diagnostic purposes, it is the detection of joint involvement and the pattern of involved joints that are of importance.[93] US may be used to monitor treatment effects in PsA lesions, such as synovitis, tenosynovitis, erosions, and enthesitis.[95–97] Several scoring systems have been proposed for this purpose,[92,97–99] including different reduced joint sets and combination of structures, also including US evaluation of skin and nails.[99] As in RA, subclinical synovitis is frequent both at time of diagnosis and in a state of clinical remission[94] and may lead to structural

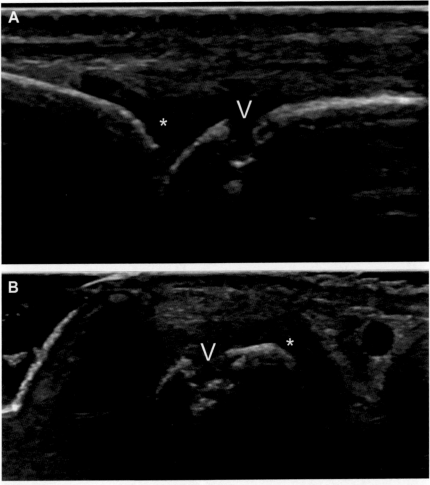

Fig. 17. (*A*) Longitudinal and (*B*) transverse US views of the second MCP joint in RA with minimal synovial hypertrophy (*) and a bone erosion (v) in the metacarpal head.

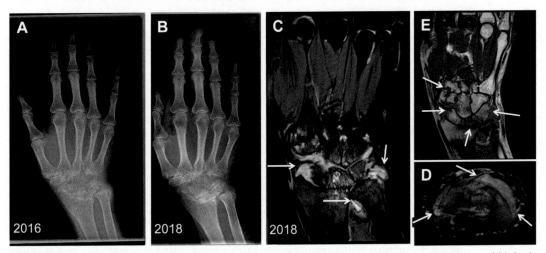

Fig. 18. A 33-year-old woman with seropositive RA for 10 years. Low disease activity on DMARD and biologics (disease activity score 28 = 3.6) on methotrexate and tumor necrosis factor inhibitor but with continuous pain in the right wrist despite 2 steroid injections. Anteroposterior radiographs from (*A*) 2016 and (*B*) 2018 show no progression. MR imaging shows severe BME in all wrist bones and moderate to severe synovitis (*arrows*) in all joint compartments on the (*C*) coronal short T1 inversion recovery and (*D*) axial fat-suppressed T2-weighted MR imaging as signs of active inflammatory disease. (*E*) Coronal T1-weighted MR imaging shows moderate erosions in most wrist bones (*arrows*).

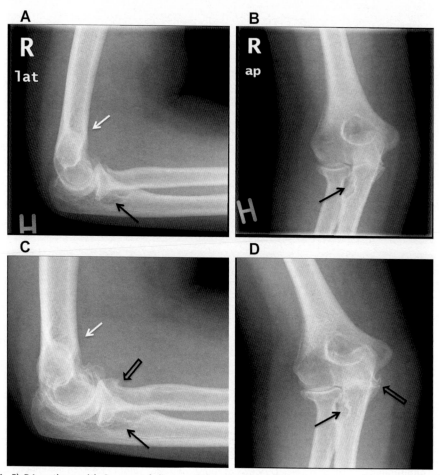

Fig. 19. (*A, B*) RA patient with 2 years of disease. (*A*) Lateral and (*B*) anteroposterior radiographs of the right elbow show elevated capsular fat pad (*white arrow*) as a sign of joint effusion, moderate erosive changes of the proximal ulnar (*black arrow*), and relatively preserved joint spaces. (*C, D*) Same patient with RA 5 years later (7 years' disease duration). (*C*) Lateral and (*D*) anteroposterior radiographs of the elbow show unchanged elevated capsular fat pad (*white arrow*) as a sign of joint effusion or synovial pannus, unchanged moderate erosive changes of the proximal ulnar (*black arrow*) but progression in uniform narrow joint spaces and secondary OA with osteophytes (*open black arrow*).

progression.[100] Although joint involvement is frequent, PsA patients tend to have more extrasynovial inflammation, including enthesitis and soft tissue changes, compared with RA patients.[101] A combination of lesions is seen in dactylitis, where the main element is tenosynovitis,[102,103] but may be combined with other components, such as synovitis, soft tissue edema, and tendon affection (swelling and/or enthesitis) of the flexor and extensor tendon (see **Fig. 27**).[102,104] Enthesitis, which is the hallmark of the disease, can be found at the insertion of the common extensor tendon and the triceps insertion of the elbow although it is more common in the lower limbs.[105] A consensus-based agreement on US definitions of enthesitis overall in spondyloarthritis (SpA), including PsA, has been reached to enable greater consistency in clinical studies.[106,107] The elementary lesions included in this definition are thickening of the enthesis, hyperechogenicity/loss of fibrillary structure, erosions, calcifications, enthesophytes, and Doppler activity at the enthesis. The latter has been shown specific for SpA, including PsA, as are erosions in this area.[108] Entheseal involvement may predict the development of SpA, including PsA,[109] and in established PsA, high synovitis scores, and active enthesitis on US at both baseline and follow-up, may indicate a poor prognosis.[100]

CT is the reference standard for erosions and bone proliferation in PsA but rarely is used as primary evaluation due to radiation issues. The introduction of DECT and cone beam CT might change

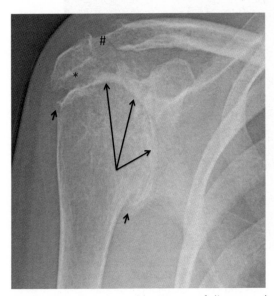

Fig. 20. RA in a patient with 15 years of disease and shoulder affection. Anteroposterior radiograph of the shoulder shows halisteresis, uniform severe joint space narrowing, and erosions in the glenohumeral joint (*arrows*). The subacromial space is also narrowed (*) and there is a widening of the acromioclavicular joint (#) as well as secondary degenerative changes with marginal osteophytes in all joint compartments (*arrowheads*).

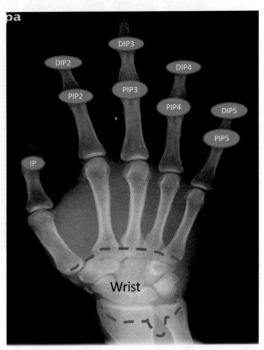

Fig. 21. Typical distribution pattern of hand PsA with asymmetric painful and swollen joints than can affect the PIP and DIP and more rarely the wrist and MCP joints.

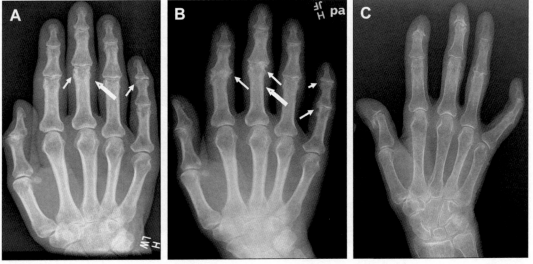

Fig. 22. (*A*) A patient with early PsA with discrete changes in the PIP and DIP joints of the right hand (*arrows*). Note the cloudy appearance of the periosteum (*thick arrow*) and sparing of the MCP and wrist joints. (*B*) Same patient 4 years later. Note preserved joint space despite moderate erosive and proliferative changes in several joints (*arrows*). Normal MCP and wrist. (*C*) Another patient with 9 years of PsA showing late stage PsA changes with generalized halisteresis, proliferative, and erosive changes in the second and third DIP joints along with pencil-in-cup appearance in the IP joint. Note also the relative sparing of the MCP and wrist joints.

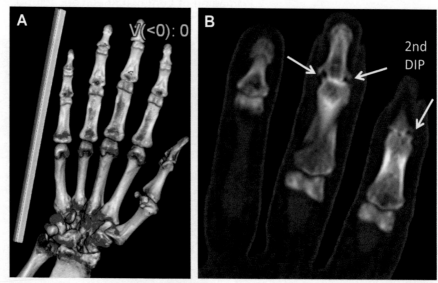

Fig. 23. (*A*) A 69-year-old man with suspected PsA shows no signs of urate deposition in a DECT scan of the right hand. (*B*) At the same time, a monochromatic CT image with bone algorithm shows signs of mouse ears configuration of the second and third DIP joint due to both erosions and bony proliferations (*arrows*) giving clues toward an underlying PsA.

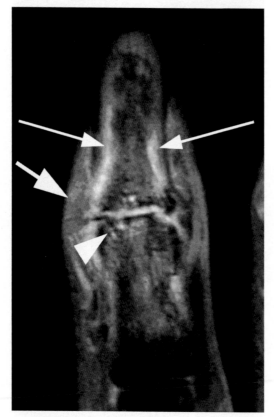

Fig. 24. Coronal fat-suppressed proton density–weighted MR imaging in patient with PsA. In contrast to EOA, PsA more commonly shows soft tissue swelling and inflammation (*short arrow*) and periostitis (*thin arrows*), which is not a feature of EOA. In PsA, erosions are commonly marginally located compared to the central location of EOA but also may be observed more centrally as in this example (*arrowhead*).

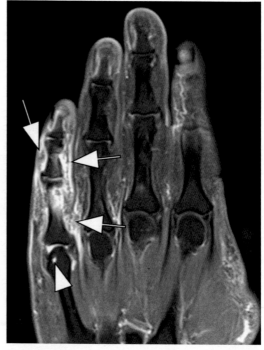

Fig. 25. A 52-year-old man patient with pain in the fifth finger. Patient has cutaneous psoriatic disease but no joint involvement so far. Coronal T1-weighted fat-suppressed contrast-enhanced MR imaging of the hand shows diffuse soft tissue inflammation reflected as marked subcutaneous contrast enhancement (*arrows*). Finding represents psoriatic dactylitis. In addition, there is a small bony erosion at the metacarpal head (*arrowhead*).

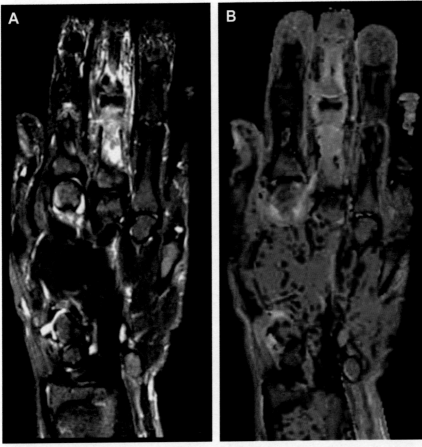

Fig. 26. (A) A 55-year-old man with clinical signs of dactylitis in the third finger coronal short T1 inversion recovery of the hand shows diffuse soft tissue inflammation reflected as marked subcutaneous edema and increased fluid signal in the capsules around the third PIP joint. (B) Corresponding coronal DCE–MR imaging of the same area shows marked contrast uptake represented as brighter shades of yellow in the soft tissues of the third digit which allows quantification of the perfusion of the various tissues as a surrogate marker of inflammation. (Created using DYNAMIKA. *Courtesy of* Dr. Olga Kubassova, Image Analysis group, London, UK.)

this because these imaging modalities also can help to exclude gout and pseudogout (see **Fig. 23**).

PsA also can affect the elbow (**Fig. 29**) and shoulder and show the same features on imaging as in hand and wrist but with more pronounced bone proliferation and erosions at tendon and ligament insertions, especially in the shoulder at the coracoclavicular ligament and the insertion of the rotator cuff tendons due to enthesitis.

GOUT

Gout is the most common arthritis in middle-aged men but can also affect women. It is caused by an accumulation of monosodium urate crystals in the soft tissues that generate an inflammatory joint response and progress to large articular and extra-articular tophi that eventually destroy nearby bone and soft tissue if not treated. The disease is associated with several metabolic, myeloproliferative, renal, and cardiovascular diseases. It also can be caused by alcohol consumption, certain chemotherapeutic drugs, or genetic error of the purine metabolism, but in a majority of cases the underlying cause is believed decreased excretion of urate metabolites in the kidney of unknown cause.[110] In the upper extremity, sudden onset of monoarthritis or oligoarthritis of wrist, MCP, and/or various finger joints in decreasing frequency can be seen causing pain, swelling, and erythema. Accompanying fever, bursitis, or tenosynovitis can give differential diagnostic challenges, because gout may resemble septic arthritis.[110,111] The symptoms typically last for 2 days and resolve spontaneously within 1 week. The disease less frequently affects the elbow and shoulder, but any tissue, including bursae and tendons, can have gout. A typical feature in the later

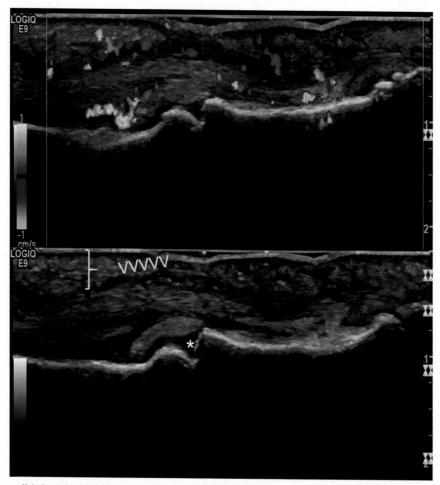

Fig. 27. Dactylitis in PsA. Longitudinal US view of the flexor tendon of the third finger with (*upper panel*) and without (*lower panel*) Doppler showing tenosynovitis (vvvvv), synovitis (*) in the PIP joint and soft tissue thickening.

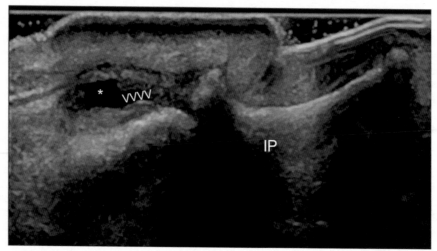

Fig. 28. Longitudinal US view of the DIP joint in PsA with synovitis (vvvv) and concomitant effusion (*). IP, intermediate phalanx.

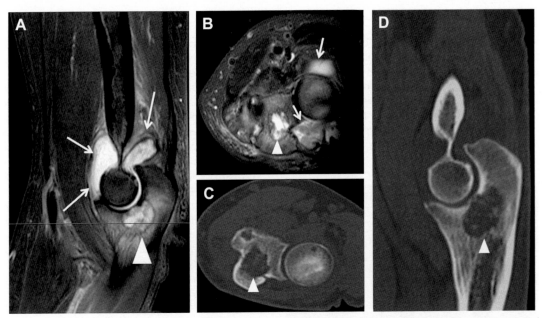

Fig. 29. A 69-year-old man with seronegative arthritis affecting the elbow, wrist, and finger joints with suspected PsA. MR imaging shows severe synovitis in all elbow compartments on both (*A*) sagittal and (*B*) axial proton density–weighted fat-suppressed sequences (*arrows*) as well as a large BME around a large erosion in the olecranon (*arrowhead*) that is much better appreciated on the (*C*) axial and (*D*) sagittal CT images.

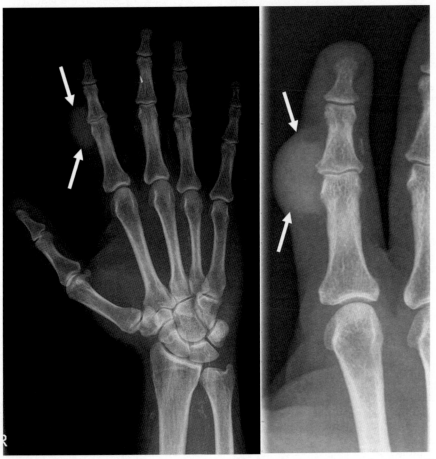

Fig. 30. A 60-year-old man on hemodialysis. (*Left*) Anteroposterior radiograph shows soft tissue swelling around the radial aspect of the second PIP joint (*arrows*) proved to be gout tophus. (*Right*) Zoomed image. First manifestation with discrete bony involvement of PIP joint.

stages of the disease is tophi formation—intra-articular, periarticular, or extraarticular. These are seen as bulky soft tissue masses with increasing radiodensity overtime due to progressive calcification (**Fig. 30**). When the joints are involved, progressive erosions are seen and in classic cases look like punched-out erosions with sclerotic borders and overhanging edges (**Fig. 31**).[112] Another

important feature is a relatively preserved joint space, even when the joint has large erosions. Gout can be treated by urate-lowering drugs, which over time can make the tophi shrink or even disappear. Casuistic evidence and small open-label studies have even shown that after successful treatment gouty erosions can heal and joints can return to near normal configuration.[110,113]

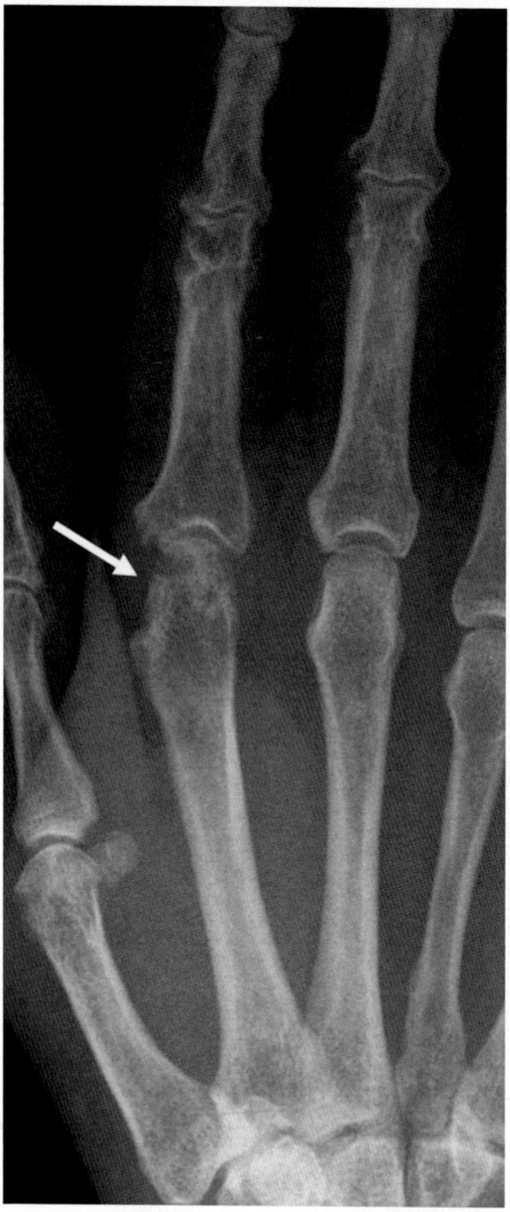

On MR imaging, tophi with a heterogeneous signal depending on the amount of calcification can be seen. Most tophi enhance homogenously after IV gadolinium administration. The distribution of intra-articular and periarticular inflammation, erosions, and the relative joint-sparing are clues toward a diagnosis of gout.

On US, deposits of monosodium urate crystals are bright, hyperechoic signals either on the surface of the cartilage or as deposits in joints and tendons. The gout-specific findings include the double contour (DC) sign (**Fig. 32**) and tophi, although aggregates and bone erosions also are listed as gout related.[114] Even though most frequently seen in the first MTP joint, urate crystal deposits also may be seen in the upper limbs—especially in wrists and the MCP joint and in the triceps tendon and with joint affection may mimic RA.[115] The US definitions for gout-specific lesions were validated in 2015 to ensure homogeneity among future studies and in clinical practice.[114,116,117] Studies have shown the DC sign highly specific (specificity ≥0.98) for gout,[118,119] and it is now part of the 2015 ACR/EULAR gout classification criteria.[120] Although highly specific for gout, the DC sign is not present in all patients with gout and especially not in very early disease. Tophus-like changes are, like the DC sign, almost exclusively found in gout,[121] and the specificity in studies are greater than or equal to 0.90.[119,122,123] The role of US for monitoring treatment effect has yet to be determined.

Fig. 31. 63-year-old man with known gout. Anteroposterior radiograph during acute phase shows chronic erosive changes with sclerotic border and concurrent soft tissue swelling around the second MCP joint (*arrow*). US confirmed hyperemia. Aspiration showed urate crystals.

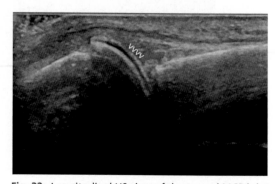

Fig. 32. Longitudinal US view of the second MCP joint in gout patient shows DC sign (vvvv).

DECT has revolutionized gout imaging. The technology can separate urate and calcium in a highly sensitive way because the tissues have different absorption spectra on 80-kiloelectron and 140/150-kiloelectron voltage. Thus, DECT has become the recommended modality to diagnose urate distribution around the joint in 3-D and even automatically calculate the volume of urate (**Fig. 33**) along with any change of urate load after treatment.[113,124,125] In addition, with a bone algorithm, conventional CT images can be used to detect potential erosive changes with better sensitivity and in more detail than either CR or MR imaging. DECT has reduced the need for aspiration of joint fluid and phase-contrast microscopic analysis to make the diagnosis and for these reasons has become part of the classification system for gout evaluation recommended by both ACR and EULAR,[120] even though the technology misclassifies several artifacts as gout[126] and lacks international agreement regarding imaging protocols and post-processing standards.

PSEUDOGOUT, OR CALCIUM PYROPHOSPHATE DEPOSITION DISEASE

CPPD is seen due to deposition of calcium crystals in the cartilage, fibrocartilage, and soft tissue around the affected joints but also can be seen in ligaments and tendons throughout the body.

CPPD is the most common crystal arthropathy associated with primary hyperparathyroidism and hemochromatosis. Most cases are seen without these conditions, however, usually in middle-aged and elderly patients and often with multiple medical comorbidities like heart disease and/or metabolic syndrome.[127] CPPD presents with a heterogeneous clinical picture ranging from asymptomatic to pseudogout syndrome with a sudden onset of 1 or several painful swollen joints that can mimic gout, infectious arthritis, neuropathic arthritis, or even RA.[128] Unlike most other inflammatory joint diseases, no specific treatment exists that can reduce or prevent deposition of crystals in the tissues.[128] In the upper extremity, the first radiocarpal (RC) joint, triangular fibrocartilage complex (TFCC), and MCP joints are predilection sites (**Fig. 34**) and in contrast to primary OA the elbow and shoulder often are affected (**Fig. 35**). On CR, fine linear or punctuate CPPD crystals can be seen distributed in the cartilage of the RC joint, TFCC, wrist ligaments, or around the MCP joints (**Fig. 36A**) that progress with large cystic changes and erosions along with asymmetric joint space narrowing, subchondral sclerosis, and osteophytes that mimic OA.[129] One distinct feature is development of hook-like osteophytes of the head of the distal metacarpal bones that should suggest CPPD or hemochromatosis (**Fig. 36B**).[130]

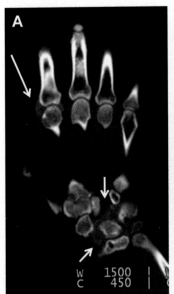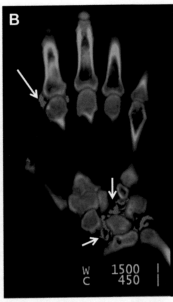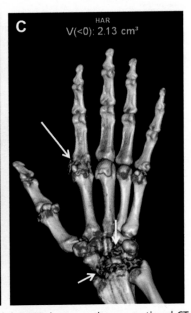

Fig. 33. A 44-year-old man with known tophi of the second MCP joint. (*A*) DECT shows on the conventional CT scan hyperdense deposits around the second MCP joint (*long arrow*) and between the wrist bones (*short arrows*). (*B*) DECT image and (*C*) volume rendering image show that these dense lesions are classified as gout crystals, seen as green spots in both images (*arrows*). (*C*) The number of green voxels can be counted and converted to a volume (V) in cm³, as shown in the top of image. (*Courtesy of* Dr. Felix Müller, Department of Radiology, Herlev Hospital, Denmark.)

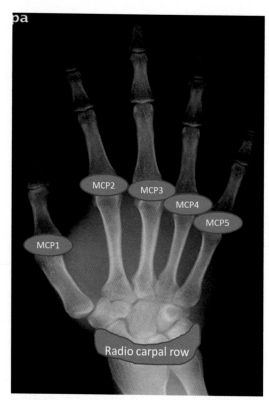

Fig. 34. Typical distribution pattern of hand CPPD with asymmetric involvement of the first RC joint, TFCC, and MCP joints as predilection sites.

MR imaging can show features similar to those seen in OA and the other inflammatory joint arthritis, including erosions, but the anatomic distribution in the CPPD points to CPPD[131] because

small calcification are difficult to detect on MR imaging (**Fig. 36**C). Similar to other types of arthritis, CT can help visualize the bony changes, and the calcifications in the cartilage, TFCC, capsule, and soft tissue especially can be appreciated in a more detailed fashion.[124] DECT can help differentiate between urate and calcium depositions (see **Fig. 33**).[112] Dedicated extremity cone beam CT also has recently been introduced to the imaging market and might have a place for assessment of this disease in peripheral joints, that is, the hand and elbow, because the technology uses very low radiation dose and high spatial resolution compared with whole-body CT scanners (**Fig. 37**). Shoulders cannot be imaged in these scanners due to their design.[132]

As with gout, US for CPPD may show the crystal deposits in the cartilage—both hyaline and fibrocartilage—as hyperechoic spots without acoustic shadowing at different joint sites.[133–135] In the upper limb, the TFCC is the most important site. Validation of US definitions for CPPD recently was published showing that it is most reliable in the TFCC and the acromioclavicular joint (**Fig. 38**).[136,137] The diagnostic value of US currently is being investigated.

HYDROXYAPATITE CRYSTAL DEPOSITION DISEASE

HADD is another common crystal deposition disease that affects primarily soft tissue and tendons and rarely affects joints. In the upper extremity it is seen as tendinitis or bursitis in the shoulder, elbow, and hand in decreasing frequency. The heterogeneous affection can be

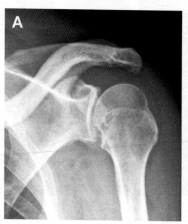
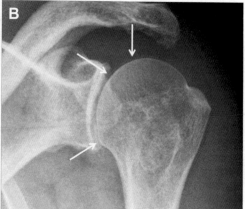

Fig. 35. A 65-year-old man with neck and shoulder pain. Subtle areas of chondrocalcinosis are seen in the glenohumeral joint, with more chondrocalcinosis in the cervical spine. (A) Anteroposterior radiograph of the left shoulder shows mild and uniform joint space narrowing. (B) An internally rotated radiograph of the same shoulder better shows the chondrocalcinosis as a fine cartilage calcification of the humeral head (*arrows*).

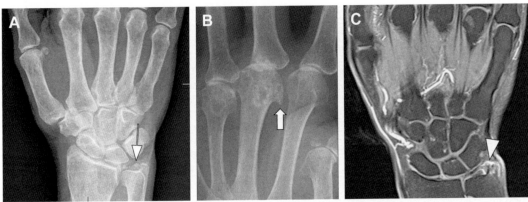

Fig. 36. A 72-year-old woman with no established diagnosis of arthritis, presenting with acute nontraumatic ulnar-sided wrist pain. (*A*) Anteroposterior radiograph of the wrist shows no relevant degenerative changes but marked calcification of the TFCC consistent with CPPD (*arrow*). (*B*) Typical hook-like osteophyte of the third metacarpal head (*arrow*) seen in CPPD and hemochromatosis. (*C*) Coronal contrast-enhanced fat-suppressed T1-weighted MR imaging of the same patients as (*A*) shows marked synovitis around the ulnar styloid process and the TFCC (*arrowhead*). Note inferior sensitivity of MR imaging for the detection of calcifications. The clinical presentation is consistent with an attack of pseudogout due to CPPD.

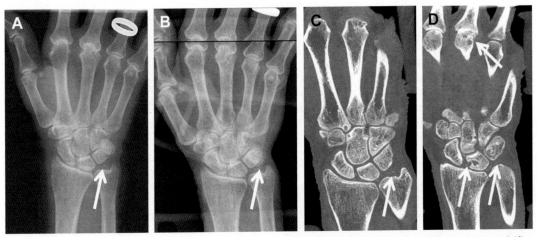

Fig. 37. (*A*) Anteroposterior radiograph of the wrist of left hand in a 70-year-old woman shows linear calcifications in the TFCC (*arrow*) that is seen equally well on the scout from the cone beam (CB) CT image (*B*). (*C, D*) At the same time, the distribution of calcium pyrophosphate deposits and corresponding erosions in the lunate and second MCP joint are better appreciated on the coronal reformats from the CBCT scan (*arrows*).

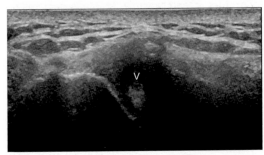

Fig. 38. US longitudinal view of the acromioclavicular joint in CPPD patient with crystal deposits (v) in the joint.

seen on CR, with periarticular calcification and linear dense depositions in soft tissue that develop to homogeneous well-delineated circular shapes, that is, in the flexor carpi ulnaris or radialis tendons around the wrist, the tendons around the elbow, or the supraspinatus tendon of the shoulder (known as calcific tendinitis) (Fig. 39).[131] Involvement of several other tendons of the rotator cuff has been described but is infrequent.[129] Patients with involvement of the shoulder tendons typically present with impingement symptoms, where US shows a hyperechoic deposition in a thickened tendon that is

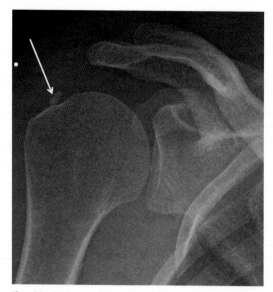

Fig. 39. Patient with pain and reporting symptoms indicative of impingement. Anteroposterior radiograph of the right shoulder shows a dense rounded deposit in the supraspinatus tendon space consistent with calcific tendinitis (*arrow*).

supraspinatus and that impinges under the acromion during abduction of the arm. If the crystals rupture into nearby subdeltoid bursa, a severe inflammatory response can occur with rapidly progressing destructive arthritis, known as Milwaukee shoulder (**Fig. 40**).

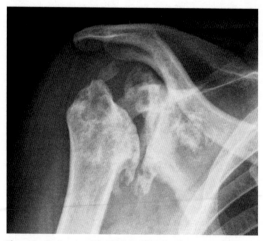

Fig. 40. Patient with HADD. The hydroxyapatite content erodes into the subacromial bursae, and aggressive arthritis with fast joint destruction develops, known as Milwaukee shoulder. Anteroposterior radiograph of the shoulder shows severe example of Milwaukee shoulder with complete joint destruction and surrounding calcified deposits.

On MR imaging, all the soft tissues and bone changes can be visualized, but, as in other inflammatory joint conditions, MR imaging findings are unspecific. Most often, the suspicion of HADD originates from either CR or US, but CT is the reference standard to depict the distribution and shape of the calcifications.

SUMMARY

Imaging findings in rheumatic conditions, especially inflammatory and degenerative joint diseases, often are nonspecific, especially in the early stages, as highlighted in this review. Thus, imaging findings should be interpreted taking into consideration the clinical context, that is, the clinical history and the clinical and paraclinical findings. To do so requires that reading radiologists be provided with a good referral that briefly states the clinical history; the main clinical findings, including involved joint(s); and disease and pain distribution as well as relevant blood tests and suspected diagnoses. This increases the likelihood of a correct diagnosis. CR is the first line of examination in all suspected arthritic conditions. Depending on the CR findings, the disease distribution, and the clinical history, the diagnostic workup can be supported by additional MR imaging, including DCE–MR imaging, US, and/or CT, including DECT and/or CBCT.

DISCLOSURES

M. Boesen is a shareholder of Image Analysis Group and has received consultancy/speaker/travel fees from Image Analysis Group, Eli Lilly, Esaote, Celgene, Pfizer, Abbvie, Carestream/Canon, Siemens, and AstraZeneca. F.W. Roemer is a shareholder of BICL. M. Østergaard has received speaker fees and/or consulting fees from Abbvie, BMS, Boehringer-Ingelheim, Celgene, Eli-Lilly, Hospira, Janssen, Merck, Novartis, Novo, Orion, Pfizer, Regeneron, Roche, and UCB and research support from Abbvie, Celgene, Centocor, Merck, and Novartis. M. Maas declares no conflict declared. L. Terslev has received speaker's fees from Roche, Pfizer, MSD, BMS, Novartis, Celgene, and GE. A. Guermazi is a shareholder of BICL and serves as a consultant to Pfizer, TissueGene, Merck Serono, AstraZeneca, Galapagos, and Roche.

ACKNOWLEDGMENTS

Thank you to the Parker Institute and Oak Foundation as well as the board of directors of Bispebjerg and Frederiksberg Hospital for supporting M. Boesen's research.

REFERENCES

1. Gholamrezanezhad A, Guermazi A, Salavati A, et al. PET-CT-MRI applications of musculoskeletal disorders, part I. PET Clin 2018;13(4):i.

2. Xie F, Kovic B, Jin X, et al. Economic and humanistic burden of osteoarthritis: a systematic review of large sample studies. Pharmacoeconomics 2016; 34(11):1087–100.

3. Allen KD, Golightly YM. State of the evidence. Curr Opin Rheumatol 2015;27(3):276–83.

4. Kloppenburg M, Kwok WY. Hand osteoarthritis–a heterogeneous disorder. Nat Rev Rheumatol 2011;8(1):22–31.

5. Belhorn LR, Hess EV. Erosive osteoarthritis. Semin Arthritis Rheum 1993;22(5):298–306.

6. Keats TE, Johnstone WH, O'Brien WM. Large joint destruction in erosive osteoarthritis. Skeletal Radiol 1981;6(4):267–9.

7. Punzi L, Ramonda R, Sfriso P. Erosive osteoarthritis. Best Pract Res Clin Rheumatol 2004;18(5): 739–58.

8. Greenway G, Resnick D, Weisman M, et al. Carpal involvement in inflammatory (erosive) osteoarthritis. J Can Assoc Radiol 1979;30(2):95–8.

9. Greenspan A. Erosive osteoarthritis. Semin Musculoskelet Radiol 2003;7(2):155–9.

10. Gazeley DJ, Yeturi S, Patel PJ, et al. Erosive osteoarthritis: a systematic analysis of definitions used in the literature. Semin Arthritis Rheum 2017;46(4): 395–403.

11. Altman RD, Gold GE. Atlas of individual radiographic features in osteoarthritis, revised. Osteoarthritis Cartilage 2007;15(Suppl A):A1–56.

12. Brower AC, Flemming DJ. 13 - osteoarthritis. In: Brower AC, Flemming DJ, editors. Arthritis in black and white. 3rd edition. Philadelphia: W.B. Saunders; 2012. p. 243–60.

13. Haugen IK, Felson DT, Englund M, et al. The association between erosive hand osteoarthritis and subchondral bone attrition of the knee: the Framingham Osteoarthritis Study. Ann Rheum Dis 2012;71(10):1698–701.

14. Olejarova M, Kupka K, Pavelka K, et al. Comparison of clinical, laboratory, radiographic, and scintigraphic findings in erosive and nonerosive hand osteoarthritis. Results of a two-year study. Joint Bone Spine 2000;67(2):107–12.

15. Ostendorf B, Mattes-Gyorgy K, Reichelt DC, et al. Early detection of bony alterations in rheumatoid and erosive arthritis of finger joints with high-resolution single photon emission computed tomography, and differentiation between them. Skeletal Radiol 2010;39(1):55–61.

16. Haugen IK, Boyesen P, Slatkowsky-Christensen B, et al. Comparison of features by MRI and radiographs of the interphalangeal finger joints in patients with hand osteoarthritis. Ann Rheum Dis 2012;71(3):345–50.

17. Boesen M, Ostergaard M, Cimmino MA, et al. MRI quantification of rheumatoid arthritis: current knowledge and future perspectives. Eur J Radiol 2009; 71(2):189–96.

18. Jans L, De Coninck T, Wittoek R, et al. 3 T DCE-MRI assessment of synovitis of the interphalangeal joints in patients with erosive osteoarthritis for treatment response monitoring. Skeletal Radiol 2013; 42(2):255–60.

19. Schraml C, Schwenzer NF, Martirosian P, et al. Assessment of synovitis in erosive osteoarthritis of the hand using DCE-MRI and comparison with that in its major mimic, the psoriatic arthritis. Acad Radiol 2011;18(7):804–9.

20. Tan AL, Grainger AJ, Tanner SF, et al. High-resolution magnetic resonance imaging for the assessment of hand osteoarthritis. Arthritis Rheum 2005; 52(8):2355–65.

21. Haugen IK, Eshed I, Gandjbakhch F, et al. The longitudinal reliability and responsiveness of the OMERACT hand osteoarthritis magnetic resonance imaging scoring system (HOAMRIS). J Rheumatol 2015;42(12). https://doi.org/10.3899/jrheum.140983.

22. Vlychou M, Koutroumpas A, Malizos K, et al. Ultrasonographic evidence of inflammation is frequent in hands of patients with erosive osteoarthritis. Osteoarthritis Cartilage 2009;17(10):1283–7.

23. Wittoek R, Jans L, Lambrecht V, et al. Reliability and construct validity of ultrasonography of soft tissue and destructive changes in erosive osteoarthritis of the interphalangeal finger joints: a comparison with MRI. Ann Rheum Dis 2011;70(2):278–83.

24. Grainger AJ, Farrant JM, O'Connor PJ, et al. MR imaging of erosions in interphalangeal joint osteoarthritis: is all osteoarthritis erosive? Skeletal Radiol 2007;36(8):737–45.

25. Kortekaas MC, Kwok WY, Reijnierse M, et al. In erosive hand osteoarthritis more inflammatory signs on ultrasound are found than in the rest of hand osteoarthritis. Ann Rheum Dis 2013;72(6):930–4.

26. Mancarella L, Addimanda O, Pelotti P, et al. Ultrasound detected inflammation is associated with the development of new bone erosions in hand osteoarthritis: a longitudinal study over 3.9 years. Osteoarthritis Cartilage 2015;23(11). https://doi.org/10.1016/j.joca.2015.06.004.

27. Kortekaas MC, Kwok WY, Reijnierse M, et al. Inflammatory ultrasound features show independent associations with progression of structural damage after over 2 years of follow-up in patients with hand osteoarthritis. Ann Rheum Dis 2015; 74(9):1720–4.

28. Mohan G, Perilli E, Kuliwaba JS, et al. Application of in vivo micro-computed tomography in the

temporal characterisation of subchondral bone architecture in a rat model of low-dose monosodium iodoacetate-induced osteoarthritis. Arthritis Res Ther 2011;13(6):R210.

29. Svensson C-M, Hoffmann B, Irmler IM, et al. Quantification of arthritic bone degradation by analysis of 3D micro-computed tomography data. Sci Rep 2017;7:44434. Available at: https://www.nature.com/articles/srep44434#supplementary-information.

30. Gabriel SE. The epidemiology of rheumatoid arthritis. Rheum Dis Clin North Am 2001;27(2):269–81.

31. Fleming A, Crown JM, Corbett M. Incidence of joint involvement in early rheumatoid arthritis. Rheumatol Rehabil 1976;15(2):92–6.

32. Schett G, Gravallese E. Bone erosion in rheumatoid arthritis: mechanisms, diagnosis and treatment. Nat Rev Rheumatol 2012;8(11):656–64.

33. Hetland ML, Stengaard-Pedersen K, Junker P, et al. Combination treatment with methotrexate, cyclosporine, and intraarticular betamethasone compared with methotrexate and intraarticular betamethasone in early active rheumatoid arthritis: an investigator-initiated, multicenter, randomized, double-blind, parallel-group, placebo-controlled study. Arthritis Rheum 2006;54(5):1401–9.

34. Horslev-Petersen K, Hetland ML, Ornbjerg LM, et al. Clinical and radiographic outcome of a treat-to-target strategy using methotrexate and intra-articular glucocorticoids with or without adalimumab induction: a 2-year investigator-initiated, double-blinded, randomised, controlled trial (OPERA). Ann Rheum Dis 2016;75(9):1645–53.

35. Smolen JS, Landewé R, Bijlsma J, et al. EULAR recommendations for the management of rheumatoid arthritis with synthetic and biological disease-modifying antirheumatic drugs: 2016 update. Ann Rheum Dis 2017;76(6):960–77.

36. Peterfy C, Strand V, Tian L, et al. Short-term changes on MRI predict long-term changes on radiography in rheumatoid arthritis: an analysis by an OMERACT Task Force of pooled data from four randomised controlled trials. Ann Rheum Dis 2017;76(6):992–7.

37. Peterfy C, Ostergaard M, Conaghan PG. MRI comes of age in RA clinical trials. Ann Rheum Dis 2013;72(6):794–6.

38. Baker JF, Conaghan PG, Emery P, et al. Validity of early MRI structural damage end points and potential impact on clinical trial design in rheumatoid arthritis. Ann Rheum Dis 2016;75(6):1114–9.

39. Ostergaard M, Peterfy CG, Bird P, et al. The OMERACT rheumatoid arthritis magnetic resonance imaging (MRI) scoring system: updated recommendations by the OMERACT MRI in arthritis working group. J Rheumatol 2017;44(11):1706–12.

40. Stomp W, Krabben A, van der Heijde D, et al. Aiming for a simpler early arthritis MRI protocol: can Gd contrast administration be eliminated? Eur Radiol 2015;25(5):1520–7.

41. Tehranzadeh J, Ashikyan O, Anavim A, et al. Enhanced MR imaging of tenosynovitis of hand and wrist in inflammatory arthritis. Skeletal Radiol 2006;35(11):814–22.

42. Boesen M, Kubassova O, Sudol-Szopinska I, et al. MR imaging of joint infection and inflammation with emphasis on dynamic contrast-enhanced MR imaging. PET Clin 2018;13(4):523–50.

43. Khalifa F, Soliman A, El-Baz A, et al. Models and methods for analyzing DCE-MRI: a review. Med Phys 2014;41(12):124301.

44. O'Connor JP, Jackson A, Parker GJ, et al. Dynamic contrast-enhanced MRI in clinical trials of antivascular therapies. Nat Rev Clin Oncol 2012;9(3):167–77.

45. Turkbey B, Thomasson D, Pang Y, et al. The role of dynamic contrast-enhanced MRI in cancer diagnosis and treatment. Diagn Interv Radiol 2009;16(3):186–92.

46. Ostergaard M, Hansen M, Stoltenberg M, et al. New radiographic bone erosions in the wrists of patients with rheumatoid arthritis are detectable with magnetic resonance imaging a median of two years earlier. Arthritis Rheum 2003;48(8):2128–31.

47. Taouli B, Guermazi A, Sack KE, et al. Imaging of the hand and wrist in RA. Ann Rheum Dis 2002;61(10):867–9.

48. Ejbjerg BJ, Vestergaard A, Jacobsen S, et al. Conventional radiography requires a MRI-estimated bone volume loss of 20% to 30% to allow certain detection of bone erosions in rheumatoid arthritis metacarpophalangeal joints. Arthritis Res Ther 2006;8(3):R59.

49. McQueen FM. Bone marrow edema and osteitis in rheumatoid arthritis: the imaging perspective. Arthritis Res Ther 2012;14(5):224.

50. Hetland ML, Ejbjerg B, Horslev-Petersen K, et al. MRI bone oedema is the strongest predictor of subsequent radiographic progression in early rheumatoid arthritis. Results from a 2-year randomised controlled trial (CIMESTRA). Ann Rheum Dis 2009;68(3):384–90.

51. Baker JF, Ostergaard M, Emery P, et al. Early MRI measures independently predict 1-year and 2-year radiographic progression in rheumatoid arthritis: secondary analysis from a large clinical trial. Ann Rheum Dis 2014;73(11):1968–74.

52. Jimenez-Boj E, Nobauer-Huhmann I, Hanslik-Schnabel B, et al. Bone erosions and bone marrow edema as defined by magnetic resonance imaging reflect true bone marrow inflammation in rheumatoid arthritis. Arthritis Rheum 2007;56(4):1118–24.

53. Szkudlarek M, Court-Payen, Jacobsen S, et al. Interobserver agreement in ultrasonography of the finger and toe joints in rheumatoid arthritis. Arthritis Rheum 2003;48(4):955–62.

54. Brown AK, Quinn MA, Karim Z, et al. Presence of significant synovitis in rheumatoid arthritis patients with disease-modifying antirheumatic drug-induced clinical remission: evidence from an imaging study may explain structural progression. Arthritis Rheum 2006;54(12):3761–73.

55. Wakefield RJ, Green MJ, Marzo-Ortega H, et al. Should oligoarthritis be reclassified? Ultrasound reveals a high prevalence of subclinical disease. Ann Rheum Dis 2004;63(4):382–5.

56. Terslev L, von der RP, Torp-Pedersen S, et al. Diagnostic sensitivity and specificity of Doppler ultrasound in rheumatoid arthritis. J Rheumatol 2008;35(1):49–53.

57. Aletaha D, Neogi T, Silman AJ, et al. 2010 rheumatoid arthritis classification criteria: an American College of Rheumatology/European League Against Rheumatism collaborative initiative. Ann Rheum Dis 2010;69(9):1580–8.

58. Aletaha D, Neogi T, Silman AJ, et al. 2010 rheumatoid arthritis classification criteria: an American College of Rheumatology/European League Against Rheumatism collaborative initiative. Arthritis Rheum 2010;62(9):2569–81.

59. Filer A, de Pablo P, Allen G, et al. Utility of ultrasound joint counts in the prediction of rheumatoid arthritis in patients with very early synovitis. Ann Rheum Dis 2011;70(3):500–7.

60. Nakagomi D, Ikeda K, Okubo A, et al. Ultrasound can improve the accuracy of the 2010 American College of Rheumatology/European League against rheumatism classification criteria for rheumatoid arthritis to predict the requirement for methotrexate treatment. Arthritis Rheum 2013;65(4):890–8.

61. Haavardsholm EA, Aga A-B, Olsen IC, et al. Ultrasound in management of rheumatoid arthritis: ARCTIC randomised controlled strategy trial. BMJ 2016;354. https://doi.org/10.1136/bmj.i4205.

62. Lillegraven S, Boyesen P, Hammer HB, et al. Tenosynovitis of the extensor carpi ulnaris tendon predicts erosive progression in early rheumatoid arthritis. Ann Rheum Dis 2011;70(11):2049–50.

63. Naredo E, Moller I, Cruz A, et al. Power Doppler ultrasonographic monitoring of response to anti-tumor necrosis factor therapy in patients with rheumatoid arthritis. Arthritis Rheum 2008;58(8):2248–56.

64. Pascual-Ramos V, Contreras-Yanez I, Cabiedes-Contreras J, et al. Hypervascular synovitis and American College of Rheumatology Classification Criteria as predictors of radiographic damage in early rheumatoid arthritis. Ultrasound Q 2009;25(1):31–8.

65. Taylor PC, Steuer A, Gruber J, et al. Ultrasonographic and radiographic results from a two-year controlled trial of immediate or one-year-delayed addition of infliximab to ongoing methotrexate therapy in patients with erosive early rheumatoid arthritis. Arthritis Rheum 2006;54(1):47–53.

66. Backhaus M, Kamradt T, Sandrock D, et al. Arthritis of the finger joints: a comprehensive approach comparing conventional radiography, scintigraphy, ultrasound, and contrast-enhanced magnetic resonance imaging. Arthritis Rheum 1999;42(6):1232–45.

67. Szkudlarek M, Narvestad E, Klarlund M, et al. Ultrasonography of the metatarsophalangeal joints in rheumatoid arthritis: comparison with magnetic resonance imaging, conventional radiography, and clinical examination. Arthritis Rheum 2004;50(7):2103–12.

68. Dohn UM, Ejbjerg BJ, Court-Payen, et al. Are bone erosions detected by magnetic resonance imaging and ultrasonography true erosions? A comparison with computed tomography in rheumatoid arthritis metacarpophalangeal joints. Arthritis Res Ther 2006;8(4):R110.

69. Dohn UM, Terslev L, Szkudlarek M, et al. Detection, scoring and volume assessment of bone erosions by ultrasonography in rheumatoid arthritis: comparison with CT. Ann Rheum Dis 2013;72(4):530–4.

70. Lillegraven S, Prince FH, Shadick NA, et al. Remission and radiographic outcome in rheumatoid arthritis: application of the 2011 ACR/EULAR remission criteria in an observational cohort. Ann Rheum Dis 2012;71(5):681–6.

71. Brown AK, Conaghan PG, Karim Z, et al. An explanation for the apparent dissociation between clinical remission and continued structural deterioration in rheumatoid arthritis. Arthritis Rheum 2008;58(10):2958–67.

72. Dale J, Stirling A, Zhang R, et al. Targeting ultrasound remission in early rheumatoid arthritis: the results of the TaSER study, a randomised clinical trial. Ann Rheum Dis 2016;75(6):1043–50.

73. Dohn UM, Ejbjerg BJ, Hasselquist M, et al. Detection of bone erosions in rheumatoid arthritis wrist joints with magnetic resonance imaging, computed tomography and radiography. Arthritis Res Ther 2008;10(1):R25.

74. Jans L, De Kock I, Herregods N, et al. Dual-energy CT: a new imaging modality for bone marrow oedema in rheumatoid arthritis. Ann Rheum Dis 2018;77(6):958–60.

75. Wu H, Zhang G, Huang X, et al. Use of dual-energy CT to detect and depict bone marrow oedema in rheumatoid arthritis: is it ready to substitute MRI? Ann Rheum Dis 2018. https://doi.org/10.1136/annrheumdis-2018-213892.

76. Ogdie A, Weiss P. The epidemiology of psoriatic arthritis. Rheum Dis Clin North Am 2015;41(4): 545–68.

77. Tevar-Sanchez MI, Navarro-Compan V, Aznar JJ, et al. Prevalence and characteristics associated with dactylitis in patients with early spondyloarthritis: results from the ESPeranza cohort. Clin Exp Rheumatol 2018;36(5):879–83.

78. Sudol-Szopinska I, Matuszewska G, Kwiatkowska B, et al. Diagnostic imaging of psoriatic arthritis. Part I: etiopathogenesis, classifications and radiographic features. J Ultrason 2016;16(64):65–77.

79. Jacobson JA, Girish G, Jiang Y, et al. Radiographic evaluation of arthritis: inflammatory conditions. Radiology 2008;248(2):378–89.

80. Jadon DR, Shaddick G, Tillett W, et al. Psoriatic arthritis mutilans: characteristics and natural radiographic history. J Rheumatol 2015;42(7):1169–76.

81. Anandarajah A. Imaging in psoriatic arthritis. Clin Rev Allergy Immunol 2013;44(2):157–65.

82. Poggenborg RP, Østergaard M, Terslev L. Imaging in psoriatic arthritis. Rheum Dis Clin North Am 2015;41(4):593–613.

83. Sudol-Szopinska I, Pracoń G. Diagnostic imaging of psoriatic arthritis. Part II: magnetic resonance imaging and ultrasonography. J Ultrason 2016; 16(65):163–74.

84. Tan AL, Fukuba E, Halliday NA, et al. High-resolution MRI assessment of dactylitis in psoriatic arthritis shows flexor tendon pulley and sheath-related enthesitis. Ann Rheum Dis 2015;74(1): 185–9.

85. Healy PJ, Groves C, Chandramohan M, et al. MRI changes in psoriatic dactylitis–extent of pathology, relationship to tenderness and correlation with clinical indices. Rheumatology (Oxford) 2008;47(1): 92–5.

86. Ostergaard M, McQueen F, Wiell C, et al. The OMERACT psoriatic arthritis magnetic resonance imaging scoring system (PsAMRIS): definitions of key pathologies, suggested MRI sequences, and preliminary scoring system for PsA hands. J Rheumatol 2009;36(8):1816–24.

87. Glinatsi D, Bird P, Gandjbakhch F, et al. Validation of the OMERACT psoriatic arthritis magnetic resonance imaging score (PsAMRIS) for the hand and foot in a randomized placebo-controlled trial. J Rheumatol 2015;42(12):2473–9.

88. Ostergaard M, Eshed I, Althoff CE, et al. Whole-body magnetic resonance imaging in inflammatory arthritis: systematic literature review and first steps toward standardization and an OMERACT scoring system. J Rheumatol 2017;44(11):1699–705.

89. Zabotti A, Bandinelli F, Batticciotto A, et al. Musculoskeletal ultrasonography for psoriatic arthritis and psoriasis patients: a systematic literature review. Rheumatology (Oxford) 2017;56(9):1518–32.

90. Delle Sedie A, Riente L, Filippucci E, et al. Ultrasound imaging for the rheumatologist. XXXII. Sonographic assessment of the foot in patients with psoriatic arthritis. Clin Exp Rheumatol 2011;29(2): 217–22.

91. Riente L, Delle Sedie A, Sakellariou G, et al. Ultrasound imaging for the rheumatologist XXXVIII. Sonographic assessment of the hip in psoriatic arthritis patients. Clin Exp Rheumatol 2012;30(2):152–5.

92. Schafer VS, Fleck M, Kellner H, et al. Evaluation of the novel ultrasound score for large joints in psoriatic arthritis and ankylosing spondylitis: six month experience in daily clinical practice. BMC Musculoskelet Disord 2013;14:358.

93. Wiell C, Szkudlarek M, Hasselquist M, et al. Ultrasonography, magnetic resonance imaging, radiography, and clinical assessment of inflammatory and destructive changes in fingers and toes of patients with psoriatic arthritis. Arthritis Res Ther 2007;9(6): R119.

94. Freeston JE, Coates LC, Nam JL, et al. Is there subclinical synovitis in early psoriatic arthritis? A clinical comparison with gray-scale and power Doppler ultrasound. Arthritis Care Res 2014;66(3): 432–9.

95. Naredo E, Batlle-Gualda E, Garcia-Vivar ML, et al. Power Doppler ultrasonography assessment of entheses in spondyloarthropathies: response to therapy of entheseal abnormalities. J Rheumatol 2010;37(10):2110–7.

96. Fraser AD, van Kuijk AW, Westhovens R, et al. A randomised, double blind, placebo controlled, multicentre trial of combination therapy with methotrexate plus ciclosporin in patients with active psoriatic arthritis. Ann Rheum Dis 2005;64(6): 859–64.

97. Backhaus M, Ohrndorf S, Kellner H, et al. Evaluation of a novel 7-joint ultrasound score in daily rheumatologic practice: a pilot project. Arthritis Rheum 2009;61(9):1194–201.

98. Ficjan A, Husic R, Gretler J, et al. Ultrasound composite scores for the assessment of inflammatory and structural pathologies in Psoriatic Arthritis (PsASon-Score). Arthritis Res Ther 2014; 16(5):476.

99. Gutierrez M, Di Geso L, Salaffi F, et al. Development of a preliminary US power Doppler composite score for monitoring treatment in PsA. Rheumatology (Oxford) 2012;51(7):1261–8.

100. El Miedany Y, El Gaafary M, Youssef S, et al. Tailored approach to early psoriatic arthritis patients: clinical and ultrasonographic predictors for structural joint damage. Clin Rheumatol 2015; 34(2):307–13.

101. Fournie B, Margarit-Coll N, Champetier de Ribes TL, et al. Extrasynovial ultrasound abnormalities in the psoriatic finger. Prospective

comparative power-doppler study versus rheumatoid arthritis. Joint Bone Spine 2006;73(5):527–31.

102. Kane D, Greaney T, Bresnihan B, et al. Ultrasonography in the diagnosis and management of psoriatic dactylitis. J Rheumatol 1999;26(8):1746–51.

103. Gutierrez M, Filippucci E, De Angelis R, et al. A sonographic spectrum of psoriatic arthritis: "the five targets. Clin Rheumatol 2010;29(2):133–42.

104. Olivieri I, Barozzi L, Favaro L, et al. Dactylitis in patients with seronegative spondylarthropathy. Assessment by ultrasonography and magnetic resonance imaging. Arthritis Rheum 1996;39(9):1524–8.

105. Balint PV, Kane D, Wilson H, et al. Ultrasonography of entheseal insertions in the lower limb in spondyloarthropathy. Ann Rheum Dis 2002;61(10):905–10.

106. Terslev L, Naredo E, Iagnocco A, et al. Defining enthesitis in spondyloarthritis by ultrasound: results of a Delphi process and of a reliability reading exercise. Arthritis Care Res (Hoboken) 2014;66(5):741–8.

107. Balint PV, Terslev L, Aegerter P, et al. Reliability of a consensus-based ultrasound definition and scoring for enthesitis in spondyloarthritis and psoriatic arthritis: an OMERACT US initiative. Ann Rheum Dis 2018;77(12):1730–5.

108. McGonagle D, Wakefield RJ, Tan AL, et al. Distinct topography of erosion and new bone formation in achilles tendon enthesitis: implications for understanding the link between inflammation and bone formation in spondylarthritis. Arthritis Rheum 2008;58(9):2694–9.

109. Tinazzi I, McGonagle D, Biasi D, et al. Preliminary evidence that subclinical enthesopathy may predict psoriatic arthritis in patients with psoriasis. J Rheumatol 2011;38(12):2691–2.

110. Pascart T, Liote F. Gout: state of the art after a decade of developments. Rheumatology (Oxford) 2018. https://doi.org/10.1093/rheumatology/key002.

111. Ragab G, Elshahaly M, Bardin T. Gout: an old disease in new perspective - a review. J Adv Res 2017;8(5):495–511.

112. Omoumi P, Zufferey P, Malghem J, et al. Imaging in gout and other crystal-related arthropathies. Rheum Dis Clin North Am 2016;42(4):621–44.

113. Dalbeth N, Doyle AJ. Imaging tools to measure treatment response in gout. Rheumatology (Oxford) 2018;57(suppl_1):i27–34.

114. Gutierrez M, Schmidt WA, Thiele RG, et al. International Consensus for ultrasound lesions in gout: results of Delphi process and web-reliability exercise. Rheumatology (Oxford) 2015;54(10):1797–805.

115. Slot O, Terslev L. Ultrasonographic signs of gout in symmetric polyarthritis. Arthritis Rheum 2010;62(11):3487.

116. Chowalloor PV, Keen HI. A systematic review of ultrasonography in gout and asymptomatic hyperuricaemia. Ann Rheum Dis 2013;72(5):638–45.

117. Terslev L, Gutierrez M, Christensen R, et al. Assessing elementary lesions in gout by ultrasound: results of an OMERACT patient-based agreement and reliability exercise. J Rheumatol 2015;42(11):2149–54.

118. Filippucci E, Riveros MG, Georgescu D, et al. Hyaline cartilage involvement in patients with gout and calcium pyrophosphate deposition disease. An ultrasound study. Osteoarthritis Cartilage 2009;17(2):178–81.

119. Ottaviani S, Richette P, Allard A, et al. Ultrasonography in gout: a case-control study. Clin Exp Rheumatol 2012;30(4):499–504.

120. Neogi T, Jansen TL, Dalbeth N, et al. 2015 gout classification criteria: an American College of Rheumatology/European League Against Rheumatism collaborative initiative. Ann Rheum Dis 2015;74(10):1789–98.

121. Naredo E, Uson J, Jimenez-Palop M, et al. Ultrasound-detected musculoskeletal urate crystal deposition: which joints and what findings should be assessed for diagnosing gout? Ann Rheum Dis 2014;73(8):1522–8.

122. Thiele RG, Schlesinger N. Diagnosis of gout by ultrasound. Rheumatology (Oxford) 2007;46(7):1116–21.

123. Wright SA, Filippucci E, McVeigh C, et al. High-resolution ultrasonography of the first metatarsal phalangeal joint in gout: a controlled study. Ann Rheum Dis 2007;66(7):859–64.

124. Wong WD, Shah S, Murray N, et al. Advanced musculoskeletal applications of dual-energy computed tomography. Radiol Clin North Am 2018;56(4):587–600.

125. Bayat S, Baraf HSB, Rech J. Update on imaging in gout: contrasting and comparing the role of dual-energy computed tomography to traditional diagnostic and monitoring techniques. Clin Exp Rheumatol 2018;36:53–60. Suppl 114(5).

126. Mallinson PI, Coupal T, Reisinger C, et al. Artifacts in dual-energy CT gout protocol: a review of 50 suspected cases with an artifact identification guide. Am J Roentgenol 2014;203(1):W103–9.

127. Sattui SE, Singh JA, Gaffo AL. Comorbidities in patients with crystal diseases and hyperuricemia. Rheum Dis Clin North Am 2014;40(2):251–78.

128. Rosenthal AK, Ryan LM. Calcium pyrophosphate deposition disease. N Engl J Med 2016;374(26):2575–84.

129. McQueen FM, Doyle A, Dalbeth N. Imaging in the crystal arthropathies. Rheum Dis Clin North Am 2014;40(2):231–49.

130. Magarelli N, Amelia R, Melillo N, et al. Imaging of chondrocalcinosis: calcium pyrophosphate

dihydrate (CPPD) crystal deposition disease – imaging of common sites of involvement. Clin Exp Rheumatol 2012;30(1):118–25.

131. Buckens CF, Terra MP, Maas M. Computed tomography and MR imaging in crystalline-induced arthropathies. Radiol Clin North Am 2017;55(5): 1023–34.

132. Carrino JA, Al Muhit A, Zbijewski W, et al. Dedicated cone-beam CT system for extremity imaging. Radiology 2014;270(3):816–24.

133. Filippou G, Adinolfi A, Cimmino MA, et al. Diagnostic accuracy of ultrasound, conventional radiography and synovial fluid analysis in the diagnosis of calcium pyrophosphate dihydrate crystal deposition disease. Clin Exp Rheumatol 2016;34(2):254–60.

134. Filippou G, Filippucci E, Tardella M, et al. Extent and distribution of CPP deposits in patients affected by calcium pyrophosphate dihydrate

deposition disease: an ultrasonographic study. Ann Rheum Dis 2013;72(11):1836–9.

135. Zufferey P, Valcov R, Fabreguet I, et al. A prospective evaluation of ultrasound as a diagnostic tool in acute microcrystalline arthritis. Arthritis Res Ther 2015;17:188.

136. Filippou G, Scire CA, Damjanov N, et al. Definition and reliability assessment of elementary ultrasonographic findings in calcium pyrophosphate deposition disease: a study by the OMERACT calcium pyrophosphate deposition disease ultrasound subtask force. J Rheumatol 2017;44(11):1744–9.

137. Filippou G, Scire CA, Adinolfi A, et al. Identification of calcium pyrophosphate deposition disease (CPPD) by ultrasound: reliability of the OMERACT definitions in an extended set of joints-an international multiobserver study by the OMERACT calcium pyrophosphate deposition disease ultrasound subtask force. Ann Rheum Dis 2018;77(8): 1194–9.

Imaging of Upper Limb Tumors and Tumorlike Pathology

Timothy Woo, MBChB, MA, FRCR[a], Radhesh Lalam, MBBS, MRCS, FRCR[a,*],
Victor Cassar-Pullicino, LRCP, MRCS, DMRD, FRCR, MD[a],
Bert Degrieck, MD[b], Koenraad Verstraete, MD[b],
Davide Maria Donati, MD[c,d], Giuseppe Guglielmi, MD[e],
Daniel Vanel, MD[f], Alberto Bazzocchi, MD, PhD[g]

KEYWORDS

- Bone tumor • Magnetic resonance imaging • Sarcoma • Tumor mimic • Upper limb

KEY POINTS

- Bone and soft tissue lesions may be found anywhere on the body, but some tumors and pathologies have an affinity for the upper extremity.
- Bone tumors are often first imaged with plain radiographs and soft tissue lesions with ultrasound. These appearances should help guide the need for further imaging.
- Many pathologies such as trauma, infection, and connective tissue disease can mimic tumors and it is important to keep the typical imaging characteristics of these lesions in mind when forming a differential diagnosis.
- Despite advanced imaging techniques, some soft tissue lesions are nonspecific in appearance and will warrant at least short-term follow-up or biopsy.
- All management of suspected soft tissue and bone sarcomas should be conducted through a specialized tertiary sarcoma service to optimize treatment and functional outcomes.

INTRODUCTION

This article covers the imaging strategy for characterization of common soft tissue and bony tumors of the upper limb, also taking into account commonly encountered pathology, such as inflammation or trauma, which may mimic malignancy. As well as more common imaging modalities, the role of newer options such as PET and elastography are also discussed.

The most common bone lesions are most usefully divided by patient age and tumor site, with a significantly different group of lesions more commonly found in the proximal humerus than more distally in the upper limb due to its retained red marrow.

Soft tissue lesions may be more difficult to diagnose accurately on imaging, but differentials often can be narrowed by the appearance of the lesion

Disclosure Statement: The authors report no conflicts of interest.
[a] Department of Radiology, Robert Jones and Agnes Hunt Orthopaedic Hospital NHS Foundation Trust, Oswestry SY10 7AG, UK; [b] Department of Radiology, Ghent University UZ-Gent, MR -1 K12, C. Heymanslaan 10, Gent B-9000, Belgium; [c] Department of Orthopaedic Oncology, IRCCS Istituto Ortopedico Rizzoli, Via G. C. Pupilli 1, Bologna 40136, Italy; [d] Department of Biomedical and Neuromotor Sciences, University of Bologna, Via U. Foscolo 7, Bologna 40123, Italy; [e] Department of Radiology, University of Foggia, Viale Luigi Pinto 1, Foggia 71100, Italy; [f] Department of Pathology, IRCCS Istituto Ortopedico Rizzoli, Via di Barbiano 1/10, Bologna 40136, Italy; [g] Diagnostic and Interventional Radiology, IRCCS Istituto Ortopedico Rizzoli, Via G.C. Pupilli 1, Bologna 40136, Italy
* Corresponding author.
E-mail address: radhesh.lalam@nhs.net

Radiol Clin N Am 57 (2019) 1035–1050
https://doi.org/10.1016/j.rcl.2019.03.008
0033-8389/19/Crown Copyright © 2019 Published by Elsevier Inc. All rights reserved.

on ultrasound, the presence of macroscopic fat or calcium, and anatomic associations.

BONE TUMORS

Bony tumors of the upper limb often present either symptomatically as bone pain or masses, or they can be discovered incidentally as a lesion on radiographs done for different indications. In either case, the first investigation acquired is often a radiograph. Appearances on the plain radiograph are often very helpful in the initial assessment of a bone lesion: determining whether it appears nonaggressive or aggressive and the lesional matrix if evident. The incidence of different bone lesions varies at different sites within the upper limb and age is also an important factor (**Fig. 1**). Unfortunately, drawbacks of radiographs are that some malignant tumors, such as low-grade chondrosarcoma, can appear relatively nonaggressive, and a variety of nonmalignant processes, such as Langerhans cell histiocytosis, subacute trauma, and infection, can appear relatively aggressive. Other facts to keep in mind are that primary bone sarcomas are rare, on the order of less than 1:100,000 incidence[1] and nonaggressive bone tumors and tumor mimics are much more

common.[2] The most common malignant bone lesion overall is metastasis, although in the pediatric population it is exceedingly rare to present with a bone metastasis without known malignancy,[3] and the most likely cause for an aggressive bony lesion in this age group is infection.

MR imaging of a bone lesion should always include at least a T1-weighted sequence and a fat-saturated fluid-sensitive sequence such as T2-weighted short tau inversion recovery (STIR) or proton density done in axial and long axis planes, including the whole bone and adjacent joints.[4] Gadolinium chelates are given in some institutions, but are most helpful for problem solving and follow-up posttreatment. Computed tomography (CT) is often complementary and can be helpful to demonstrate lesional matrix and periosteal reaction (although this can be evident on radiograph) and can be helpful if MR imaging is contraindicated or in difficult anatomic regions, for example, small bones of the hand. Diffusion-weighted (DWI) MR imaging, PET with fluorodeoxyglucose ([18]FDG-PET) and dynamic contrast-enhanced (DCE) MR imaging have been shown in multiple studies to be correlated with chemotherapy response in osteosarcoma.[5,6] DWI and DCE–MR imaging have been used in some

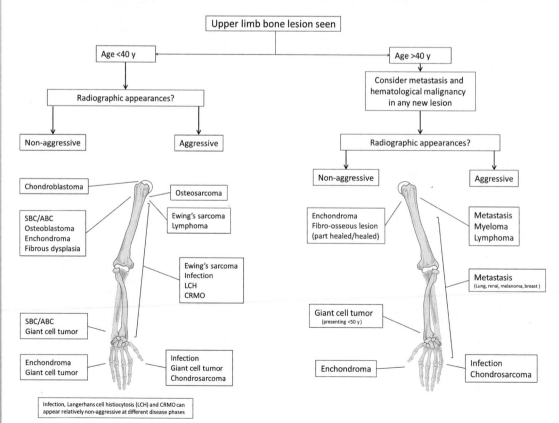

Fig. 1. Common bone lesions according to age and location in the upper limb.

studies to aid primary diagnosis, but cannot usually preclude biopsy and are not currently recommended as routine.[7] [18]FDG-PET is not currently routine for primary assessment, but recent studies have shown some benefit to staging accuracy in high-grade lesions[8] over chest CT alone[9] and both PET and DCE–MR imaging have been used in selected cases to indicate tumor extent and locate the most cellular and active parts of tumor for biopsy.[7] Many centers also use [18]FDG-PET to assess for local and distant recurrence where it has established benefit.[10] Na[18]F-PET has been used in the detection of bony metastases from osteosarcoma as well as other nonskeletal primaries, and demonstrates potentially better sensitivity compared with [18]FDG-PET for blastic lesions and conventionally FDG nonavid tumors, such as metastases from thyroid tumors. There is also better accuracy in the skull because of the absence of brain uptake.[11] However, it is poorer at detection of small lytic metastases and can demonstrate multiple false-positive areas due to benign causes of bone turnover (eg, degenerative disease).

Radiographically Nonaggressive Tumors

A nonaggressive radiographic appearance is characterized classically by a geographic lesion with narrow zone of transition to normal bone, benign, if any, periosteal reaction, and often a sclerotic border with no soft tissue component or cortical destruction.[4] Certain lesions, such as osteoid osteomas, are typical in appearance regardless of site. Primary bone tumors are vanishingly rare in those older than 40 years, and as such initial

discussion focuses on lesions presenting in the younger skeleton. Any new bone lesion found in a patient older than 40 should be considered malignant regardless of radiographic appearances, but benign lesions such as enchondromas can persist into older age and these are also discussed.

Patients younger than 40 years

Pathognomonic lesions Lesions such as osteoid osteomas are common in the upper limb and have a classic pathognomonic appearance of thick periosteal reaction on radiograph with a radiolucent nidus often more evident on CT. Lesions arising in the subcortical bone or medulla can lack the classic periosteal reaction, but the nidus is visible on CT (**Fig. 2**). MR imaging usually demonstrates profuse marrow, periosteal, and soft tissue edema. They can present in any bone of the upper extremity, but are slightly more common in the hand and carpus.[12] The differential for this appearance in the lower limb would be a stress fracture, which is not uncommon in active adolescents. Although a less common site, upper extremity stress fractures have been reported in weight lifters and throwing athletes,[13] and without this typical history, it should not be a routine consideration. Osteochondromas are another relatively common lesion that can occur anywhere in the upper limb, but that favor the proximal humerus and hand bones. The key features of a bony protuberance demonstrating continuity with marrow cavity pointing away from joint line is pathognomonic in most cases. The cartilage cap may demonstrate variable chondroid-type

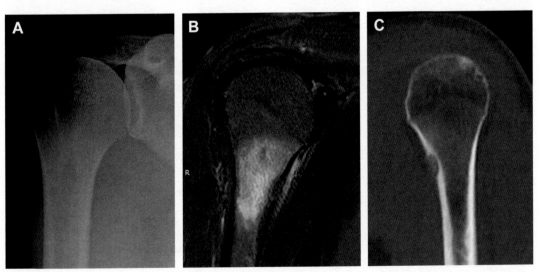

Fig. 2. Well-defined nonaggressive lytic lesion in the proximal humerus on radiograph lacking periosteal reaction (*A*), but MR imaging (*B*) and CT (*C*) demonstrate the typical radiodense nidus and intense bone marrow edema of an osteoid osteoma.

calcification, which can mimic other juxtacortical ossifying lesions, such as maturing myositis ossificans and parosteal osteosarcoma. In these cases, CT is helpful to demonstrate marrow continuity, although MR imaging and ultrasound are required to assess and follow up the cartilage cap thickness.

Distal upper limb lesions In the bones of the wrist and hand, a lytic lesion with a narrow zone of transition is most likely to represent an enchondroma, and approximately half of all enchondromata arise in the hands and feet.[1] Small bone enchondromas behave differently from other body sites: they rarely have matrix calcification, they can be expansile and/or exophytic in growth habit, and rarely transform into chondrosarcoma. Pathologically, hand enchondromata are more cellular and commonly demonstrate atypia, making correlation with radiological features more important. Features raising suspicion for malignancy include progressive bony destruction or cortical breakthrough, change of MR imaging characteristics/enhancement, development of a soft tissue mass, or clinical increase in pain. We follow-up these tumors at 1 and 3 years initially, with further follow-up dependent on interval change (**Fig. 3**). Surgical intervention is considered if interval growth exceeds 6 mm in one plane.[14] In some

studies, DCE–MR imaging has been used in this respect, but cannot reliably differentiate between a cellular active enchondroma and low-grade chondrosarcoma.[15]

Less common differentials for a lytic lesion in the wrist and hand bones include giant cell tumor (GCT) of bone in skeletally mature patients and simple and aneurysmal bone cysts (SBC/ABC) in the pediatric age group. In the upper limb, GCT is most common in the distal radius. GCT is an intermediate-grade tumor, which can be locally aggressive and has potential for metastasis, usually to lung. However, histologically, metastases are not malignant. GCT of the tubular bones of the hand is a distinct immunohistochemical subtype that occurs in a younger age group (<20 years) and often exhibits aggressive behavior with expansile growth pattern, extraosseous soft tissue, and a higher propensity for local recurrence[16] (**Fig. 4**). ABCs can be a primary tumor or secondarily associated with any bone tumor (most commonly GCT). Primary and secondary ABC can be distinguished histologically by fluorescence in situ hybridization for a specific genetic rearrangement in the USP6/CDH11 proto-oncogenes absent in secondary lesions.[17]

Although these lesions may appear similar radiographically, the lobulated fluidlike signal of enchondromata on MR imaging is reliably

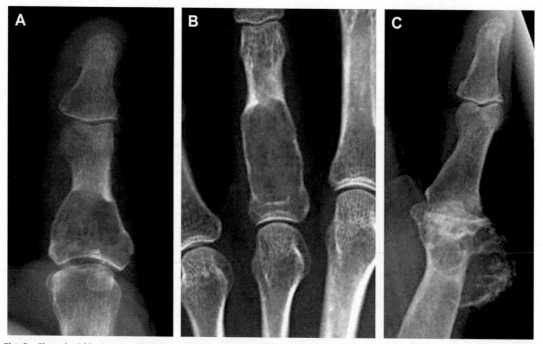

Fig. 3. Chondroid lesions in the tubular bones of the hands behave differently in other areas. They often show no matrix calcification (*A*) and can be markedly expansile (*B*) due to the small marrow space. Conversion to chondrosarcoma is thought to be rarer than at other sites, but cortical breach or associated calcifying soft tissue mass (*C*) should raise suspicion.

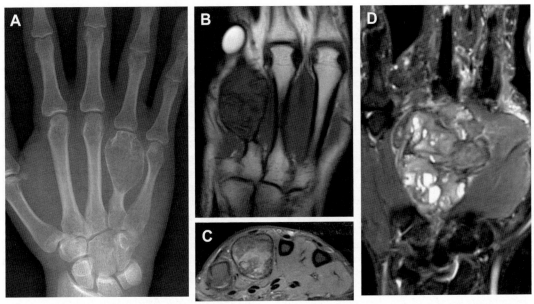

Fig. 4. Expansile and relatively aggressive-appearing lesion in the fourth metacarpal (*A*) demonstrating low signal on T1 (*B*) and intermediate-low signal on fat-saturated proton-density sequence (*C*) in keeping with GCT of bone. Six months following fourth ray amputation, coronal STIR (*D*) images demonstrate large soft tissue recurrence with ABC component.

differentiated from the intermediate to low inhomogeneous signal more commonly seen in GCT. The fluid-fluid levels of ABC are usually pathognomonic (**Fig. 5**). Gadolinium is not often required for diagnosis, but can be useful following curettage to demonstrate any recurrent or residual tumor. Other nonmalignant bone neoplasms, such as osteoblastoma, fibrous dysplasia, and chondroblastoma, also affect the distal upper limb, but are more common proximally.[18]

Proximal upper limb lesions A radiographically nonaggressive lesion in the unfused proximal humerus would include ABC and SBC for which it is the most common upper limb site. However, at this site, ABC-like components are seen in other

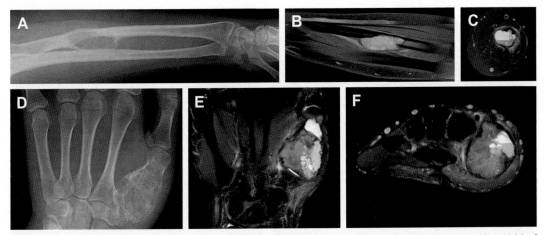

Fig. 5. Two cases demonstrating aneurysmal bone cyst formation. A well-marginated lucency in the midshaft radius (*A*) demonstrates fluid-fluid levels on sagittal fat-saturated proton density (*B*) and T2-weighted (*C*) images with no soft tissue component in keeping with a primary ABC. Radiograph demonstrates an expansile lucent lesion in the first metacarpal (*D*) showing fluid-fluid levels on coronal (*E*) and axial (*F*) fat-saturated proton-density images, but also a large soft tissue component. Biopsy of the soft tissue component demonstrated an osteoblastoma with secondary ABC change.

tumors, including telangiectatic osteosarcoma. Such lesions should be scrutinized for any evidence of aggressiveness: for example, cortical destruction or enhancing nodular tumor components, as the proximal humerus is also the most common site for osteosarcoma in the upper limb.

Osteoblastomas are usually lytic in nature with variable osseous matrix and can be associated with ABC. They are less common in the upper limb, but when they do occur usually involve the metadiaphyseal humerus more than the forearm or hand.[19] A lytic lesion involving the epiphysis or subchondral bone of the humeral head is suggestive of chondroblastoma in this age group. These 2 lesions may demonstrate alarmingly intense surrounding marrow and/or soft tissue edema on MR imaging, but can usually be differentiated by anatomic site and matrix calcification if present (**Fig. 6**). Nonossifying fibromas are common lesions of the immature skeleton, but are much rarer in the upper extremity compared with the lower in nonsyndromic patients.[20] However, the cortically based, often scalloped, and clearly defined radiographic appearance is often pathognomonic. Fibrous dysplasia is a common lesion found in any age group and in the upper limb is most commonly found in the proximal humerus. It can demonstrate a wide variety of appearances on radiograph and MR imaging, and demonstrates variable contrast enhancement and tracer avidity; however, its radiographic appearance is nonaggressive,[21] and it is nearly always medullary in location.

Patients older than 40 years

In older patients, these lesions are much less commonly encountered, as they have either been treated or have spontaneously healed; therefore, a new lytic lesion should be treated with suspicion for malignant pathology (most commonly metastasis or myeloma) until proven otherwise. Enchondromas are very common in the proximal humerus and can persist to adulthood, often incidentally demonstrated on shoulder investigations. CT is sometimes required to demonstrate matrix calcification and detail any cortical destruction that would suggest conversion to chondrosarcoma (**Fig. 7**). Well-defined sclerotic lesions are often seen, which are thought to represent healed areas of fibro-osseous lesions or bone cysts. MR imaging often demonstrates a mix of fluid and remodeled bone with marrow fat signal and no edema or destructive characteristics.

Radiographically Aggressive Tumors

Aggressive radiographic features include ill-defined margins and cortical destruction, often associated with complex periosteal reaction and soft tissue mass.[4] In the pediatric age group, this is most likely to represent infection, even in the absence of clinical signs of sepsis. In older patients, metastasis and myeloma are more common, especially if multifocal. The most common pathologies are discussed, with imaging strategies to differentiate tumor mimics.

Younger age group (<40 years)

Proximal upper limb lesions An aggressive tumor in the humerus in a young patient, especially

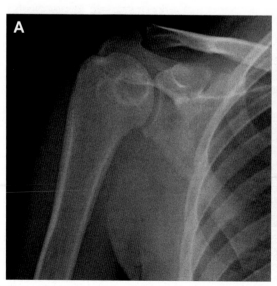
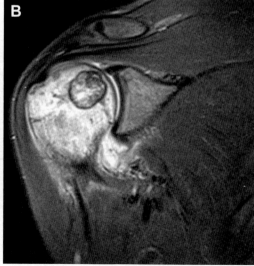

Fig. 6. Radiograph (*A*) demonstrates a well-circumscribed epiphyseal lesion in the humeral head with faint calcification. STIR (*B*) coronal image demonstrates the intense marrow edema typical for chondroblastoma.

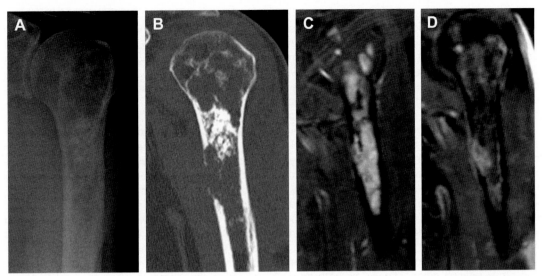

Fig. 7. A 65-year-old patient presents with an incidental finding of lytic lesion of the proximal humerus on radiograph (*A*), with typical ring-and-arc calcification in keeping with chondroid lesion. However, endosteal scalloping of the lateral cortex on radiograph corresponded with an area of cortical break on CT (*B*) and coronal STIR (*C*). On the postcontrast T1-weighted images, enhancing tumor nodule is seen. Biopsy proved focus of dedifferentiation within an enchondroma (*D*).

younger than 30 is most likely to represent an osteosarcoma. The humerus is the most common upper limb site representing 10% to 15% of cases, with other distal sites making up fewer than 2%.[22,23] One or more of the features of osteoid matrix, ossifying soft tissue mass, and aggressive periosteal reaction is present in 90% of cases of conventional-type osteosarcoma (**Fig. 8**). Staging MR imaging of the limb for skip lesions and CT of the chest for metastases (sometimes ossifying) is routine. Several studies have demonstrated utility for [18]FDG-PET in staging and DWI- and DCE–MR imaging in predicting chemotherapy response rates, but this is not currently established routine practice.[5,6] Other differentials for an aggressive lytic lesion in this group are Ewing sarcoma and lymphoma, which also favor the proximal humerus. These can be indistinguishable from osteosarcoma on imaging, although calcification of the soft tissue mass is seen only in the latter.

The main differential for osteosarcoma in this age group is infection. Osteomyelitis is also most commonly seen in the humerus in the upper limb, favoring the distal metaphysis and can demonstrate similarly aggressive imaging appearances. Inflammatory markers and white cell counts are only raised in approximately three-quarters of patients, and not all patients

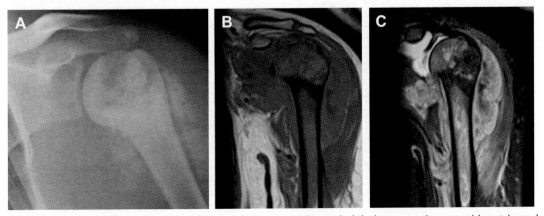

Fig. 8. Aggressive-appearing proximal humeral lesion on radiograph (*A*) demonstrating osteoid matrix and osteoid-type calcification in the soft tissue mass typical of conventional osteosarcoma. T1 (*B*) and STIR (*C*) coronal MR imaging acquisitions demonstrate the full extent of the bone and soft tissue involvement.

are febrile.[24] The presence of soft tissue abscesses on cross-sectional studies is more suggestive of infection, whereas calcification/ossification of the soft tissue mass is very unlikely in acute osteomyelitis and more suggestive of osteosarcoma. Extension of signal changes across a joint implies infection with concurrent septic arthritis.

Langerhans cell histiocytosis (LCH) also can appear aggressive in early stages, with rapid osseous destruction and soft tissue mass and cannot be reliably differentiated from infection or tumor on imaging, therefore necessitating biopsy in some cases (Fig. 9). It is more often monoostotic (50%–75%), but whole-body bone imaging with MR imaging or bone scan can reveal subclinical lesions[25]

A mineralizing juxtacortical soft tissue mass can prove difficult diagnostically, as both parosteal osteosarcomas and myositis ossificans can present in this way. Early parosteal osteosarcomas can also mimic stress fractures due to apparent localized cortical thickening. Myositis ossificans is a nonaggressive process of mineralization and eventually heterotopic bone and cartilage formation in the soft tissues, often without recalled trauma. In the upper extremity, both are most commonly observed around the humerus, although parosteal osteosarcoma is relatively rare in the upper limb. At certain stages of each disease, these 2 lesions can be very difficult to tell apart, presenting as partially mineralized masses that can demonstrate periosteal reaction, radiotracer uptake, and marrow edema. The bone maturation pattern of these lesions is the most sensitive

feature for diagnosis, with myositis ossificans demonstrating more mature bone on the lesional periphery (see Fig. 15), and the osteoid matrix of osteosarcomas tending to ossify centrally and in a disorganized fashion. This is often best seen on CT, with MR imaging and nuclear medicine being less specific.[26]

Distal upper limb In the forearm and hand, a radiographically aggressive lesion is by far most likely to represent infection, as all malignant primary bone neoplasms are rare distally except chondrosarcoma[1,27] (see Fig. 3). Inflammatory markers also may be raised in malignancy, mimicking infection. When the clinical picture is uncertain, biopsy is often required (see Fig. 9). Chondrosarcomas favor the proximal humerus and tubular hand bones, reflecting the common sites for enchondroma from which it is sometimes indistinguishable on imaging, as previously discussed. They are more common in older patients, but can arise at any age.[28]

Multifocal lesions Multifocal aggressive lesions in young patients are less likely to represent metastases than in patients older than 40, although a multifocal/metastatic presentation of osteosarcoma, Ewing tumor, or lymphoma, as well as polyostotic LCH could be considered. Chronic relapsing multifocal osteomyelitis is also a consideration, which can demonstrate imaging findings similar to infection. It is classically multifocal in distribution, but can involve a single site at presentation in approximately 20%.[29] The humerus is again the most common site in the upper limb (affected

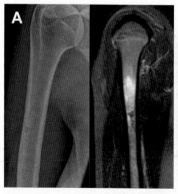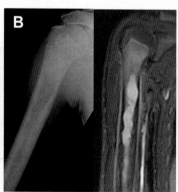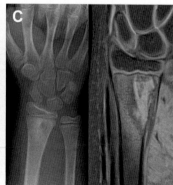

Fig. 9. Radiographs and coronal STIR images demonstrating aggressive radiographic appearances in 3 pediatric patients mimicking tumor. (A) Humeral diaphyseal lesion biopsy proven to represent a focus of LCH. Subsequent whole-body MR imaging demonstrated multifocal asymptomatic lesions. (B) Ill-defined medullary lesion with cortical thickening and scalloping with soft tissue edema and periosteal reaction in a patient with acute osteomyelitis. Temperature and inflammatory markers were found to be raised after the study. (C) Distal radial metaphyseal aggressive lesion with marked soft tissue edema with biopsy subsequently proving a focus of chronic recurrent multifocal osteomyelitis. Whole-body imaging demonstrated this was a solitary lesion.

in 14% of cases), but the forearm and hand may be affected in approximately 4%.[30]

Older age group (>40 years)

The most likely causes of single or multifocal bone lesions in an older patient are metastases and hematogenous malignancy, most often myeloma. Due to its retained red marrow, the proximal humerus is again the most common site of disease. Lesional pathology can be divided by radiographic appearances, with expansile lesions favoring thyroid or renal metastases or myeloma, and sclerotic lesions favoring prostate or breast metastases and lymphoma. Distal or acrometastases are much less common (<0.1% of bony metastases), with lung (33%) and renal cell (20%) accounting for more than half of lesions[31] (**Fig. 10**). Lesions from multiple myeloma or solitary plasmacytomas are not uncommon in the proximal humerus (17% of plasmacytomas), although they tend to favor the axial skeleton. They are extremely rare in the more distal upper limb.[32] This diagnosis is favored by the classic "punched out" lesion on radiograph, which can demonstrate cortical thinning/breakthrough and be mildly expansile. Investigation for systemic disease and whole-body imaging for further lesions with [18]FDG-PET or MR imaging is essential.

SOFT TISSUE TUMORS
Presentation and Imaging Strategy

Soft tissue tumors and tumorlike processes usually present as painless lumps, but less commonly patients may complain of painful masses or symptoms secondary to impingement of nearby neurovascular structures. They are approximately 20 times more common than bony lesions.[33]

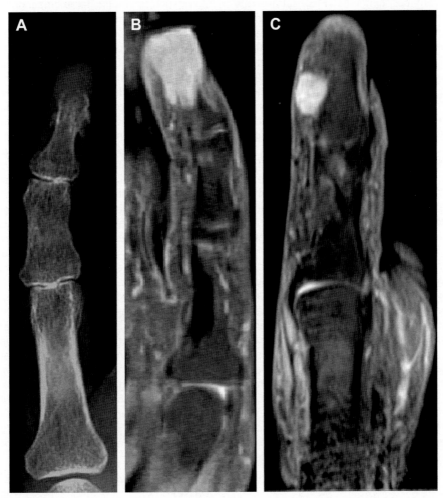

Fig. 10. Patient presenting with lump on little finger pulp demonstrated subtle tuft erosion on radiograph (*A*). Coronal STIR MR imaging images of the hand demonstrated a large destructive soft tissue lesion here (*B*) but also a second similar lesion adjacent to the thumb distal phalanx (*C*). Biopsy demonstrated metastasis from an occult lung adenocarcinoma primary.

Ultrasound is the initial imaging modality of choice, as it allows definitive diagnosis of certain pathologies such as lipomas, ganglion cysts, and chronic hematomas/seromas in most cases, precluding or guiding the need for further investigation.[34] Ultrasonographic elastography is used extensively for breast malignancy, but despite potential, a recent study found limited evidence for its use in soft tissue tumors; however, it may have some use in delineating lesional extent, investigating postexcision recurrence and identifying cellular areas of tumor for biopsy.[35]

MR imaging of soft tissue lesions must consist of at least one T1-weighted spin-echo sequence and fluid-sensitive, fat-saturated/STIR sequence done parallel to the tumor long axis, as well as an axial fluid-sensitive sequence. A gradient-echo sequence also can be added if looking for blood breakdown products; for example, in tenosynovial giant cell tumor (GCTTS). Intravenous gadolinium contrast is currently recommended for most nonfatty soft tissue lesions.[36] However, in the upper limb, most lesions are relatively superficial and vascularity often can be accurately determined by ultrasound, precluding the need for contrast in some cases. Postcontrast acquisitions also can be useful to differentiate cystic components from solid tumor in necrotic tumors and lesions typically demonstrating fluidlike signal, such as myxomas.

Plain radiographs are useful to ascertain the presence and quality/shape of calcification, as well as subtle bony changes. In some cases, CT can be used to demonstrate subtle calcifications not well demonstrated on radiographs.

[18]FDG-PET is not currently routine for assessment of soft tissue lesions but some studies have demonstrated that it may upstage a small proportion of high-grade tumors (eg, undifferentiated pleomorphic sarcoma) compared with current convention of chest CT only,[8] given that metastases should be expected in up to 60% of grade 3 cases and 10% of metastases are to bone.[36,37] However, it has yet to be determined whether this is clinically beneficial, given the markedly increased dose. Several studies have demonstrated a use for PET, DCE–MR imaging, and DWI–MR imaging in demonstrating pretreatment response to chemotherapy, as well as monitoring and assessing recurrent disease.[7,37,38] This is not undertaken routinely but may be of use in select cases.

Ultrasound Assessment of Soft Tissue Masses

Ultrasound is a cost-effective and accurate method of triaging and stratifying risk of soft tissue lesions, especially in the upper extremity where it is known that the great majority are benign (>99%[33,34]) and tumors are relatively superficial and accessible.

Several lesions are diagnostic on ultrasound and have pathognomonic benign appearances that preclude further imaging.

Lipomas can be dismissed if they are small (<5 cm), superficial to the deep fascia, and of similar, homogeneous echogenicity to the surrounding fat with sparse, if any, vascularity. Any atypical features should be investigated with MR imaging with a protocol including fat-saturated or STIR sequences (**Fig. 11**).

Ganglia or synovial cysts make up approximately a quarter of presentations[39] and tend to favor the wrist in the upper limb. This diagnosis can be made with confidence if communication with a joint is demonstrated. Other purely cystic lesions, such as chronic hematomas, postoperative seromas, and some abscesses also can be confidently diagnosed, especially if there is a corroborative clinical history.

Morel-Lavalee–type degloving lesions are rare in the upper extremity, but have been reported around the shoulder and elbow.[40] However, a fluid echogenicity lesion deep to the deep fascia and not associated with joint or tendon sheath may represent a myxoma and should prompt consideration for MR imaging. Glomus tumors are uncommon lesions but have a major predisposition for the fingertip (75% of lesions) demonstrated on ultrasound as an intensely vascular nailbed nodule.

Synovial pathology, such as localized joint synovitis and tenosynovitis, as well as vascular pathologies, such as thrombophlebitis, certain vascular malformations,[41] and aneurysms/pseudoaneurysms, are also best seen and diagnosed on targeted ultrasound.

A study by Lakkaraju and colleagues[34] of 358 soft tissue masses demonstrated excellent correlation of benign ultrasound appearances to histology. Suspicion for malignancy should be raised if ultrasound demonstrates a solid, nonfatty mass, especially if deep to the fascia. Power Doppler flow may be negative in malignant lesions, but disorganized vascularity is a concerning feature. Rapid enlargement, lesional size, and pain are other clinical features that can prompt further imaging in the absence of radiological concern.

MR Imaging Characterization of Soft Tissue Masses

The strength of MR imaging in the assessment of masses in the upper limb is twofold, in that it can suggest the internal soft tissue composition of a

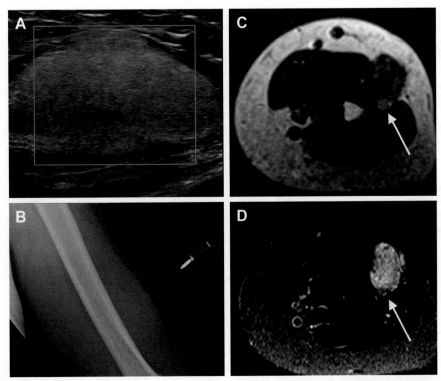

Fig. 11. Patient presenting with soft tissue mass demonstrating diffusely hyperechoic appearances on ultrasound (*A*) and no calcification (*B*). MR images were not typical of a simple lipoma, but T1-weighted (*C*) and STIR (*D*) axial images demonstrated a mass with focal areas of increased T1 signal (*arrow*), which suppress relative to the rest of the tumor indicating the presence of macroscopic fat. Excision demonstrated a spindle cell lipoma.

lesion as well as give a much clearer picture of anatomic structures that the lesion is arising from or in close proximity to.

MR imaging has a greater sensitivity for malignant soft tissue lesions than ultrasound as surrounding soft tissue edema, central necrosis, destruction of tissue planes, and involvement of adjacent structures and bones is clearly delineated. Regional lymphadenopathy in the epitrochlea or axilla can sometimes be seen. In these lesions, referral to a sarcoma service is warranted and MR imaging can help to ascertain viable areas of the lesion for targeted biopsy.

In other lesions, MR imaging features can be less specific, although certain features can assist in limiting a differential or even giving a specific diagnosis.

High T1-Signal Lesions

Macroscopic fat within a lesion on fat-saturated/STIR sequences imply a limited subset of lesions, most commonly lipomas (if completely saturating) and atypical lipomatous tumors/liposarcomas (if incompletely saturating, see **Fig. 11**). Cavernous hemangiomas can demonstrate variable or no macroscopic fat, but the presence of fat on MR

imaging and linear vascular flow on ultrasound is usually sufficient for diagnosis.[41] Neural fibrolipoma is a rare lesion that almost exclusively occurs in the upper limb and of which 80% involve the median nerve. MR imaging demonstrates a pathognomonic fusiform enlargement of the nerve with nerve bundles separated by fat signal soft tissue.

High signal on T1-weighted images also can indicate hemorrhage, and a common diagnostic problem is differentiation of benign hemorrhage from a hemorrhagic soft tissue sarcoma as high T1 signal on fat-saturated postcontrast images complicates assessment of enhancement and subacute lesions often demonstrate heterogeneous signal. Follow-up MR imaging may be required to definitively demonstrate the thin peripheral enhancement of a hematoma and to rule out an underlying lesion. In some cases, close follow-up (3–6 weeks) with serial ultrasound is helpful to demonstrate resolution (**Fig. 12**).

Low T2 Signal Lesions

Low signal on fluid-sensitive sequences can be due to several causes, which can help to narrow the differential.

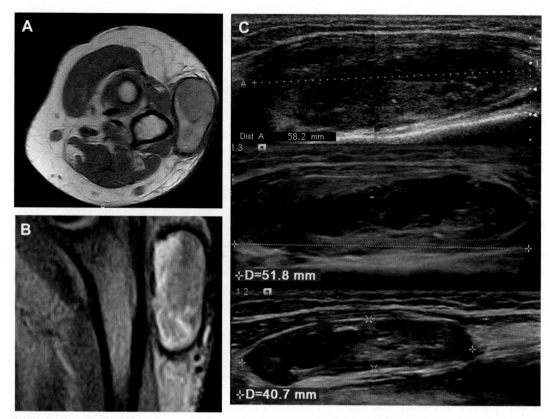

Fig. 12. Patient presented with enlarging mass on the forearm with no history of trauma. T1-weighted (*A*) and fat-saturated proton density (*B*) images demonstrate a heterogeneous signal subcutaneous lesion with low-signal rim and foci of nonsuppressing high T1 signal. Encapsulated hematoma was suspected. Serial ultrasound studies (*C*) at 6-month intervals demonstrate reassuring slow resolution of the lesion.

In the upper limb, the most common lesion is GCTTS, which is the extra-articular pathologic equivalent to pigmented villonodular synovitis (PVNS). It has a marked tropism for the finger flexor tendon sheaths, most commonly affecting the proximal first and third digits.[39] MR imaging usually demonstrates a lobulated peritendinous mass containing areas of low T2 signal, and in this tumor this is thought to represent hemosiderin deposition. Blooming artifact on gradient-echo sequences can be seen, but this is less common than in articular PVNS. As it is a slow-growing mass, pressure erosion into adjacent bone and sometimes periostitis is seen, especially if it arises on the extensor aspect (**Fig. 13**).

Other causes of low T2 signal include fibrous lesions due to high collagen content. In this case, low-signal areas can often be focal or striated, and there is often avid contrast enhancement. In the upper limb, the most common lesion is palmar fibromatosis (Dupuytren disease), although in this case ultrasound is usually diagnostic. Tendon sheath fibromas are uncommon fibrous lesions

also favoring the flexor tendons of the hand and wrist that can be confused with GCTTS, as the latter also can demonstrate low-signal fibrous septae.

Certain subtypes of neurofibromas (diffuse type) are collagen rich and can demonstrate central areas of low signal, but are usually seen on a background of neurofibromatosis.[42]

Calcification

Low-signal foci also can represent calcification, and comparison with plain radiographs (or CT in some cases) is required to ascertain presence and type of calcification (**Fig. 14**). For example, osteoid calcification may occur in myositis ossificans and juxtacortical osteosarcoma (**Fig. 15**). Common differentials for "ring-and-arc"–type chondroid calcifications include loose cartilage bodies in a joint, which can be due to degenerative or inflammatory disease or secondary to synovial chondromatosis. The latter commonly involves tendon sheaths in the hand and the shoulder, and elbow joints in the upper limb.[43] Periosteal

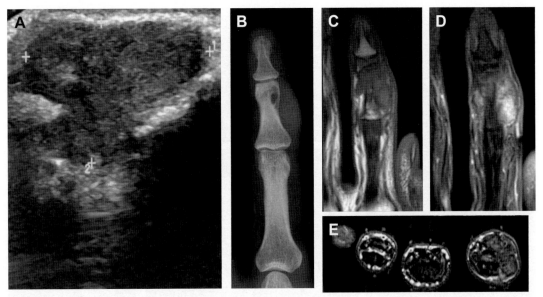

Fig. 13. Patient presenting with slow-growing lump on the index finger. This demonstrated a lobulated and hypovascular appearance on ultrasound (*A*), with pressure erosion of the middle phalanx on radiograph (*B*). T1-weighted (*C*) and fat-saturated proton density (*D*) coronal and axial T2-weighted (*E*) images demonstrate a relatively low T2 signal lesion that is enveloping the flexor tendon typical for GCTTS, which was proven on excision.

and extraosseous chondromas are much rarer, although soft tissue chondromas exhibit a major tropism for the fingers. Typically, spherical phleboliths often demonstrate radiolucent centers on radiographs and are easily distinguishable from other types of calcification, implying an underlying varicosity or vascular malformation.

Nonspecific calcification in a superficial lesion is most commonly related to previous trauma/fat necrosis, but the upper extremity is also the second most common site for pilomatricoma, a skin appendage tumor commonly demonstrating fine calcification. Inflammatory nodules, such as gouty

tophi, often calcify, with rheumatoid nodules calcifying uncommonly. Usually, a typical location (eg, at the extensor surface of the elbow) and the presence of adjacent joint or bursal disease facilitates diagnosis in these cases, but occasionally biopsy is required.

However, calcification is not always a benign phenomenon and is also seen in some of the soft tissue sarcomas. Epithelioid sarcoma and synovial sarcoma both favor the extremities and can variably calcify (20% and 33% respectively[1,39]). Synovial sarcomas, in particular, can appear relatively innocuous on imaging when of a small size, and

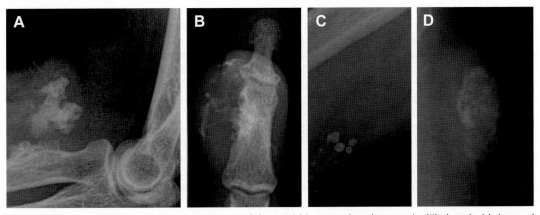

Fig. 14. Different soft tissue calcification patterns: (*A*) osteoid in osteochondromatosis, (*B*) chondroid ring-and-arc in soft tissue chondroma, (*C*) phlebolith in venous malformation, (*D*) sandlike dystrophic calcification in pilomatricoma.

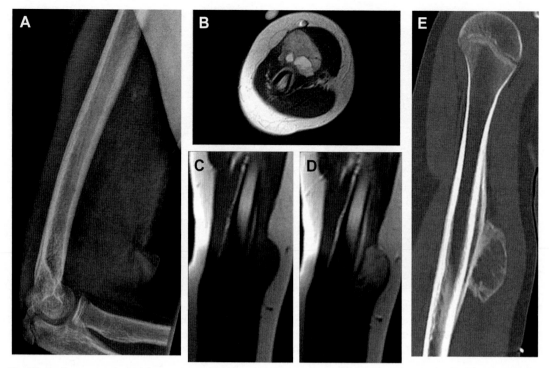

Fig. 15. Patient presented with growing clinically evident mass in the upper arm. Initial radiograph demonstrated ill-defined osteoid-type mineralization and aggressive-appearing periosteal reaction adjacent to the humerus (*A*). T2-weighted axial (*B*) and precontrast (*C*) and postcontrast (*D*) T1-weighted MR imaging 2 weeks later demonstrate an enhancing soft tissue juxtacortical mass with periosteal and soft tissue edema with ABC component, and osteosarcoma was initially suggested. However, CT (*E*) done at tertiary sarcoma center demonstrates the reassuring typical peripheral to central mineralization pattern of myositis ossificans. Patient reported no history of trauma.

should be considered a differential in any enhancing juxta-articular nodule, especially if calcified.

Nonspecific Appearances

Differentials for lesions demonstrating nonspecific features on MR imaging can be narrowed by anatomic position, patient age, and clinical history. An enhancing fascial-based mass with surrounding edema, for example, would be a typical location for a myxofibrosarcoma. A mass positioned along a neurovascular bundle may commonly represent a peripheral nerve sheath tumor (PNST), such as a schwannoma, for example, but aggressive MR imaging features in this location would favor leiomyosarcoma[44] or malignant PNST.

In older patients with concurrent or past malignancy, soft tissue metastases may be considered within the differential; however, in patients presenting with soft tissue mass in one large study, only 1.3% of these were a metastasis and even considering patients with known malignancy, soft tissue masses were 5 times more likely to be a new soft tissue sarcoma than a metastasis.[45] The most common primary sites were lung (31%) and melanoma (19%) and the upper limb was the presenting site in 34%, making it a common site for an uncommon pathology.

Nonvisualization of a mass on imaging despite clinically evident abnormality is another possible scenario. The most common cause of this is a localized inflammatory pathology, cellulitis and other pyogenic soft tissue infection being the most prevalent, but systemic conditions causing panniculitis, such as sarcoidosis and rheumatoid arthritis, and malignancy, such as cutaneous lymphoma, also can present similarly, with nonmarginated superficial edemalike signal on MR imaging (**Fig. 16**). In these cases, dermatology referral and skin biopsy can be diagnostic. The rare myxoinflammatory fibrosarcoma also may present as poorly marginated subcutaneous signal change, and is most commonly found in the fingers and hand.[46]

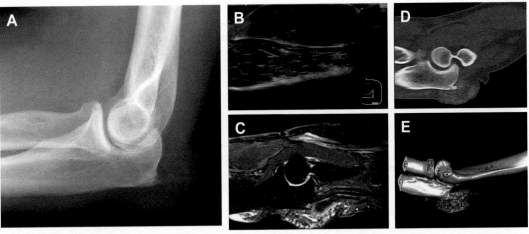

Fig. 16. Patient presented with mass on the extensor aspect of the elbow discrete on clinical examination demonstrating no definite calcification on radiograph (*A*). Ultrasound (*B*) and proton-density sagittal plane MR imaging (*C*) demonstrated an ill-defined soft tissue abnormality centered on the subcutaneous tissue with a fluid center, and the possibility of a necrotic soft tissue tumor was raised. However, CT acquired at tertiary sarcoma center (*D*) demonstrates diffuse mineralization, and dual-energy CT (*E*) proved deposition of urate crystals in keeping with olecranon bursitis associated with gout.

SUMMARY

In this article, we have discussed the common lesions arising from bone and soft tissue, with particular focus on lesions with a tropism for the upper extremity and common locations where these tumors can arise. The radiologist should have a structured approach to the investigation and differential diagnosis of these lesions, but ultimately, any lesions with suspicious features suggestive of atypia should be referred to a tertiary sarcoma center for management.

REFERENCES

1. Manaster BJ. Diagnostic imaging. Musculoskeletal: non-traumatic disease. Salt Lake City (UT): Amirsys; 2010.
2. Link TM, Brinkschmidt C, Lindner N, et al. Primary bone tumors and "tumor-like lesions" of the shoulder. Their histopathology and imaging. Rofo 1999; 170(5):507–13 [in German].
3. Shapeero LG, Couanet D, Vanel D, et al. Bone metastases as the presenting manifestation of rhabdomyosarcoma in childhood. Skeletal Radiol 1993; 22(6):433–8.
4. Lalam R, Bloem JL, Noebauer-Huhmann IM, et al. ESSR consensus document for detection, characterization, and referral pathway for tumors and tumor-like lesions of bone. Semin Musculoskelet Radiol 2017;21(5):630–47.
5. Byun BH, Kim SH, Lim SM, et al. Prediction of response to neoadjuvant chemotherapy in osteosarcoma using dual-phase (18)F-FDG PET/CT. Eur Radiol 2015;25(7):2015–24.
6. Wang CS, Du LJ, Si MJ, et al. Noninvasive assessment of response to neoadjuvant chemotherapy in osteosarcoma of long bones with diffusion-weighted imaging: an initial in vivo study. PLoS One 2013;8(8):e72679.
7. Costa FM, Canella C, Gasparetto E. Advanced magnetic resonance imaging techniques in the evaluation of musculoskeletal tumors. Radiol Clin North Am 2011;49(6):1325–58. vii-viii.
8. Macpherson RE, Pratap S, Tyrrell H, et al. Retrospective audit of 957 consecutive. Clin Sarcoma Res 2018;8:9.
9. Ciccarese F, Bazzocchi A, Ciminari R, et al. The many faces of pulmonary metastases of osteosarcoma: retrospective study on 283 lesions submitted to surgery. Eur J Radiol 2015;84(12): 2679–85.
10. Garner HW, Kransdorf MJ, Peterson JJ. Posttherapy imaging of musculoskeletal neoplasms. Radiol Clin North Am 2011;49(6):1307–23, vii.
11. Bastawrous S, Bhargava P, Behnia F, et al. Newer PET application with an old tracer: role of 18F-NaF skeletal PET/CT in oncologic practice. Radiographics 2014;34(5):1295–316.
12. Themistocleous GS, Chloros GD, Benetos IS, et al. Osteoid osteoma of the upper extremity. A diagnostic challenge. Chir Main 2006;25(2): 69–76.
13. Anderson MW. Imaging of upper extremity stress fractures in the athlete. Clin Sports Med 2006; 25(3):489–504, vii.
14. Sampath Kumar V, Tyrrell PN, Singh J, et al. Surveillance of intramedullary cartilage tumours in long bones. Bone Joint J 2016;98-B(11):1542–7.

15. Geirnaerdt MJ, Hogendoorn PC, Bloem JL, et al. Cartilaginous tumors: fast contrast-enhanced MR imaging. Radiology 2000;214(2):539–46.

16. Yanagisawa M, Okada K, Tajino T, et al. A clinicopathological study of giant cell tumor of small bones. Ups J Med Sci 2011;116(4):265–8.

17. Oliveira AM, Perez-Atayde AR, Inwards CY, et al. USP6 and CDH11 oncogenes identify the neoplastic cell in primary aneurysmal bone cysts and are absent in so-called secondary aneurysmal bone cysts. Am J Pathol 2004;165(5):1773–80.

18. Kularatne U, James SL, Evans N, et al. Tumours and tumour mimics in the olecranon. Clin Radiol 2015; 70(7):760–73.

19. Berry M, Mankin H, Gebhardt M, et al. Osteoblastoma: a 30-year study of 99 cases. J Surg Oncol 2008;98(3):179–83.

20. Betsy M, Kupersmith LM, Springfield DS. Metaphyseal fibrous defects. J Am Acad Orthop Surg 2004;12(2):89–95.

21. Biermann JS. Common benign lesions of bone in children and adolescents. J Pediatr Orthop 2002; 22(2):268–73.

22. Pradhan A, Reddy KI, Grimer RJ, et al. Osteosarcomas in the upper distal extremities: are their oncological outcomes similar to other sites? Eur J Surg Oncol 2015;41(3):407–12.

23. Sforzo CR, Scarborough MT, Wright TW. Bone-forming tumors of the upper extremity and Ewing's sarcoma. Hand Clin 2004;20(3):303–15, vi.

24. Street M, Crawford H. Pediatric humeral osteomyelitis. J Pediatr Orthop 2015;35(6):628–33.

25. Arkader A, Glotzbecker M, Hosalkar HS, et al. Primary musculoskeletal Langerhans cell histiocytosis in children: an analysis for a 3-decade period. J Pediatr Orthop 2009;29(2):201–7.

26. Tyler P, Saifuddin A. The imaging of myositis ossificans. Semin Musculoskelet Radiol 2010;14(2): 201–16.

27. Iwamoto Y. Diagnosis and treatment of Ewing's sarcoma. Jpn J Clin Oncol 2007;37(2):79–89.

28. Giuffrida AY, Burgueno JE, Koniaris LG, et al. Chondrosarcoma in the United States (1973 to 2003): an analysis of 2890 cases from the SEER database. J Bone Joint Surg Am 2009;91(5):1063–72.

29. Falip C, Alison M, Boutry N, et al. Chronic recurrent multifocal osteomyelitis (CRMO): a longitudinal case series review. Pediatr Radiol 2013;43(3):355–75.

30. Borzutzky A, Stern S, Reiff A, et al. Pediatric chronic nonbacterial osteomyelitis. Pediatrics 2012;130(5): e1190–7.

31. Stomeo D, Tulli A, Ziranu A, et al. Acrometastasis: a literature review. Eur Rev Med Pharmacol Sci 2015; 19(15):2906–15.

32. Dores GM, Landgren O, McGlynn KA, et al. Plasmacytoma of bone, extramedullary plasmacytoma, and multiple myeloma: incidence and survival in the United States, 1992-2004. Br J Haematol 2009; 144(1):86–94.

33. Zyluk A, Mazur A. Statistical and histological analysis of tumors of the upper extremity. Obere Extrem 2015;10(4):252–7.

34. Lakkaraju A, Sinha R, Garikipati R, et al. Ultrasound for initial evaluation and triage of clinically suspicious soft-tissue masses. Clin Radiol 2009;64(6): 615–21.

35. Winn N, Lalam R, Cassar-Pullicino V. Sonoelastography in the musculoskeletal system: current role and future directions. World J Radiol 2016;8(11):868–79.

36. Noebauer-Huhmann IM, Weber MA, Lalam RK, et al. Soft tissue tumors in adults: ESSR-approved guidelines for diagnostic imaging. Semin Musculoskelet Radiol 2015;19(5):e1.

37. Issels RD, Lindner LH, Verweij J, et al. Neo-adjuvant chemotherapy alone or with regional hyperthermia for localised high-risk soft-tissue sarcoma: a randomised phase 3 multicentre study. Lancet Oncol 2010;11(6):561–70.

38. Tewfik JN, Greene GS. Fluorine-18-deoxyglucose-positron emission tomography imaging with magnetic resonance and computed tomographic correlation in the evaluation of bone and soft-tissue sarcomas: a pictorial essay. Curr Probl Diagn Radiol 2008;37(4):178–88.

39. Khaled W, Drapé JL. MRI of wrist and hand masses. Diagn Interv Imaging 2015;96(12):1238–46.

40. Cochran GK, Hanna KH. Morel-Lavallee lesion in the upper extremity. Hand (N Y) 2017;12(1):NP10–3.

41. Rimondi E, Mavrogenis AF, Errani C, et al. Biopsy is not necessary for the diagnosis of soft tissue hemangiomas. Radiol Med 2018;123(7):538–44.

42. Song YS, Lee IS, Choi KU, et al. Soft tissue masses showing low signal intensity on T2-weighted images: correlation with pathologic findings. Journal of the Korean Society of Magnetic Resonance in Medicine 2014;18(4):279.

43. Murphey MD, Vidal JA, Fanburg-Smith JC, et al. Imaging of synovial chondromatosis with radiologic-pathologic correlation. Radiographics 2007;27(5): 1465–88.

44. Abed R, Abudu A, Grimer RJ, et al. Leiomyosarcomas of vascular origin in the extremity. Sarcoma 2009;2009:385164.

45. Abed R, Grimer RJ, Carter SR, et al. Soft-tissue metastases: their presentation and origin. J Bone Joint Surg Br 2009;91(8):1083–5.

46. Narváez JA, Martinez S, Dodd LG, et al. Acral myxoinflammatory fibroblastic sarcomas: MRI findings in four cases. AJR Am J Roentgenol 2007;188(5): 1302–5.

MR Imaging of the Upper Limb: Pitfalls, Tricks, and Tips

Federico Bruno, MD[a], Francesco Arrigoni, MD[a], Raffaele Natella, MD[b],
Nicola Maggialetti, MD[c], Silvia Pradella, MD[d], Marcello Zappia, MD[c],
Alfonso Reginelli, MD[b], Alessandra Splendiani, MD[a], Ernesto Di Cesare, MD[a],
Giuseppe Guglielmi, MD[e], Vittorio Miele, MD[d], Andrea Giovagnoni, MD[f],
Luca Brunese, MD[c], Carlo Masciocchi, MD[a], Antonio Barile, MD[a,*]

KEYWORDS

• MR imaging • Shoulder • Elbow • Wrist • Artifacts • Pitfalls

KEY POINTS

• MR imaging is one of the most widely used imaging tools to assess several pathologic conditions in the upper limb, especially around the shoulder, elbow, and wrist joint.
• Several anatomic variants and imaging artifacts can show unusual appearance and mimic pathologic entities.
• Knowledge of the possible imaging pitfalls encountered in MR imaging of the upper limb, and the available tips and tricks to recognize them, is essential to avoid significant diagnostic errors.

INTRODUCTION

MR imaging, together with ultrasound, is one of the most widely used imaging tools both in the diagnostic and interventional musculoskeletal fields, suitable for different conditions affecting both the upper and lower limb.[1–20] This imaging technique carries an excellent diagnostic accuracy thanks to its high intrinsic spatial and contrast resolution; however, there are different kinds of anatomic variants and artifacts that can be confused with pathologic entities.[21,22] This article reviews the main conditions that can lead to diagnostic pitfalls in the imaging of the upper limb (mainly the shoulder, elbow, and wrist joints), together with possible tips to solve these equivocal cases.

SHOULDER

Labrum

The glenoid labrum, besides different types of lesions, can present several anatomic variants in morphology, shape, and thickness (triangular being the most common, but frequently round, cleaved, thinned, until the cases of aplasia) that can be a source of diagnostic errors mimicking a tear, especially when encountered posteriorly, where they are less frequent.[23] However, the supraequatorial labrum (between 11 and 3 o'clock) is the area with the greatest anatomic variation, especially involving the biceps labral complex (BLC).[24,25]

Disclosure Statement: The authors have nothing to disclose.
[a] Department of Biotechnological and Applied Clinical Sciences, University of L'Aquila, via Vetoio 1, L'Aquila 67100, Italy; [b] Department of Precision Medicine, University of Campania "Luigi Vanvitelli," via Pansini 5, Napoli 80131, Italy; [c] Department Life and Health "V. Tiberio," University of Molise, Via Francesco De Sanctis 1, Campobasso 86100, Italy; [d] Department of Radiology, Careggi University Hospital, Largo Brambilla 3, Florence 50134, Italy; [e] Department of Radiology, University of Foggia, Viale Luigi Pinto 1, Foggia 71100, Italy; [f] Department of Radiology, Ospedali Riuniti, Università Politecnica delle Marche, via Conca 71, Ancona 60121, Italy
* Corresponding author.
E-mail address: antonio.barile@cc.univaq.it

Radiol Clin N Am 57 (2019) 1051–1062
https://doi.org/10.1016/j.rcl.2019.03.010

Sublabral sulcus or recess

This is the most common BLC anatomic variant of the superior labrum labral bicipital complex. It can be visualized on routine MR scans but is best characterized with fat-saturated T1-weighted MR arthrogram images as a contrast-outlined linear structure that follows the contour of glenoid articular hyaline cartilage and extends medially beneath the labrum between 11 and 1 o'clock.[23] The diagnostic pitfall is that it can mimic a type II superior labral anteroposterior (SLAP) lesion. Tips to help in the differential diagnosis are mainly the smooth profile, the orientation directed medially and parallel to the glenoid cartilage, and the localization, confined to the superior insertion of the long head of the biceps tendon (LHBT).[26]

Sometimes this area at the labrum-glenoid interface can show intermediate signal intensity, secondary to a histologic transition between cartilage and fibrocartilage, magic angle (with short echo time [TE] sequences) and partial volume effect, but this is another normal finding to keep in mind when looking for a lesion in this region.[25,27]

Sublabral foramen or hole

Sublabral foramen or hole (**Fig. 1**) is another congenital anatomic labral variant, appearing as discontinuation between the anterosuperior labrum and the underlying glenoid, creating communication with the subscapularis recess.[23] The typical location is anterior to the BLC, at 2 o'clock. As for sublabral sulcus, there are some tricks to differentiate a sublabral hole from a tear. The main clues are represented by the size (usually not more than 15 mm in sublabral foramen, and without significant labrum displacement), the direction (the sublabral hole does not extend posteriorly past the insertion of the LHBT tendon), and

the localization (at the labral base and not within the labral substance, as the case of real labral lesions). Moreover, isolated tears of the labrum at this level are rare.[27,28]

Meniscoid-type superior labrum

This is another normal variant of the labrum near the BLC, and refers to a congenital detachment of the base of the superior labrum from the glenoid, therefore having a meniscus shape protruding into the joint.[29]

Buford complex

A well-known but sometimes overlooked congenital labral variant characterized by the absence of the anterosuperior glenoid labrum, associated with a thickened and cordlike middle glenohumeral ligament that attaches to the anterosuperior labrum, anterior to the BLC.[27]

Cartilage

Articular cartilage undercutting

It is the undercutting of the labrum by the articular glenoid cartilage; subsequently, the high signal intensity of the hyaline cartilage may lead to the misleading diagnosis of a labral or SLAP tear.[23] The trick to avoiding this pitfall is to recognize the course of the alteration parallel to the glenoid cortex, whereas labral tears are directed laterally. Moreover, the cartilage signal intensity is lower than fluid on fluid-sensitive sequences, and this can also help in the diagnosis[25,30]

Cartilage bare areas

In the shoulder there are some typical areas devoid of articular cartilage, important to recognize, as they can appear as a chondral defect (**Fig. 2**). The most common pitfall of this type is central bare of the glenoid fossa, in which

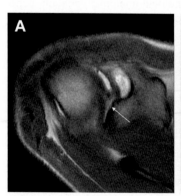 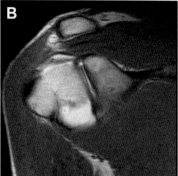 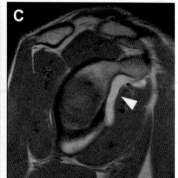

Fig. 1. Axial (*A*), coronal (*B*), and sagittal (*C*) MR angiography images of the shoulder showing a sublabral foramen (*arrow*). Note the localization of the foramen between the labral base and the glenoid bone, not extending posteriorly past the insertion of the LHBT tendon. Due to communication through the foramen, there is distention on the subscapularis recess (*arrowhead*).

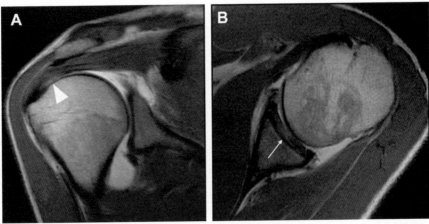

Fig. 2. Cartilage bare areas at the level of the supraspinatus footprint (*arrowhead* in *A*) and in the central glenoid (*arrow* in *B*).

the cartilage thinning is often associated with a subchondral bone thickening (the so-called tubercle of Assaki), and the bare area at the posterolateral humeral head profile. A useful trick not to call an osteochondral lesion or a Hill-Sachs lesion in these cases is the absence of subchondral bone marrow alterations and intra-articular loose bodies.[31]

Another bare area can be encountered at the level of the supraspinatus footprint. This bare area usually measures up to 1.5 to 2.0 mm and must be distinguished from a partial articular surface tendon tear.[25]

Glenohumeral Ligaments

The superior, middle, and inferior glenohumeral ligaments are best depicted using MR arthrography and have significant variation in anatomy.[32] The *superior glenohumeral ligament,* despite its variants in origin and shape, does not usually cause significant diagnostic pitfalls.[33]

The *middle glenohumeral ligament* (MGHL) is the most variable regarding size, thickness, and constancy, and is also affected by the arm (internal rotation will cause a wavy appearance, external rotation will stretch it toward the capsule). Most common variants involve its insertion to the anterosuperior labrum or to the anterior scapular neck (where can mimic a capsular tear). In up to 30% of individuals it may be not visualized; in these cases, there is concurrent enlargement of the subscapularis bursa (due to joint communication).[25]

The major diagnostic pitfall is that the ligament course along the labrum may be misdiagnosed as a labral tear or an intra-articular loose body; in such doubtful cases, following the entire ligament through several consecutive slices or in different planes can solve the dilemma[31] (**Fig. 3**).

The *inferior glenohumeral ligament* can sometimes be a source of diagnostic pitfall, as its inferior variable insertion to the neck of the humerus where it may have a jagged appearance mimicking

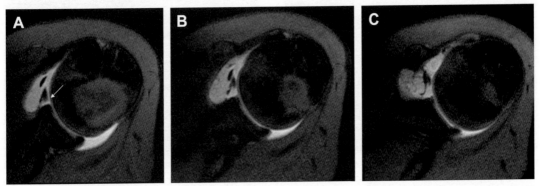

Fig. 3. Axial MR angiography slices of the shoulder showing MGHL mimicking a labral tear (*arrow* in *A*). Following the ligament, through consecutive lower slices (*B, C*) we recognize the presence of a double MGHL.

a tear, or to the labrum where it may show a focal area of increased T2 signal as a result of partial volume averaging. The abduction and external rotation (ABER) position can solve the dilemma, stretching the capsule inferiorly.

The inferior capsule also can be a frequent location for synovial folds mimicking intra-articular inclusion bodies (careful evaluation of signal intensity signs of magnetic susceptibility or a dependent position are possible clues for loose bodies).[25]

The anterior capsular insertion region, with its 3 insertional variants, can be an area of diagnostic pitfalls during MR arthrography, in which overdistension of the capsule or an internally rotated arm may produce a false appearance of a redundant type II/III capsular insertion.[34]

Bony Structures

Os acromiale is an accessory bone resulting from incomplete fusion of the acromial epiphysis and can be possibly confused with a distal fracture of the acromion. Differential diagnosis includes clinical history (isolated fractures of the acromion are rare) and evaluation of the bony margins (os acromial is well corticated)[34]

The humeral head has a physiologic flattening at the level of the head-shaft junction on the posterolateral profile (**Fig. 4**). This appearance could be a diagnostic pitfall mimicking a Hill-Sachs lesion. However, this alteration lies below the level of the coracoid process, where Hill-Sachs fracture occurs.

Sometimes the *insertion of the coracoacromial ligament* or the insertion of the deltoid muscle to the inferolateral aspect of the acromion can have an osteophytelike appearance, and multiple slice/plane views can be useful for the characterization.[34]

Bone marrow signal alterations can be quite frequent at the level of the humeral head of the humeral shaft.[34] Typical marrow abnormalities encountered are represented by focalities of red marrow along with the subchondral articular surface or the physeal plate (in adolescents) of the humerus; differential diagnosis of bone marrow reconversion/infiltration patterns should be kept in mind (**Fig. 5**)

Muscles and Tendons

One of the most frequent diagnostic pitfalls around the shoulder on routine MR examinations is represented by the magic angle effect. This artifact, caused by the increased signal intensity on short TE sequences when anisotropic imaging structures oriented at 55° to the B0 magnetic field, is particularly frequent at the level of the supraspinatus crescent area and can be mistaken for an area of tendinosis.[35]

Tips and tricks to reduce the magic angle effect are repositioning of the patient, increasing of the TE to 37 ms, and comparison of findings with T2 sequences.

The LHBT can be congenitally doubled, mimicking a tendon split. Unlike true tears, however, cases of double LHBT show homogeneous hypointense signal with flat morphology, without

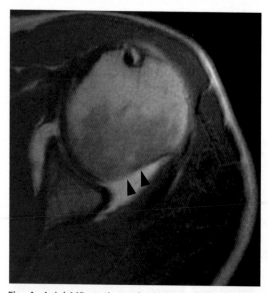

Fig. 4. Axial MR angiography image of the shoulder showing the physiologic flattening of the humeral head at the level of the head-shaft junction on the posterolateral profile (*arrowheads*).

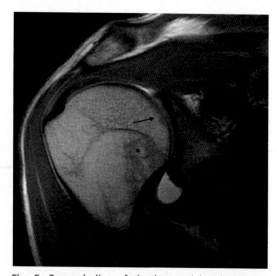

Fig. 5. Coronal slice of the humeral head showing areas of red marrow at the level of the subcortical profile (*arrow*) and below the physeal line (*asterisk*).

the wavy, jagged, and hyperintense appearance seen in tendinosis and tendon lesions.[35]

LHBT also can have abnormal signal intensity in its intracapsular segment due to magic angle artifact. Moreover, it also may appear medially displaced, as the intra-articular portion of the tendon runs superiorly and posteriorly from the bicipital groove to the biceps anchor. There can be other misleading findings within the bicipital groove, such as the biceps vincula (synovial bands) between the tendon and the synovial sheath, blood vessels, and anomalous supraspinatus insertions (aponeurotic expansion of the supraspinatus tendon).[36]

Position and Other Diagnostic Pitfalls

Some diagnostic pitfalls and artifacts may be driven by an incorrect patient positioning. For example, the rotator cuff is best imaged with the arm in slight external rotation, to obtain the best in-plane position of the supraspinatus and infraspinatus muscle fibers, minimizing magic angle effects and overlapping artifacts of tendons and capsular structures.[37,38]

Knowledge of the normal and abnormal anatomic relationships is essential when performing dedicated sequences such as ABER positioning; in such position, the proximal LHBT may have a wavy appearance that should not be mistaken for a tear.[39]

Performing MR arthrography, the unintentional intra-articular injection of little air may cause areas of abnormal signal intensity, potential diagnostic pitfalls for loose bodies, tendon tears, or synovitis. There are, however, some clues that can help to identify small air bubbles, such as the blooming effect on susceptibility sequences and the nondependent location.[35]

Another minor source of diagnostic errors in shoulder MR imaging described in the literature is represented by abnormally *prominent blood vessels* that may course through tendons, muscle, and bone (eg, spinoglenoid notch), mimicking tendon/labral tears and cysts.[37]

Postoperative Shoulder MR Pitfalls

Knowledge of the postsurgical tissue and anatomy modifications is essential to avoid misdiagnosis of normal findings as pathologic.[40,41] For example, following rotator cuff repair surgery, areas of intermediate-high signal intensity or low signal intensity within the tendon are normal, representing physiologic granulation or fibrotic tissue. Also, the presence of fluid or even obliteration of the subacromial-subdeltoid space are normal postsurgical findings, not to address as retear.

Similarly, contrast leakage through a repaired tendon in the healing phase is not indicative of failed surgery[25] (**Fig. 6**).

A normal finding encountered after glenohumeral instability surgery can be a mild superior subluxation of the humeral head.[42]

ELBOW
Bone

Pseudodefect of the capitellum

The pseudodefect of the capitellum (**Fig. 7**) is a diagnostic pitfall encountered only in MR imaging (not evident on conventional radiographs), especially on coronal and sagittal cuts. It is the appearance of an interruption in the capitellar surface that occurs at the posterior aspect of the joint and is caused by the peculiar morphology of the capitellum, characterized by a progressive decrease in width from anterior to posterior and the presence of the adjacent rough surface of the groove and lateral epicondyle.[43] Pseudodefect of the capitellum can be mistaken for an osteochondral injury. Sometimes, a low signal intensity line can be seen extending within the subchondral bone from the pseudodefect and should not be mistaken for a fracture.[44] To distinguish a pseudodefect from true pathology, the main tricks are to look for the localization of the defect (pseudodefect is posterior, osteochondral defects tend to locate anteriorly) and to scroll the axial images, where the articular surface should appear smooth

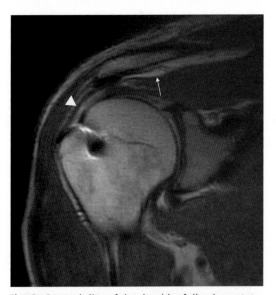

Fig. 6. Coronal slice of the shoulder following rotator cuff surgical reconstruction. Note the intermediate-high signal intensity (*arrowhead*) and contrast leakage through the repaired tendon (*arrow*), to be considered as normal postoperative findings.

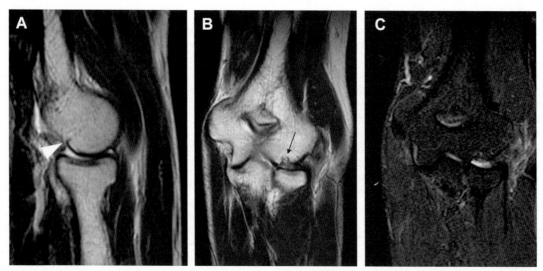

Fig. 7. MR imaging appearance of a pseudodefect of the capitellum as an interruption in the cortical surface at the posterior aspect on sagittal (*arrowhead* in *A*) and coronal (*arrow* in *B*) cuts. Note there are no subchondral bone marrow abnormalities suggestive for an osteochondral injury or fracture (as evident in fat-suppressed sequence in *C*).

and without evidence of bone marrow alterations in the case of a pseudodefect.[45]

Trochlear groove
The ulnar side is also at risk for diagnostic pitfalls on sagittal MR images. On the articular surface of the coronoid process, there is a bony ridge devoid of articular cartilage, not to be misdiagnosed as an osteophyte. More medially, the articular surface may show the presence of a well-defined central defect, the trochlear groove, possibly mistaken for a chondral lesion (**Fig. 8**); the absence of bone marrow edema confirms the benignity of the process.[46]

Bone marrow alterations
As in the shoulder, several bone segments in the elbow (mainly the distal metaphysis of the humerus and the radial neck) can be affected by bone marrow changes, such as marrow reconversion.[47]

Supracondylar process of the humerus
This a bone process (probably a development remnant) arising from the distal anteromedial humerus and extending downward. The MR appearance can be misleading sometimes, while the radiographic picture is quite characteristic. The primary differential diagnosis is the osteochondroma that typically grows away from the epiphysis.[45]

Synovia
Synovial folds/plicae are normal variations of the articular synovial lining characterized by synovial tissue projection and reflections within the joint cavity. Although asymptomatic, they can undergo

thickening, inflammation, and impingement syndromes and be a source of diagnostic errors being similar to loose articular bodies.[46]

Ligaments
Ligaments around the elbow can represent a potential diagnostic pitfall in MR imaging, as they

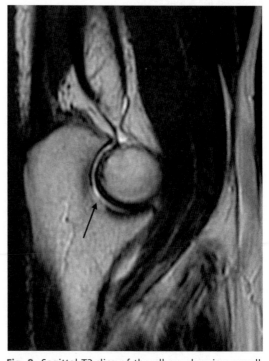

Fig. 8. Sagittal T2 slice of the elbow showing a well-defined central articular surface defect of the trochlea (*arrow*, trochlear groove).

may show abnormal signal intensity even in physiologic situations.[44] For example, the ulnar collateral ligament may have such appearance due to the presence of interspersed fat within its proximal insertion (where the ligament is relatively wider). Also, the radial collateral ligament can be subjected to partial volume cuts and magic angle effects (**Fig. 9**). Another case of abnormal signal intensity of the medial collateral ligament is in children before the physeal plate closure. For these reasons, the diagnosis of a tear should take into account also clinical data and technical acquisition parameters.[46]

Tendons

The *triceps tendon* is the one potentially causing diagnostic pitfalls in the elbow, due to its variable insertion of the 3 tendon heads (lateral, long, and medial), and the presence of physiologic intratendinous fat infiltration, that can mimic tendon degeneration and tears[47] (**Fig. 10**).

Cubital Tunnel

Anatomic variations of the cubital tunnel have been described. The main one is the medial subluxation/dislocation of the ulnar nerve over the tip of the medial epicondyle. This is not always

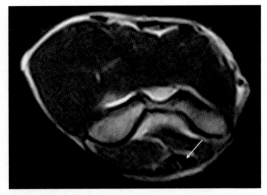

Fig. 10. Axial slice of the elbow at the level of the triceps tendon insertion showing intratendinous areas of high signal intensity (*arrow*), due to the presence of physiologic intratendinous fat infiltration but mimicking intratendinous tears.

associated with clinical symptoms or signs of neuropathy, and the imaging evidence of a displaced ulnar nerve should not lead to that diagnosis straightforward.[47]

Ulnar nerve subluxation is caused by interaction among groove anatomy, dynamic stability, and stresses. Imaging the elbow in even light flexion, the nerve will appear flattened.[48] Due to magic angle effect, the ulnar nerve also can show a high signal in fluid-weighted images; if the segment of abnormal signal intensity is short and focal (less than 4 axial slices), it is more likely to represent true pathology. Also, minor enlargement of the nerve is not specific for a pathologic involvement. The MR imaging features of ulnar nerve disease include signal alterations, change in diameter of the nerve, and secondary findings such as muscle edema and atrophy. The absence of these features, as well as the lack of symptoms related to friction neuritis, are reliable signs of the presence of asymptomatic ulnar nerve dislocation.[46]

The *anconeus epitrochlearis* (the fourth head of the triceps) is a small accessory muscle, potentially misdiagnosed as a mass within the cubital tunnel.[44]

There are also other structures that can mimic masses in the cubital tunnel; sometimes blood vessels (ulnar artery and accompanying venous channels) may show increased T2 signal and engorgement; these findings may be misinterpreted as signs of neuritis or nerve injury[44] (**Fig. 11**).

WRIST

The anatomy of the carpal and metacarpal bones is complex.[49] Recognizing the normal anatomy, let alone the pathologic disease processes, is challenging enough.

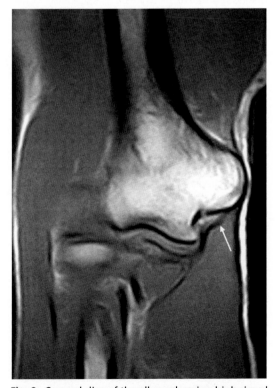

Fig. 9. Coronal slice of the elbow showing high signal intensity area of the ulnar collateral ligament (*arrow*) at the level of its proximal insertion.

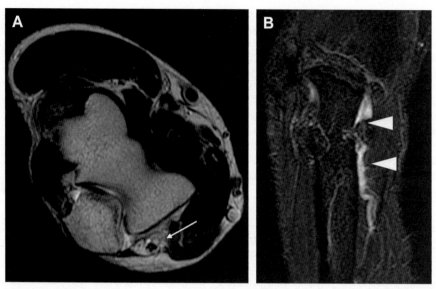

Fig. 11. Axial (*A*) slice of the elbow showing areas of increased T2 signal and engorgement at the cubital tunnel (*arrow*); coronal short tau inversion recovery cuts demonstrate this anomaly to be caused by the presence of blood vessels (*arrowheads* in *B*), without signs of ulnar nerve involvement.

Bone

One of the main MR pitfalls in wrist imaging is caused by patient positioning. Most patients are not imaged with the arm at the patient's side but with the so-called superman position, to locate the wrist with the isocenter of the magnet. However, the position is less comfortable; moreover, a "pseudo DISI/VISI configuration" may result from a different biomechanical load in this position.[50]

Such a diagnosis should be made with caution in these cases to avoid diagnostic pitfalls, mainly if we do not have radiographic correlation or evidence of ligament injury.

Incidental carpal cysts are a frequent cause of diagnostic uncertainty, especially when studying a patient with an inflammatory disease in which bone erosions are suspected. In such cases, a clear imaging distinction between the 2 entities is necessary. Simple carpal cysts arise at the level of ligamentous attachment either in the center of at the periphery throughout the carpus[49] (**Fig. 12**).

The capitate also has volar and dorsal grooves, normal cortical irregularities as found at the base of the second metacarpal bone and the bare area of the triquetrum (**Fig. 13**), that can be misdiagnosed as erosions. Another imaging pitfall mimicking erosions are cortical nutrient artery channels. In all these cases, image interpretation in light of clinical and laboratory picture, as well as research of typical rheumatoid arthritis imaging findings of synovitis, are of paramount importance.[49]

The *carpal boss* is a bony outgrowth at the level of the dorsal wrist (second or third metacarpal, or capitate or trapezoid), a known but often underdiagnosed cause of wrist pain, especially in MR imaging.

Another potential imaging pitfall of the bony wrist is the medial articular lunate facet with the hamate (type II lunate), a common lunate configuration that may be associated in some cases with subchondral edema and chondromalacia.[49]

Tendons

As for other joint tendons, flexor and extensor tendons of the wrist are subject to magic angle effect and can display increased signal intensity on MR imaging, with a false tendinosis appearance. The most frequently affected tendons are the flexor pollicis longus tendon distally in the carpal tunnel and the extensor pollicis longus and extensor carpi ulnaris tendons. The absence of additional imaging findings consistent with tendon disease (eg, tendon sheath synovitis) and normal appearance on long TE sequences are useful clues to recognize alterations due to magic angle effect[50] (**Fig. 14**).

Another cause of apparent abnormal intrasubstance tendon signal intensity is the presence of multiple tendon slips and fat interposed between the tendinous fascicles, usually affecting the abductor pollicis longus tendon and mimicking longitudinal tears.[50]

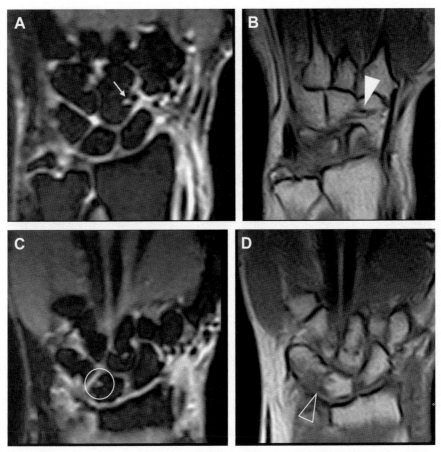

Fig. 12. Coronal short tau inversion recovery slices of the wrist showing small cystic bone alterations at the level of the carpal bones (*arrow* in *A*; *circle* in *C*); morphologic T1 images demonstrate these alterations to be simple carpal cysts at the level of ligamentous attachment (*arrowheads* in *B* and *D*).

The abductor pollicis longus tendon may also have a similar behavior due to its multiple bundle architecture.

Last, wrist position within the coil (neutral position, protonation, or supination) may affect tendon alignment of the extensor carpi ulnaris tendon within its ulnar styloid groove, with a tendency to subluxation in supination (pseudosubluxation).

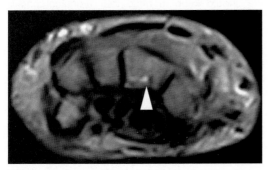

Fig. 13. Axial slice of the wrist showing a volar groove of the capitate (*arrowhead*).

Triangular Fibrocartilage Complex

The triangular fibrocartilage complex (TFCC) can lead to some diagnostic pitfalls owing to its anatomic architecture; the space between the proximal and distal lamina (ligamentum subcruentum), often shows intermediate to high signal intensity and can be misinterpreted as a tear.[51] Also, the radial and especially ulnar attachments of the TFCC often show increased signal intensity[50] (**Fig. 15**).

Ligaments

Intrinsic and extrinsic wrist ligaments often contribute to the challenging imaging interpretation of wrist MR imaging, thanks to their variable shape and configuration. In particular, the scapholunate ligament can show a triangular configuration, but less frequently appears as a linear structure.[49] The volar portion of the scapholunate ligament, with its bandlike ligamentous structure separated by loose vascular connective tissue,

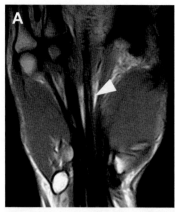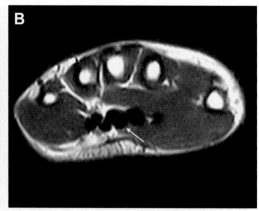

Fig. 14. Coronal (*A*) T1-weighted slice of the wrist showing increased signal intensity with a false tendinosis appearance of a flexor tendon (*arrowhead*) due to magic angle effect; the T2-weighted axial slice confirms the normal appearance of the tendon (*arrow* in *B*).

demonstrates striated heterogeneous increased signal intensity. Also, the lunotriquetral ligament shapes vary from a delta configuration to a linear or amorphous appearance. The high flexibility of the lunotriquetral ligament is also responsible for the high variability of shape and signal intensity of this ligament on different wrist positions during imaging.[50]

Moreover, ligament signal intensity also can be inconstant, with the possible presence of central or linear vertical intermediate signal areas instead of homogeneous low signal intensity. This increased signal intensity can lead to a misdiagnosis of a ligament tear, but the absence of a fluid signal at the interface or through the ligament can be a clue to avoid this pitfall.[50]

Carpal Tunnel

Among the carpal tunnel structures, the median nerve is the one leading most to diagnostic pitfalls due to its course variants (eg, a high division of the median nerve, bifid median nerve, split median nerve by a persistent median artery, or an aberrant muscle) and accessory branches.

As for other wrist structures, the anatomic alignment of the median nerve is highly dependent on wrist positioning, so the relationship to other structures should be considered as a unique parameter to assess a median nerve involvement of carpal tunnel syndrome.[50]

Many muscle anomalies also have been described within the carpal tunnel, such as the reversed palmaris longus muscle, the accessory palmaris profundus, the accessory flexor digitorum superficialis, and aberrant origins of the thenar and lumbrical muscles.

Last, in the assessment of cartilage thickness, we should keep in mind that technical pitfalls may derive by chemical shift artifacts at the cartilage-bone marrow interface, leading to possible errors in the evaluation of cartilage thickness.[50]

SUMMARY

The complexity in anatomy and pathologic conditions of upper limb structures can lead to several errors in the interpretation of MR imaging findings. Knowledge of these possible pitfalls is essential to achieve a correct diagnosis of normal and pathologic findings.

Fig. 15. Coronal cut of the wrist showing increased signal intensity of the TFCC at the level of the ulnar attachment (*arrowhead*); this appearance can be misinterpreted as a tear.

REFERENCES

1. Valentini G, Marcoccia A, Cuomo G, et al. Early systemic sclerosis: marker autoantibodies and videocapillaroscopy patterns are each associated with distinct clinical, functional and cellular activation markers. Arthritis Res Ther 2013. https://doi.org/10.1186/ar4236.

2. Perrotta FM, Astorri D, Zappia M, et al. An ultrasonographic study of enthesis in early psoriatic arthritis patients naive to traditional and biologic DMARDs treatment. Rheumatol Int 2016;36(11):1579–83.

3. Caranci F, Briganti F, La Porta M, et al. Magnetic resonance imaging in brachial plexus injury. Musculoskelet Surg 2013. https://doi.org/10.1007/s12306-013-0281-0.

4. Masciocchi C, Barile A, Lelli SCV. Magnetic resonance imaging (MRI) and arthro-MRI in the evaluation of the chondral pathology of the knee joint. Radiol Med 2004;108(3):149–58.

5. Barile A, Conti L, Lanni G, et al. Evaluation of medial meniscus tears and meniscal stability: weight-bearing MRI vs arthroscopy. Eur J Radiol 2013;82(4):633–9.

6. Barile A, Bruno F, Arrigoni F, et al. Emergency and trauma of the ankle. Semin Musculoskelet Radiol 2017;21(3). https://doi.org/10.1055/s-0037-1602408.

7. Zoccali C, Arrigoni F, Mariani S, et al. An unusual localization of chondroblastoma: the triradiate cartilage; from a case report a reconstructive technique proposal with imaging evolution. J Clin Orthop Trauma 2017. https://doi.org/10.1016/j.jcot.2017.07.011.

8. Bruno F, Barile A, Arrigoni F, et al. Weight-bearing MRI of the knee: a review of advantages and limits. Acta Biomed 2018;89. https://doi.org/10.23750/abm.v89i1-S.7011.

9. Arrigoni F, Bruno F, Zugaro L, et al. Developments in the management of bone metastases with interventional radiology. Acta Biomed 2018;89. https://doi.org/10.23750/abm.v89i1-S.7020.

10. De Filippo M, Russo U, Papapietro VR, et al. Radiofrequency ablation of osteoid osteoma. Acta Biomed 2018;89. https://doi.org/10.23750/abm.v89i1-S.7021.

11. Arrigoni F, Bruno F, Zugaro L, et al. Role of interventional radiology in the management of musculoskeletal soft-tissue lesions. Radiol Med 2018. https://doi.org/10.1007/s11547-018-0893-4.

12. Barile A, Arrigoni F, Bruno F, et al. Present role and future perspectives of interventional radiology in the treatment of painful bone lesions. Future Oncol 2018. https://doi.org/10.2217/fon-2017-0657.

13. Cazzato RL, Arrigoni F, Boatta E, et al. Percutaneous management of bone metastases: state of the art, interventional strategies and joint position statement of the Italian College of MSK Radiology (ICoMSKR) and the Italian College of Interventional Radiology (ICIR). Radiol Med 2018;1(0123456789):3.

14. Masciocchi C, Conchiglia A, Gregori LM, et al. Critical role of HIFU in musculoskeletal interventions. Radiol Med 2014;119(7):470–5.

15. Masciocchi C, Zugaro L, Arrigoni F, et al. Radiofrequency ablation versus magnetic resonance guided focused ultrasound surgery for minimally invasive treatment of osteoid osteoma: a propensity score matching study. Eur Radiol 2016;26(8):2472–81.

16. Barile A, Lanni G, Conti L, et al. Lesions of the biceps pulley as cause of anterosuperior impingement of the shoulder in the athlete: potentials and limits of MR arthrography compared with arthroscopy. Radiol Med 2013;118(1):112–22.

17. Barile A, La Marra A, Arrigoni F, et al. Anaesthetics, steroids and platelet-rich plasma (PRP) in ultrasound-guided musculoskeletal procedures. Br J Radiol 2016. https://doi.org/10.1259/bjr.20150355.

18. Barile A, Regis G, Masi R, et al. Musculoskeletal tumours: preliminary experience with perfusion MRI. Radiol Med 2007;112(4):550–61.

19. Barile A, Arrigoni F, Bruno F, et al. Computed tomography and MR imaging in rheumatoid arthritis. Radiol Clin North Am 2017. https://doi.org/10.1016/j.rcl.2017.04.006.

20. Barile A, Arrigoni F, Zugaro L, et al. Minimally invasive treatments of painful bone lesions: state of the art. Med Oncol 2017;34(4). https://doi.org/10.1007/s12032-017-0909-2.

21. Masciocchi C, Conti L, D'Orazio F, et al. Errors in musculoskeletal MRI. In: Romano L, Pinto A, editors. Errors in radiology. Milano: Springer; 2012. p. 209–17.

22. Mandato Y, Reginelli A, Galasso R, et al. Errors in the radiological evaluation of the alimentary tract: Part I. Semin Ultrasound CT MR 2012;33(4):300–7.

23. Kaplan A, Stinson W, Bryans KC, et al. MRI imaging of normal shoulders variants and pitfalls. Radiology 1992;184(2):519–24.

24. Massengill D, Shnie C, Shapiro S, et al. Labrocapsular mentous complex of the shoulder: normal anatomy, anatomic variation, and of MR imaging pitfalls and MR. Radiographics 1994;1211–23.

25. Pierce JL, Nacey NC, Jones S, et al. Postoperative shoulder imaging: rotator cuff, labrum, and biceps tendon. RadioGraphics 2016;36(6):1648–71.

26. Dunham KS, Bencardino JT, Rokito AS. Anatomic variants and pitfalls of the labrum, glenoid cartilage, and glenohumeral ligaments. Magn Reson Imaging Clin N Am 2012;20(2):213–28.

27. Beltran J, Bencardino J, Mellado J, et al. MR arthrography of the shoulder: variants and pitfalls. RadioGraphics 1997;17(6):1403–12.

28. Modarresi S, Motamedi D, Jude CM. Superior labral anteroposterior lesions of the shoulder: part 2, mechanisms and classification. Am J Roentgenol 2011;197(3):604–11.

29. Farid N, Bruce D, Chung CB. Miscellaneous conditions of the shoulder: anatomical, clinical, and pictorial review emphasizing potential pitfalls in imaging diagnosis. Eur J Radiol 2008;68(1):88–105.

30. Patel K. MRI of shoulder trauma. Semin Musculoskelet Radiol 2007;1(C):1–34.

31. Vinson EN, Wittstein J, Garrigues GE, et al. MRI of selected abnormalities at the anterior superior aspect of the shoulder: potential pitfalls and subtle diagnoses. Am J Roentgenol 2012;199(3):534–45.

32. Pouliart N, Boulet C, De Maeseneer M, et al. Advanced imaging of the glenohumeral ligaments. Semin Musculoskelet Radiol 2014;18(4):374–97.

33. Park YH, Lee JY, Moon SH, et al. MR arthrography of the labral capsular ligamentous complex in the shoulder: imaging variations and pitfalls. Am J Roentgenol 2000;175(3):667–72.

34. Felix G, Setor De Radiologia M, Por D. Artifacts and pitfalls in shoulder magnetic resonance imaging. Radiol Bras 2015;48(4):242–8.

35. Rudez J, Zanetti M. Normal anatomy, variants and pitfalls on shoulder MRI. Eur J Radiol 2008;68(1): 25–35.

36. Goh CK, Peh WCG. Pictorial essay: pitfalls in magnetic resonance imaging of the shoulder. Can Assoc Radiol J 2012;63(4):247–59.

37. Carool KW, Helms CA. Magnetic resonance imaging of the shoulder: a review of potential sources of diagnostic errors. Skeletal Radiol 2002;31(7): 373–83.

38. Beltran LS, Adler R, Stone T, et al. MRI and ultrasound imaging of the shoulder using positional maneuvers. Am J Roentgenol 2015;205(3):W244–54.

39. Fitzpatrick D, Walz DM. Shoulder MR imaging normal variants and imaging artifacts. Magn Reson Imaging Clin N Am 2010;18(4):615–32.

40. Reginelli A, Zappia M, Barile A, et al. Strategies of imaging after orthopedic surgery. Musculoskelet Surg 2017;101. https://doi.org/10.1007/s12306-017-0458-z.

41. Barile A, Bruno F, Mariani S, et al. What can be seen after rotator cuff repair: a brief review of diagnostic imaging findings. Musculoskelet Surg 2017;101. https://doi.org/10.1007/s12306-017-0455-2.

42. White LM, Bancroft LW. Postoperative imaging of the knee and shoulder. In: Hodler J, von Schulthess GK, Zollikofer CL, editors. Musculoskeletal diseases 2013–2016. Milano: Springer; 2013. p. 73–84.

43. Chung CB, Stanley AJ, Gentili A. Magnetic resonance imaging of elbow instability. Semin Musculoskelet Radiol 2005;9(1):67–76.

44. Rosenberg S. MR imaging of the elbow: normal variant and potential pitfalls of the trochlear groove and cubital. Radiology 1995;415–8. https://doi.org/10.1111/j.1469-0691.2009.03066.x.

45. Sampaio ML, Schweitzer ME. Elbow magnetic resonance imaging variants and pitfalls. Magn Reson Imaging Clin N Am 2010;18(4):633–42.

46. Sonin AH, Tutton SM, Fitzgerald SW, et al. MR imaging of the adult elbow. RadioGraphics 1996;16(6): 1323–36.

47. Rosenberg ZS, Bencardino J, Beltran J. MRI of normal variants and interpretation pitfalls of the elbow. Semin Musculoskelet Radiol 1998;2(2): 141–55.

48. Husarik DB, Saupe N, Pfirrmann CW, et al. Elbow nerves: MR findings in 60 asymptomatic subjects—normal anatomy, variants, and pitfalls. Radiology 2009;252(1):148–56.

49. Malone WJ, Snowden R, Alvi F, et al. Pitfalls of wrist MR imaging. Magn Reson Imaging Clin N Am 2010; 18(4):643–62.

50. Pfirrmann CWA, Zanetti M. Variants, pitfalls and asymptomatic findings in wrist and hand imaging. Eur J Radiol 2005;56(3):286–95.

51. Burns JE, Tanaka T, Ueno T, et al. Musculoskeletal imaging TFCC pitfalls. Radiographics 2011;31: 63–78.

Imaging of Peripheral Nerves of the Upper Extremity

Vivek Kalia, MD, MPH, MS[a],*, Jon A. Jacobson, MD[b]

KEYWORDS

• Peripheral nerves • Ultrasound • Ultrasonography • MR imaging • Nerve imaging

KEY POINTS

- A combination of clinical examination, electrodiagnostic testing, and imaging studies, chiefly MR imaging and ultrasonography, are often needed to identify a specific diagnosis for an individual patient.
- The most common upper extremity peripheral neuropathies include carpal tunnel syndrome, cubital tunnel syndrome, and cervical radiculopathy, which can all be assessed by both MR imaging and ultrasonography.
- Ultrasound evaluation of peripheral nerves should use high-resolution 15- to 18-MHz transducers, attempt to evaluate nerves along their short axis, compare with the contralateral extremity as appropriate, and use color Doppler technique to distinguish small peripheral nerves from regional vasculature.
- MR imaging of peripheral nerves should use high spatial resolution while maintaining a reasonable scan-acquisition time, use as high a field strength as possible for diagnostic imaging, use a high matrix (>256) to achieve in-plane resolution of 0.3 to 0.4 mm, use low slice thickness of 2 to 3 mm in the distal extremity, and use fat-suppressed highly T2-weighted sequences to evaluate for nerve pathology and muscular denervation edema.
- With MR imaging evaluation of nerves, 3D iso-voxel acquisitions are ideal but are time consuming. Fat suppression with Dixon technique is preferred over STIR sequences.

INTRODUCTION
Discussion of Problem/Clinical Presentation

Peripheral neuropathy of the upper extremity is a common clinical scenario encountered by a wide variety of medical care providers. Diseases of the peripheral nerves can be broadly categorized as mononeuropathies, polyneuropathies, and mononeuropathy multiplex. Weakness or sensory loss seen in one extremity only most often denotes a peripheral neuropathy rather than a central nervous system issue.[1] Common clinical presentations include focal sensory loss of weakness in the involved nerve distribution, although the presence of pain in the associated extremity may cause confusion, as pain may limit the action and mobility of an involved limb. Weakness in the presence of pain thus does not always indicate true neurologic dysfunction.[1]

The most common upper extremity mononeuropathy involves the median nerve as carpal tunnel syndrome, with an incidence of approximately

---

Disclosure Statement: The authors have no commercial or financial conflicts of interest.
[a] Department of Radiology, Division of Musculoskeletal Radiology, University of Michigan Hospital, Main Campus, 1500 East Medical Center Drive, Taubman Center 2910D, Ann Arbor, MI 48109-5326, USA;
[b] Department of Radiology, Division of Musculoskeletal Radiology, University of Michigan Hospital, Main Campus, 1500 East Medical Center Drive, Taubman Center 2910L, Ann Arbor, MI 48109-5326, USA
* Corresponding author.
E-mail address: kaliavi@med.umich.edu

3.4% in one population-based study in the Netherlands.[2] Cervical radiculopathy is also common, with incidence highest in persons aged 50 to 54 years, involving the C6 and C7 nerve roots up to 64% of the time.[3] Brachial plexopathy has a reported incidence of about 1.6 per 100,000 population.[4] Cubital tunnel syndrome is the second most common nerve entrapment of the upper extremity, with an incidence of 21 to 25 per 100,000 population.[5]

A combination of clinical examination, electrodiagnostic testing, and imaging studies is often needed to identify a specific diagnosis for an individual patient. In particular scenarios, such as entrapment neuropathies, imaging is helpful in identifying the cause, severity, etiology, and location of the entrapment. Recent years have availed considerable advances in techniques for imaging of peripheral nerves. This article reviews imaging techniques and pathologies of the peripheral nerves of the upper extremity.

Although in many cases MR imaging remains the gold standard for nerve imaging, ultrasonography has become increasingly important for numerous reasons, including its ability to offer dynamic information while a patient moves his or her upper extremity and attempts to recreate symptomatology, its availability when contraindications to MR imaging exist, and its more widespread availability and lower cost profile. A further advantage of ultrasonography is its ability to readily and quickly image the entire extremity, including the contralateral side, which in many clinical scenarios is asymptomatic and provides a superb internal control to variant anatomy between individuals. Ultrasonography also offers superb spatial resolution to depict morphologic changes in nerves or individual fascicles. Lastly, when preoperative MR imaging reveals a nerve abnormality that will be addressed surgically, ultrasonography allows mapping of the location of an abnormality on the skin surface, which may be of tremendous help to surgeons.[6] Limitations of ultrasonography include limited evaluation of deep nerves, susceptibility to anisotropy, and small field of view.

NORMAL ANATOMY AND IMAGING TECHNIQUE
Discussion of Important Anatomic Considerations

Brachial plexus
Imaging evaluation of the brachial plexus, which innervates the upper extremity, is chiefly performed by a combination of MR imaging and ultrasonography; however, this is true only for the postganglionic brachial plexus and for peripheral neuropathy. The preganglionic brachial plexus is optimally evaluated with computed tomography myelography. Ultrasonography and high-field-strength, small-field-of-view MR neurography are capable of evaluating other regional nerve structures at the level of the proximal brachial plexus, including the suprascapular nerve, long thoracic nerve, and spinal accessory nerve.

The anatomy of the brachial plexus has been described from proximal to distal as roots, trunks, divisions, cords, and then branches. The 4 primary locations evaluated in the postganglionic brachial plexus are the paravertebral, interscalene, supraclavicular, and infraclavicular segments.[6] The C5 to C8 brachial plexus roots are visualized as they exit their neural foramina adjacent to the vertebral transverse processes. In the interscalene triangle, the brachial plexus roots and trunks are seen between the anterior and middle scalene muscles, and in the supraclavicular region the brachial plexus divisions are seen. In the infraclavicular region with the patient positioned in the arm abduction and external rotation position, the brachial plexus cords are seen around the axillary artery. Compared with MR imaging, ultrasonography has some limitations when evaluating the areas of the brachial plexus obscured by the clavicle or rib, such as the divisions.

The suprascapular nerve, originating from the upper trunk of the brachial plexus, can be traced inferolaterally and be detected distally within the suprascapular and spinoglenoid notches on both ultrasonography and MR imaging.

The spinal accessory nerve, which innervates the sternocleidomastoid (SCM) and trapezius muscles, can be traced along the posterolateral margin of the SCM muscle. The spinal accessory nerve may be injured iatrogenically during lymph node biopsy in this region (the posterior triangle).

The long thoracic nerve, which innervates the serratus anterior muscle, can be seen at the level of the scalene muscles and into the supraclavicular fossa. The long thoracic nerve pierces through the middle scalene muscle[7] and traverses lateral to the suprascapular nerve.

Median nerve
The median nerve originates from spinal nerve roots C6 to T1, specifically from the medial and lateral cords of the brachial plexus. It descends down the arm starting lateral to the brachial artery and about midway down the arm becomes situated medially. The median nerve then courses distally and enters the anterior forearm compartment in the cubital fossa, where it travels between flexor digitorum profundus and flexor digitorum superficialis (FDS) muscles and gives off two major

branches in the forearm: the anterior interosseous nerve (AIN) and the palmar cutaneous nerve. The median nerve then enters the hand via the carpal tunnel. The median nerve terminates by dividing into a recurrent branch and the palmar digital branches.

Ulnar nerve

The ulnar nerve originates from spinal nerve roots C8 to T1 and is a continuation of the medial cord of the brachial plexus. The ulnar nerve descends down the medial aspect of the upper arm and passes just posterior to the medial epicondyle of the humerus at the level of the elbow, and travels into the cubital tunnel at the level of the elbow. In the proximal forearm, the ulnar nerve pierces the 2 heads of the flexor carpi ulnaris (FCU) and travels alongside the ulna, deep to the FCU muscle. It gives off 3 main branches in the forearm: (1) muscular branch, (2) palmar cutaneous branch, and (3) dorsal cutaneous branch. At the wrist, the ulnar nerve travels superficial to the flexor retinaculum and medial to the ulnar artery. It enters the hand via the Guyon or ulnar canal and terminates in the hand into superficial and deep branches.

Radial nerve

The radial nerve originates from spinal nerve roots C5 to T1 and is the terminal continuation of the posterior cord of the brachial plexus. At the level of the axilla, it is located posterior to the axillary artery. The radial nerve descends down the upper arm, traveling in the shallow spiral groove posterior to the humerus. It divides into a superficial sensory branch and a deep motor branch, which enters the radial tunnel. The motor branch then runs between the superficial and deep heads of the supinator muscle and becomes the posterior interosseous nerve (PIN) as it exits the supinator posteriorly. The PIN then courses along the dorsal interosseous membrane and divides into smaller branches for the extensor musculature of the forearm. The superficial branch courses distally through the forearm, eventually moving dorsally, crossing over the radius and first extensor wrist compartment tendons in a subcutaneous location.

Musculocutaneous nerve

The musculocutaneous nerve (MCN) arises from the lateral cord of the brachial plexus, traverses through the coracobrachialis muscle, and descends along the lateral aspect of the arm between the biceps brachii and brachialis muscles. The MCN continues into the forearm as the lateral antebrachial cutaneous nerve, traveling behind the cephalic vein. MCN entrapment is rare but may occur as a result of weightlifting (eg, excessive hypertrophy of the biceps brachii and brachialis muscles), with patients presenting painless weakness of elbow flexion and forearm supination.

IMAGING PROTOCOLS

Boxes 1 and 2 list the main aspects of the imaging protocols.

IMAGING FINDINGS AND PATHOLOGY
Brachial Plexus

Brachial plexus abnormalities may require both MR imaging and ultrasound evaluation depending on the etiology, for example, whether or not it is related to trauma. Trauma-related brachial plexus injuries include nerve root avulsion, nerve laceration/transection, and the formation of neuromas in the setting of traction injuries. Nontraumatic causes of brachial plexus abnormalities include Parsonage-Turner syndrome (PTS)/amyotrophic neuralgia and thoracic outlet syndrome. PTS may present as segmental nerve swelling or focal nerve constriction,[10] often involving the suprascapular nerve,[6] evaluated well by both ultrasonography and appropriate MR imaging protocols. Traumatic injury to the suprascapular nerve may cause changes in acute and eventually chronic denervation such as muscular atrophy and fatty infiltration of the supraspinatus and infraspinatus muscles, which are best evaluated on MR imaging.

Entrapment Neuropathies

Ultrasonography is helpful in identifying causes of entrapment neuropathies such as fibrous bands, ganglion cysts, anomalous muscles, and osseous deformities.[11–13] External compression on nerves

---

Box 1
Ultrasound evaluation of peripheral nerves

- High-resolution 15- to 18-MHz transducers are recommended when imaging the extremity nerves

- Peripheral nerves are more conspicuous when imaged in their short axis

- Cine sweeps of areas of interest often provide better spatial information than solely relying on still images

- Comparison with contralateral upper extremity is helpful in cases of subtle abnormality, when symptoms are only present on one side

- Color Doppler technique is useful to distinguish small nerves from regional vasculature

- Direct correlation with symptoms elicited during transducer pressure further localizes nerve pathology

---

Box 2
MR imaging evaluation of peripheral nerves

- Must balance the need for high spatial resolution to view peripheral nerves of diameter typically <5 mm with the cost of lower signal-to-noise ratio (SNR) and longer acquisition time

- Imaging at 3.0 T preferable because of inherent higher SNR

- Field of view should be kept minimum over the region of interest with use of surface coils to reduce empty space around extremity

- High matrix of >256 recommended to achieve in-plane resolution of 0.3 to 0.4 mm

- Low slice thickness of 2 to 3 mm in distal extremity and 4 to 5 mm in proximal extremity

- Minimal to no interslice gap

- Recommend fat-suppressed highly T2-weighted sequences to demonstrate nerve pathology and muscular denervation edema

- 3D iso-voxel acquisitions are ideal but are time consuming → major benefit is thinner slices and multiplanar reconstruction of the curved courses of nerves

- Fat suppression may be achieved optimally with the Dixon technique, which suffers slightly more from susceptibility effects compared with short-tau inversion recovery sequences, but benefits from increased SNR and postcontrast compatibility.[8,9] Parallel imaging techniques may be used to shorten the acquisition time

---

causes a predictable sequence of abnormalities that can be evaluated on imaging, particularly early perineural and endoneural (eg, fascicular) edema, and more chronically, perineural fibrosis.[14–16] Such extrinsic compression may appear on imaging as[5]:

- Abrupt caliber changes in the nerve along its course

- Flattened appearance of nerve at site of compression

- Focal or diffuse enlargement of nerve at and proximal to the entrapment resulting from fascicular edema

- Loss of normal fascicular architecture of nerve (ie, loss of "honeycomb" appearance)

- Nerve sheath (epineurium) thickening, which may present as an echogenic halo around a nerve

- Hypervascularity in and around involved nerves

- Atrophy of musculature innervated by the nerve in question

Median nerve

Proximal median nerve entrapment may present as a motor-only phenomenon (also known as AIN syndrome or Kiloh-Nevin syndrome) (**Fig. 1**) or as a clinical mimicker of carpal tunnel syndrome known as pronator syndrome.[5]

Pronator syndrome results from entrapment of the median nerve at 1 or more of 4 locations: (1) by the ligament of Struthers at the level of the distal humerus; (2) by a thickened bicipital aponeurosis at the level of the proximal elbow; (3) by direct compression between the superficial and deep heads of the pronator teres muscle at the level of the elbow joint; or (4) by a thickened proximal edge of the FDS muscle or fibrous band between the pronator teres and FDS at the level of the proximal forearm.[5] Patients present with pain and paresthesias in the volar aspect of the elbow, forearm, and the first, second, and third digits as well as radial aspect of the fourth digit.

AIN syndrome results from entrapment of the AIN between the heads of the pronator teres muscle and the proximal edge of the FDS arch, whether from a hematoma, mass, thickened interosseous artery, or secondary to PTS. Patients present with weakness or inability to pinch the fingertips of the thumb and index finger together.

Distal median nerve entrapment manifests as carpal tunnel syndrome (CTS), which results from entrapment of the median nerve within the carpal tunnel (**Fig. 2**). Patients present with nocturnal wrist pain and paresthesias in the distribution of the median nerve. Imaging findings may demonstrate thickening of the overlying flexor retinaculum, increased crowding in the carpal tunnel caused by ganglion cysts or anomalous muscles (eg, palmaris longus, palmaris profundus), or tenosynovitis involving flexor tendons related to inflammatory arthritis, amyloidosis, or gout. On ultrasonography, CTS manifests as enlarged cross-sectional area of the median nerve, as determined by analysis of the nerve at 2 levels: (1) within the carpal tunnel and (2) at the level of the pronator quadratus in the distal forearm. A change of greater than 2 mm^2 in area is consistent with CTS.

Ulnar nerve Ulnar nerve entrapment at the level of the elbow occurs in the fibro-osseous cubital tunnel, which is formed by the elbow joint capsule and posterior band of the ulnar collateral ligament anteriorly, Osborne's retinaculum (and arcuate ligament) posteriorly, the medial epicondyle medially, and the olecranon process laterally. Flexion of the elbow causes a dynamic increase in pressure in the cubital tunnel, and cubital tunnel syndrome is usually elicited by and exacerbated by

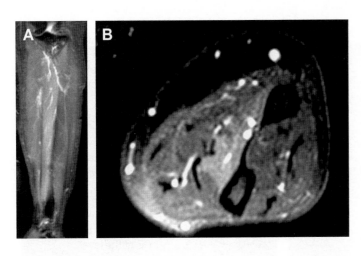

Fig. 1. A 42-year-old man with hand weakness. Coronal short-tau inversion recovery (STIR) (*A*) and axial T2-weighted fat-saturated (*B*) images of the mid-forearm demonstrate intramuscular edema in the flexor digitorum profundus muscle in the anterior forearm compartment. Imaging and clinical findings were consistent with a motor neuropathy known as anterior interosseous nerve syndrome, a rare proximal median nerve entrapment syndrome.

this position (**Figs. 3** and **4**). Patients present with pain, paresthesias, and weakness in the fifth digit and ulnar aspect of the fourth digit, as well as numbness in the dorsal ulnar aspect of the hand. On ultrasonography, the ulnar nerve will appear enlarged and hypoechoic, with loss of its normal fibrillar architecture. Both ultrasonography and MR imaging may demonstrate nerve enlargement, possible external compression by bone fragments or loose joint bodies, space-occupying lesions such as ganglion cysts, regional inflammatory change, and accessory musculature that may contribute to cubital tunnel syndrome (ie, anconeus epitrochlearis). Ulnar nerve injury may also occur by direct trauma or stretch injuries (**Fig. 5**).

In snapping ulnar nerve syndrome, the ulnar nerve may dislocate anteriorly over the medial epicondyle with elbow flexion, with or without the

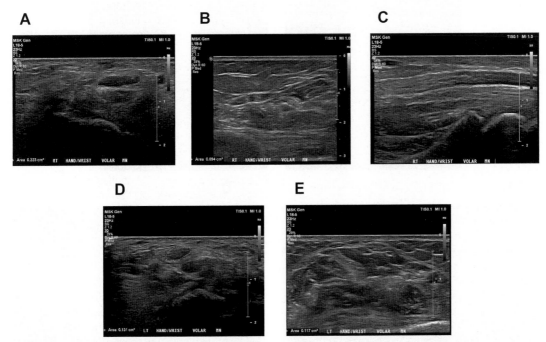

Fig. 2. A 55-year-old woman with pain and paresthesias in radial aspect of the dominant right hand, more severe at night. Transverse ultrasound images at the level of the carpal tunnel distally (*A*) and the pronator quadratus proximally (*B*) demonstrate a difference in cross-sectional area of greater than 2 mm^2, suggestive of distal median nerve entrapment or carpal tunnel syndrome. Longitudinal ultrasound image at the level of the proximal carpal tunnel (*C*) shows proximal dilatation/swelling of the nerve. Comparison transverse images (*D*, *E*) ultrasound images of the contralateral asymptomatic wrist at the same levels show a more normal appearance and size of the median nerve.

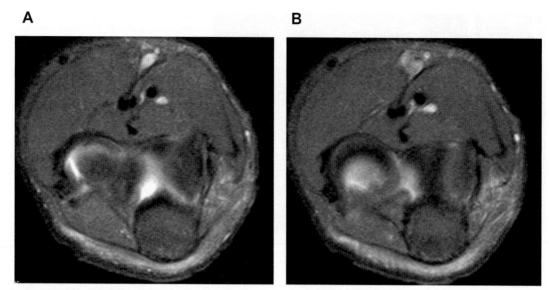

Fig. 3. Axial T2-weighted spectral presaturation with inversion recovery (SPIR) images of the left elbow of a 58-year-old man (*A*, *B*) at the level of the cubital tunnel demonstrate signal hyperintensity involving the ulnar nerve and soft tissues surrounding it.

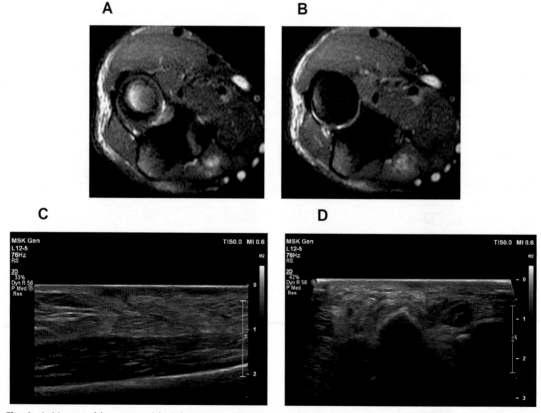

Fig. 4. A 44-year-old woman with right upper extremity paresthesias in the distribution of the ulnar nerve (small finger). Axial T2-weighted SPIR images of the right elbow (*A*, *B*) demonstrate marked signal hyperintensity of the ulnar nerve and surrounding tissues. Longitudinal (*C*) and transverse (*D*) ultrasound images of the ulnar nerve demonstrate hypoechogenicity and enlargement of the nerve, in keeping with cubital tunnel syndrome.

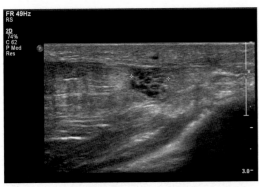

Fig. 5. A 49-year-old man with severe upper extremity pain and paresthesias after hitting his elbow on a workbench. Longitudinal ultrasound image of the ulnar nerve demonstrates several fascicular enlargement and hypoechogenicity reflecting ulnar nerve enlargement with edema, in this case caused by direct trauma.

medial head of the triceps brachii tendon. It may then spontaneously reduce to normal position, and this repetitive process that occurs with elbow flexion can lead to friction neuritis of the ulnar nerve.[5] Dynamic ultrasound evaluation during resisted elbow flexion and extension may elicit transient dislocation of the ulnar nerve in real time.

More rarely, the ulnar nerve may become entrapped at the level of the Guyon canal, an oblique fibro-osseous triangular tunnel in the wrist. The ulnar nerve divides into the superficial sensory and 2 or 3 deep motor branches within the Guyon canal. Patients present with paresthesias and eventually motor difficulties in the distribution of the fourth and fifth digits. On ultrasonography, the ulnar nerve at the level of the Guyon canal will appear thickened and hypoechoic, and a cause such as external compression by a ganglion cyst or accessory muscle (eg, accessory abductor digiti minimi) should be sought.

Radial nerve Radial nerve compression or entrapment can occur at the level of the elbow and lead to either radial tunnel syndrome or PIN (supinator) syndrome. Patients with radial tunnel syndrome present with pain at the lateral aspect of the proximal forearm, which mimics lateral epicondylitis. Patients with PIN syndrome present with painless weakness of the forearm extensor musculature, often caused by compression at the arcade of Frohse, the thickened tendinous proximal edge of the superficial head of the supinator. On ultrasound evaluation of PIN syndrome, there is enlargement and hypoechogenicity of the PIN most commonly at the arcade of Frohse.

Nerve Tumors

As previously noted, both benign and malignant peripheral nerve sheath tumors (PNSTs) have variable characteristics on ultrasonography[17] and MR imaging.[18] Despite this, some general principles apply: PNSTs are typically fusiform lesions (**Fig. 6**) seen in the distribution of a nerve. Malignant PNSTs are typically associated with major nerve trunks, whereas benign PNSTs (which

A　　　　　　　　**B**

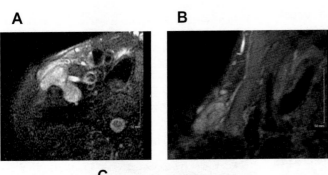

C

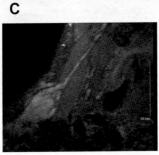

Fig. 6. A 61-year-old man with right upper extremity weakness. Axial (A) and coronal (B, C) T2-weighted fat-saturated images demonstrate a lobulated fusiform mass contiguous with nerves supplying the upper extremity, consistent with a peripheral nerve sheath tumor (PNST).

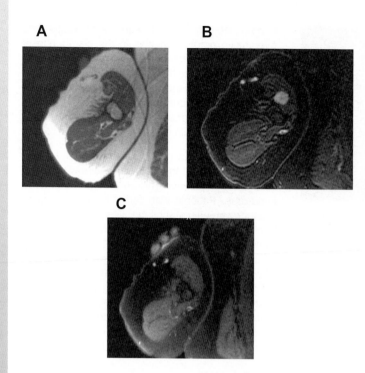

A

B

C

Fig. 7. Axial T1-weighted non–fat-saturated image (A) of the upper arm in a 56-year-old woman shows no gross abnormality. Axial T1-weighted fat-saturated precontrast (B) and postcontrast (C) images at the same level show a large avidly enhancing ovoid mass originating in the region of the musculocutaneous nerve, 1 of the 5 major branches of the brachial plexus. Pathology results demonstrated a benign PNST. Malignant PNSTs are typically associated with major nerve trunks, whereas benign PNSTs (which consist of schwannomas and neurofibromas) may be located along cutaneous or deep nerves.

consist of schwannomas and neurofibromas) may be located along cutaneous or deep nerves (**Fig. 7**). PNSTs typically show low to intermediate signal on T1-weighted images and high signal on T2-weighted images.[19] On ultrasonography, most PNSTs are hypoechoic and homogeneous, and demonstrate posterior acoustic enhancement and continuity with the peripheral nerve in question.

Some benign PNSTs may display a target appearance on sonography (centrally hyperechoic with a hypoechoic periphery)[20]; however, this may be seen in as few as 25% of cases.[17] Importantly, there are ultrasound imaging features common to both PNSTs and ganglion cysts, which may mimic PNSTs—features such as a hypoechoic and homogeneous appearance. Color Doppler flow within such a lesion can effectively exclude a ganglion cyst and suggest PNST. With MR imaging, a target sign has also been described (central low signal and peripheral high T2-weighted signal) in a benign PNST, especially a neurofibroma, and absent with a malignant PNST.[21]

Importantly, one retrospective review of 10 patients with PNSTs showed that sonography was unable to reliably distinguish among schwannoma, neurofibroma, and malignant PNSTs.[17] Size of a PNST greater than 5 cm generally portends a malignant cause, and increase in size also suggests malignant transformation.[18] MR imaging is often helpful in equivocal imaging cases: malignant PNSTs tend to be more heterogeneous[18] because of internal necrosis and hemorrhage, although this is not a 100% specific finding. Perilesional edema (demonstrated by increased T2 signal intensity) may also suggest perilesional infiltration or edema seen more commonly with malignant PNSTs.[22]

REFERENCES

1. Rutkove SB. Differential diagnosis of peripheral nerve and muscle disease. In: Shefner JM, editor. UpToDate. 2018. Available at: https://www.uptodate.com/contents/differential-diagnosis-of-peripheral-nerve-and-muscle-disease?topicRef=5282&source=see_link 2018. Accessed December 1, 2018.
2. de Krom MC, Knipschild PG, Kester AD, et al. Carpal tunnel syndrome: prevalence in the general population. J Clin Epidemiol 1992;45(4):373.
3. Radhakrishnan K, Litchy WJ, O'Fallon WM, et al. Epidemiology of cervical radiculopathy. A population-based study from Rochester, Minnesota, 1976 through 1990. Brain 1994;117(Pt 2):325.
4. Beghi E, Kurland LT, Mulder DW, et al. Brachial plexus neuropathy in the population of Rochester, Minnesota, 1970-1981. Ann Neurol 1985;18(3):320.
5. Klauser AS, Buzzegoli T, Taljanovic MS, et al. Nerve entrapment syndromes at the wrist and elbow by sonography. Semin Musculoskelet Radiol 2018;22(3):344–53.
6. Nwawka OK. Ultrasound imaging of the brachial plexus and nerves about the neck. Ultrasound Q

2018. https://doi.org/10.1097/RUQ.000000000000 0396.

7. Lieba-Samal D, Morgenbesser J, Moritz T, et al. Visualization of the long thoracic nerve using high-resolution sonography. Ultraschall Med 2015;36(3): 264–9.

8. Cha JG, Jin W, Lee MH, et al. Reducing metallic artifacts in postoperative spinal imaging: usefulness of IDEAL contrast-enhanced T1- and T2-weighted MR imaging—phantom and clinical studies. Radiology 2011;259(3):885–93.

9. Lee JB, Cha JG, Lee MH, et al. Usefulness of IDEAL T2-weighted FSE and SPGR imaging in reducing metallic artifacts in the postoperative ankles with metallic hardware. Skeletal Radiol 2013;42(2): 239–47.

10. Aranyi Z, Csillik A, Devay K, et al. Ultrasonographic identification of nerve pathology in neuralgic amyotrophy: enlargement, constriction, fascicular entwinement, and torsion. Muscle Nerve 2015;52(4): 503–11.

11. Gassner EM, Schocke M, Peer S, et al. Persistent median artery in the carpal tunnel: color Doppler ultrasonographic findings. J Ultrasound Med 2002; 21(04):455–61.

12. Peer S, Kovacs P, Harpf C, et al. High-resolution sonography of lower extremity peripheral nerves: anatomic correlation and spectrum of disease. J Ultrasound Med 2002;21(03):315–22.

13. Tagliafico A, Cadoni A, Fisci E, et al. Nerves of the hand beyond the carpal tunnel. Semin Musculoskelet Radiol 2012;16(02):129–36.

14. Koenig RW, Pedro MT, Heinen CP, et al. High-resolution ultrasonography in evaluating peripheral nerve entrapment and trauma. Neurosurg Focus 2009; 26(02):E13.

15. Martinoli C, Bianchi S, Pugliese F, et al. Sonography of entrapment neuropathies in the upper limb (wrist excluded). J Clin Ultrasound 2004;32(09):438–50.

16. Plaikner M, Loizides A, Loescher W, et al. Thickened hyperechoic outer epineurium, a sonographic sign suggesting snapping ulnar nerve syndrome? Ultraschall Med 2013;34(01):58–63.

17. Reynolds DL Jr, Jacobson JA, Inampudi P, et al. Sonographic characteristics of peripheral nerve sheath tumors. AJR Am J Roentgenol 2004;182(3): 741–4.

18. Kakkar C, Shetty CM, Koteshwara P, et al. Telltale signs of peripheral neurogenic tumors on magnetic resonance imaging. Indian J Radiol Imaging 2015; 25(4):453–8.

19. Chee DW, Peh WC, Shek TW. Pictorial essay: Imaging of peripheral nerve sheath tumors. Can Assoc Radiol J 2011;62:176–82.

20. Lin J, Jacobson JA, Hayes CW. Sonographic target sign in neurofibromas. J Ultrasound Med 1999;18: 513–7.

21. Murphey MD, Smith WS, Smith SE, et al. From the archives of the AFIP. Imaging of musculoskeletal neurogenic tumors: radiologic-pathologic correlation. Radiographics 1999;19(5):1253–80.

22. Wasa J, Nishida Y, Tsukushi S, et al. MRI features in the differentiation of malignant peripheral nerve sheath tumors and neurofibromas. AJR Am J Roentgenol 2010;194:1568–74.

Upper Limb Interventions

Luca Maria Sconfienza, MD, PhD[a,b,*], Vito Chianca, MD[a],
Carmelo Messina, MD[a,b], Domenico Albano, MD[c], Grazia Pozzi, MD[a],
Alberto Bazzocchi, MD, PhD[d]

KEYWORDS

• Shoulder • Elbow • Wrist • Hand • Ultrasound • Interventional radiology

KEY POINTS

- Ultrasound-guided procedures are effective to treat tendinopathies of the upper limb using different approaches.
- Intra-articular procedures can be performed under ultrasound guidance using either an in-plane or an out-of-plane approach.
- Rotator cuff calcific tendinopathy can be effectively treated using ultrasound-guided percutaneous irrigation.

INTRODUCTION

The upper limb is an anatomic region composed of several muscles, ligaments, tendons, and joints. Although muscular and ligamentous lesions are relatively uncommon, tendons, joints, and nerves may be affected by different pathologic conditions, which very frequently can be approached using interventional procedures,[1] with ultrasound being the preferred guidance method.[2,3] The need of imaging guidance seems justified by an increased accuracy of needle placement, which is particularly important when using those substances explicating their action only in the joint space, associated with reduced complications. However, published evidence for some of these treatments is still controversial.

This article reviews the most common ultrasound-guided procedures performed in the musculoskeletal system of the upper limb.

SHOULDER
Acromioclavicular Joint Injections

Osteoarthritis is the most common condition involving the acromioclavicular joint (ACJ) and is a frequent cause of chronic shoulder pain.[3] When performed without imaging guidance, success rates of injections are as low as 67%[4] because of a lack of space and variable morphology of the ACJ, whereas injections performed under ultrasound guidance have demonstrated excellent accuracy.[5] Intra-articular injection of steroids and/or local anesthetic is a well-accepted technique both for treatment and differential diagnosis.[5] Hyaluronic acid (HA) injection can also be associated, although literature evidence is absent.[6]

Technique

The probe is placed on a coronal plane over the ACJ to visualize the acromion, the clavicle, and the joint space. Then, with an out-of-plane approach, the needle is inserted into the joint. Joint space is very small, thus we advise not to inject more than 1 mL to avoid severe pain due to joint distension. In general, 1 mL of low-solubility steroid is enough to provide pain relief and can be followed by HA injection 2 weeks apart.

Disclosure Statement: The authors do not have any conflict of interest related to the present article.
[a] IRCCS Istituto Ortopedico Galeazzi, Via Riccardo Galeazzi 4, Milano 20161, Italy; [b] Dipartimento di Scienze Biomediche per la Salute, Università degli Studi di Milano, Via Pascal 36, Milano 20122, Italy; [c] Università degli Studi di Palermo, Dipartimento di Biomedicina, Neuroscienze e Diagnostica Avanzata, Via del Vespro, 129, 90127 Palermo, Italy; [d] Diagnostic and Interventional Radiology, IRCCS Istituto Ortopedico Rizzoli, Via G. C. Pupilli 1, Bologna 40136, Italy
* Corresponding author. IRCCS Istituto Ortopedico Galeazzi, Via Riccardo Galeazzi 4, Milano 20161, Italy.
E-mail address: io@lucasconfienza.it

Radiol Clin N Am 57 (2019) 1073–1082
https://doi.org/10.1016/j.rcl.2019.05.002
0033-8389/19/© 2019 Elsevier Inc. All rights reserved.

Gleno-Humeral Joint Injections

Gleno-humeral joint (GHJ) injections can be performed to treat different conditions such as adhesive capsulitis, osteoarthritis, and rotator cuff tear arthropathy,[6] and also to inject contrast agents for MR or computed tomography arthrography.[7]

Treatment of adhesive capsulitis, GHJ osteoarthritis, and rotator cuff arthropathy includes physical therapy and oral anti-inflammatory and analgesic medications. Intra-articular injections can be performed when other treatment is not enough to improve the clinical outcome.[8]

Technique

Intra-articular joint injections of the shoulder can be performed with an anterior or posterior approach. We prefer the posterior approach, as it more superficial, and the presence of the coracoid process anteriorly may impair needle tip visualization. The patient usually lies supine on the bed and the probe is placed on the posterior joint recess with an axial scan. Once the space between the humeral head and the glenoid bone is seen, a spinal needle is inserted oblique with lateral-to-medial direction. In patients with rotator cuff arthropathy, a higher volume of HA (up to 6 mL) may be used, which can be injected either posteriorly or directly under the acromion, placing the probe slightly lateral to the acromion on a coronal scan and inserting the needle oblique with an in-plane approach. This procedure can be repeated approximately 2 weeks apart. For GHJ osteoarthritis, we generally inject 1 mL low-solubility steroid + 1 mL lidocaine 2% followed by HA injection approximately 2 weeks apart. For adhesive capsulitis, we generally inject a mixture of 2 mL low-solubility steroid + 2 mL lidocaine 2% + 6 mL saline 0.9% NaCl to help capsule distension, repeated approximately 2 weeks apart and followed by physiokinesis therapy.

Subacromial-Subdeltoid Bursa Injections

The subacromial-subdeltoid (SASD) bursa is a very large synovial bursa covering most of the rotator cuff, having the function of reducing the friction of rotator cuff tendons during movement. Pathologic involvement of the SASD bursa is associated with most conditions affecting the rotator cuff or during inflammatory joint conditions. Direct injection of the SASD bursa may produce substantial pain relief. A recent meta-analysis reported significant difference in favor of ultrasound-guided injection versus blinded injection regarding pain score, shoulder function scores and shoulder abduction motion range at 6 weeks,[9] with pain relief decreased at 12 months regardless of injection methods.[10]

Technique

The arm should be placed in the best position to see the bursa with ultrasound. We preferably use the modified Crass position with the probe aligned along the supraspinatus tendon, although neutral arm and other probe positions also are acceptable. Then, the needle is inserted obliquely with an in-plane approach, up to placing the needle tip into the bursa. We usually inject 1 mL low-solubility steroid. In cases of chronic bursitis, the addition of a small amount of saline (up to 5 mL) may help stretching synovial adhesions. An example of this procedure is reported in **Fig. 1**.

Calcific Tendinopathy

Rotator cuff calcific tendinopathy is a frequent condition caused by calcium deposits in the rotator cuff and is particularly common in women between 40 and 50 years of age.[11] Asymptomatic calcifications do not require treatment; however, when they become painful, percutaneous irrigation of calcific tendinopathy (ultrasound-PICT) can be proposed as first-line treatment,[12] providing significant pain relief and a low rate of minor complications.[13] A meta-analysis[11] demonstrated an estimated 55% pain reduction at 11 months on average after ultrasound-PICT procedure. de Witte and colleagues[14] compared ultrasound-PICT combined with SASD steroid injection versus SASD injection alone. At 1 year, clinical results were significantly better in patients who underwent ultrasound-PICT. Bazzocchi and colleagues[15] reported 147 patients and stated that in 70% of shoulders, the treatment resulted in a quick and significant reduction of symptoms.

Technique

The patient is placed in supine position with the arm of the affected shoulder in the best position to achieve an optimal visualization of the calcification. Under ultrasound guidance, up to 10 mL of lidocaine into the SASD and around the calcification are injected. Different approaches have been reported in the literature using 1[16] or 2 needles[17] of variable size to inject and retrieve fluid and dissolve calcium deposits. Recently, the double-needle approach was reported as more appropriate when treating harder deposits, whereas 1 needle can be used for fluid calcifications.[18] Under ultrasound guidance, needles are inserted with an in-plane approach inside the calcification.[19] If the double-needle technique is used, the deeper needle must be inserted first, while the second is inserted superficially and on the same plane, with

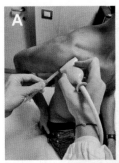

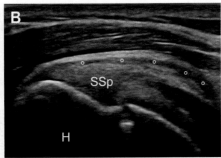

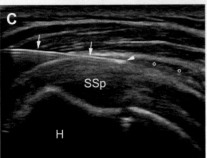

Fig. 1. Subacromial-subdeltoid bursa injection. (*A*) Simulation of patient, probe, and needle position. (*B*) Patient with degenerative tendinopathy of the supraspinatus tendon (SSp). Chronic bursitis (*circles*) is seen. H, humerus. (*C*) A 21-gauge needle (*arrows*) is positioned into the bursa (*arrowhead*, needle tip) and 1 mL of low-solubility steroid is injected.

the bevel in the opposite direction to the first needle to create a flushing circuit.[20,21] Then, a fluid is used to dissolve and aspirate the calcium. Some reported the use of lidocaine; however, we prefer to use warm saline, as we found it reduces procedure duration and improves calcium deposit fragmentation, particularly in cases of harder consistency.[22] At the end of the procedure, SASD bursa is injected with 1 mL low-solubility steroid.[23] After the procedure, we suggest patients not to raise the arm over the shoulder for approximately 1 week and to undergo a cycle of physiokinesis therapy.

Long Head of Biceps Tendinopathy

Degenerative long head of biceps (LHB) tendinopathy is quite a common condition and can be associated with tenosynovitis. Simple fluid distension of the sheath is also commonly encountered in patients without degenerative tendinopathy, as the sheath is in communication with the GHJ cavity and acts as a reservoir for intra-articular effusion. Treatment of these conditions is initially conservative, but intrasheath injections of steroids can be performed to provide faster pain relief.[24] Blinded injections have lower accuracy compared with injection with ultrasound guidance.[25] Blinded procedures also may result in intratendinous injection, which is not advisable when steroids are involved.[26] Studies report an accuracy rate between 87% and 93% of tendon sheath injections when performed with ultrasound guidance.[27]

Technique

The LHB tendon is visualized on an axial scan on the anterior aspect of the humerus. Then, a 21-gauge to 23-gauge needle is inserted with an in-plane approach. The sheath can be accessed with either a lateral or medial approach, taking care to the presence of a small recurrent branch of the anterior circumflex humeral artery that frequently runs on the medial side of the sheath itself. Once in the sheath, 1 mL low-solubility steroid is injected, avoiding intratendinous injection. The injection also can be performed at the level of rotator interval, especially if the sheath is not distended.[25] An example of this procedure is reported in **Fig. 2**.

ELBOW
Epicondylitis/Epitrochleitis

Epicondylitis and epitrochleitis are degenerative conditions caused by continuous overload over a prolonged period that causes repetitive microtears predominantly at the insertional hypovascular areas of extensor and flexor tendons of the elbow, respectively.[28]

Peritendinous and intratendinous steroid injections have been traditionally performed, either blinded or under ultrasound guidance. However, these procedures may lead to tendon damage and to subcutaneous fat atrophy. A systematic review showed that intratendinous corticosteroid injection performed better than placebo, local anesthetic, and conservative management in relation to pain relief and improved grip strength at

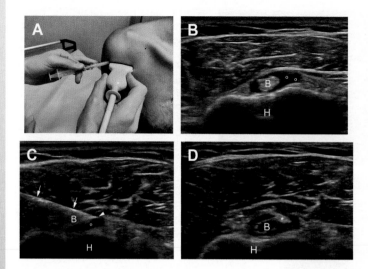

Fig. 2. LHB sheath injection. (*A*) Simulation of patient, probe, and needle position. (*B*) Patient with bicipital pain and fluid sheath distension (*circles*). B, biceps; H, humerus. (*C*) A 21-gauge needle (*arrows*) is positioned into the sheath (*arrowhead*, needle tip) and 1 mL of low-solubility steroid is injected. (*D*) After injection, the hyperechoic appearance of the injected steroid can be seen (*asterisk*).

6 weeks, with no significant differences at 6 months and more.[29] Other procedures include dry needling (series of repeated punctures performed in the degenerated portions of the tendon), platelet-rich plasma (PRP) injection, prolotherapy (injection of an irritant substance into the degenerative areas), and sclerotherapy (injection of sclerosing agents that cause thrombosis and vessel occlusion).[30] In a randomized trial comparing dry needling with or without PRP, no differences in pain scores were noted at 12 weeks. At 24 weeks, however, patients treated with PRP performed better compared with the control group.[31]

Technique

The procedure is performed similarly regardless of the injected substance. For lateral epicondylitis, the patient is seated opposite to the operator with the elbow 90° flexed. For medial epicondylitis, the patient lies prone on the bed with the elbow 90° flexed over his or her back. The common flexor or extensor tendons are visualized on a longitudinal scan. For prolotherapy or sclerotherapy, some local anesthetic can be injected around the tendon, while it should not be used for dry needling and PRP. A 21-gauge needle is inserted into the degenerated area of tendon with an in-plane approach. There, a series of 15 to 20 punctures is performed in case of dry needling, or the selected substance is injected. After the procedure, oral painkillers may be used to control post-procedural pain. Phisiokinesis therapy is also recommended.

Olecranon Bursitis

Olecranon bursitis is an inflammatory process characterized by increased fluid volume within

the bursal space associated with hypertrophic synovium, either aseptic or septic. Most patients respond to conservative treatment, which includes ice, rest, oral anti-inflammatory drugs, and antibiotics.[32] In nonresolving cases, ultrasound-guided drainage with a small amount of steroid injection can be performed.

Weinstein and colleagues[33] reported a group of 47 patients with noninfected, aspirated olecranon bursitis; only 25 patients with bursitis were then injected with steroid 7 days after aspiration. Pain reduction was significant for the steroid group compared with the control group. Smith and colleagues[34] reported a prospective trial of 42 patients with aseptic olecranon bursitis, reporting no clinical benefit when adding oral anti-inflammatory drugs to the treatment regimen, except for shorter symptom duration.

Technique

The patient lies prone on the bed with the arm along his or her body. The bursitis is visualized using axial or longitudinal scans. Then, a wide-bore needle (16–18 gauge) is inserted into the bursa and fluid is aspirated. After aspiration, the bursa can be injected with 1 mL low-solubility steroid, which is contraindicated in case of suspected or known septic origin. A compressive bandage is then applied.

Intra-Articular Injection

Intra-articular elbow injections can be performed for different conditions. Steroids can be injected for inflammatory conditions (such as rheumatoid arthritis, crystal-induced arthropathies, or osteoarthritis), HA (in case of osteoarthritis), or local anesthetic (to confirm the intra-articular origin of pain).[35] In patients with osteoarthritis, we usually inject 1 mL of low-solubility steroid followed by HA approximately 2 weeks apart.

Cunnington and colleagues[36] showed that accuracy of ultrasound guidance was 91% compared with 64% of landmark guidance. Kim and colleagues[37] reported higher accuracy rate of ultrasound-guided (100%) versus palpation guidance (77.5%).

Technique

The elbow can be injected with different accession routes. Often, patients needing elbow injections have very advanced joint degeneration, so the best access should be carefully searched. In general, direct anterior access is not recommended, as the distal biceps tendon, the brachial artery, and the median nerve run on that side. We prefer to use a lateral accession route. The patient is seated in front of the operator with the elbow 90° flexed placed on the examination table. The ultrasound probe is aligned longitudinally to visualize the humeral-radial joint space. Then, a 21-gauge needle is inserted vertically with an out-of-plane approach, transfixing the common extensor tendon if needed.

An example of this procedure is reported in **Fig. 3**.

WRIST AND HAND
Joint Injection

Joints around the wrist may be affected by degenerative (eg, trapezio-metacarpal osteoarthritis) or inflammatory conditions (eg, rheumatoid arthritis). When not responding to conservative treatments, intra-articular injections may be beneficial.[38] Of note, except for the radiocarpal, most of the joints around the wrist are quite small. Thus, the amount of injected substance should not exceed 0.5 to 0.7 mL to avoid pain induced by capsular distension. In case of monoarthritides, intra-articular injection of low-solubility steroid is indicated. In degenerative conditions, it can be followed by

intra-articular injection of HA approximately 2 weeks apart. Dubreuil and colleagues[39] published a meta-analysis including 10 eligible studies, concluding that steroid ultrasound-guided injection results in greater reduction of pain than palpation-guided injection at 1 to 6 weeks of follow-up.

Technique

All joints around the wrist should be injected with an out-of-plane approach, as joint space is very small and periarticular osteophytes may further reducing the available space. To inject the radiocarpal joint, the patient is seated in front of the operator and the hand placed on the bed with palm down. The probe should be aligned longitudinally on a para-median scan on the radial side of the wrist, over the free space between the extensor carpi radialis longus and the second extensor digitorum longus tendon. For the trapezio-metacarpal joint, the wrist is placed on the bed with the ulnar side facing down and the probe aligned longitudinally along the major axis of the first metacarpal bone. For the metacarpophalangeal and interphalangeal joints, the hand is placed on the bed with palm down and the probe is placed longitudinally on a para-median scan over the selected joint. In all cases, the needle is then inserted vertically out-of-plane. Due to the sensitivity and superficial location of this area, small and short needles (eg, 25–27 gauge, 1 cm length) can be used, except for HA, where larger bores are needed.[40]

De Quervain Disease and Other Tenosynovitis

De Quervain disease is a chronic stenosing tenosynovitis of the tendons of the first dorsal extensor compartment of the wrist. Conservative management includes activity modifications, rest, oral or topical anti-inflammatory drugs, and bracing.[38] When failing, ultrasound-guided injections can be proposed as an alternative to surgical

A   **B**

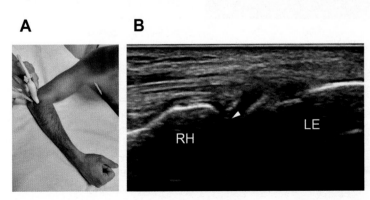

Fig. 3. Intra-articular elbow injection. (*A*) Simulation of patient, probe, and needle position. (*B*) With the probe centered on the humeral-radial joint (LE, lateral epicondyle; RH, radial head), the needle is inserted vertically with an out-of-plane approach, and the needle tip (*arrowhead*) is visible inside the joint.

debridement. Orlandi and colleagues[41] showed that intrasheath injection of low-solubility steroids followed by HA injections 2 weeks apart improve the outcome compared with steroid injection only. Other studies reported pain relief in 89% to 97% of patients at 6-week follow-up 15% to 30% recurrence rate.[42,43]

Technique

The patient should be seated in front of the examiner with the wrist placed on the examination table with ulnar side facing down. The first extensor compartment should be visualized by placing the probe on an axial scan on the lateral aspect of the radius. A small needle (23–25 gauge) is inserted laterally and superficially with an in-plane approach to reach the tendon sheath. Before injection, it is important to detect the presence of an accessory vertical septum in the retinaculum, so both subcompartments should be injected.[44] Caution should be taken to avoid the radial artery (running on the volar side) and the superficial branches of the radial nerve (running on both sides). Thus, the use of local anesthetic is not recommended, as a shock sensation reported by the patient is an indirect sign of nerve puncture. An example of this procedure is reported in **Fig. 4**.

Other tenosynovitis around the wrist may occur in association with inflammatory conditions, such as rheumatoid arthritis, and may clinically present as dorsal lumps[45] or carpal tunnel syndrome (CTS), because of the compression of the median nerve in the carpal tunnel given by sheath distension. In these cases, intrasheath injection of low-solubility steroids may help. Technical approach varies according to the anatomic location of tendons.

Carpal Tunnel Syndrome

CTS is the most common entrapment neuropathy in the upper limb, caused by compression of the median nerve at the level of the wrist within the fibro-osseous tunnel formed by the carpal bones and the flexor retinaculum.[46] When conservative treatment with rest, physical therapy, bracing, and oral anti-inflammatory drugs fails, ultrasound-guided injection may be proposed as an option before surgical release. Ultrasound-guided injection appears to improve clinical and neurophysiological outcomes.[47] A decrease of flattening ratio and cross-sectional area of the median nerve ultrasound parameters compared with blind injection technique is also reported.[48]

Technique

The patient is seated in front of the operator with the wrist placed on the examination table with the palm facing up. The median nerve is visualized on a short-axis scan under the flexor retinaculum. A 23-gauge needle is then inserted lateral to the probe with an in-plane approach. Either radial or ulnar approach is feasible, although particular

A   **B**

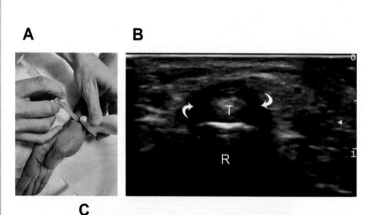

C

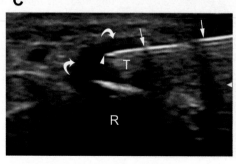

Fig. 4. Treatment of De Quervain disease. (*A*) Simulation of patient, probe, and needle position. (*B*) Tendons of the first extensor compartments (T) are thickened and entrapped by a very thick retinaculum (*curved arrows*). R, radius. (*C*) A 23-gauge needle (*arrows*) is inserted between the tendon and the retinaculum (*arrowhead*, needle tip) and the chosen substance is injected.

caution should be taken avoiding the radial artery and the ulnar neurovascular bundle, respectively. The needle tip should be placed under the retinaculum around the nerve. The purpose is to create a circumferential spread of the drug, visualizing a hypoechoic halo surrounding the nerve itself (so-called "doughnut" or "target" signs).[49] The best way to accomplish this is to inject half the drug on the superficial side of the nerve and the other half on the deep side. Usually, 1 mL of low-solubility steroid is used, occasionally diluted with lidocaine. It is important not to exceed with the amount of the injected fluid to avoid transient pressure increase in the carpal tunnel and temporary symptom worsening. An example of this procedure is reported in **Fig. 5**.

Ganglia

Ganglia are the most common benign soft tissue lesions of the wrist.[50] They are generally asymptomatic and tend to increase and decrease in size cyclically, thus treatment is not required unless for cosmetic or compressive concerns. Ganglia can be treated with surgery or with percutaneous drainage, with a recurrence rate between 20% and 50%.[51] Ganglion aspiration with or without injection of corticosteroid has variable success rates ranging from 27% to 89%.[52,53] Zeidenberg and colleagues[54] reported follow-up data of 39 patients treated with percutaneous drainage; a recurrence rate of 20% and a pain resolution rate of 87% were reported.

Technique
The patient is seated in front of the operator with the hand on the examination table, positioned according to the location of the ganglion. The scan plane is generally chosen to maximize the visibility of the ganglion and to avoid surrounding structures. A small amount of cutaneous anesthesia

can be injected with a small needle (23 gauge). Large-bore needles should be used, as ganglion content is generally very dense. We prefer 16-gauge needles, although 18 gauge is also acceptable. We also suggest injecting a small amount of anesthetic inside the ganglion, to help dilute the dense content, especially if smaller needles are used. Then, the needle is advanced into the ganglion and the content should be aspirated with a small syringe: the smaller the syringe, the higher the suction force exerted. Last, 0.5 mL of low-solubility steroid can be injected into the ganglion. Note that, if the same large needle is used, high local compression should be applied immediately when removing the needle itself to avoid steroid reflux. After procedure, a compression taping is applied for 5 to 10 days to minimize the probability of recurrence.

Trapezio-Metacarpal Joint Injection

Osteoarthritis is the most common condition involving the trapezio-metacarpal joint and is a frequent cause of chronic wrist pain. Intra-articular injections may provide temporary pain relief. One issue of this location is that joint space is particularly narrow and osteophytes may further reduce joint space. Thus, ultrasound guidance seems to be mandatory, especially when HA is used.

In cases of steroid injection, significant pain reduction was observed at short-term follow-up; however, this improvement was not maintained after a few months.[55] Swindells and colleagues[56] also noted a median pain score reduction from 68 to 16 at 1 month for almost all patients. Another study reported that high molecular weight HA injections may be effective in decreasing local inflammation and pain, although significant decrease in the synovial hypertrophy score was not observed.[57] Data reported a higher success

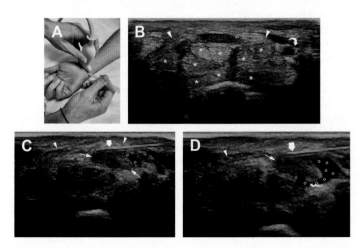

Fig. 5. Carpal tunnel injection (*A*) Simulation of patient, probe, and needle position. (*B*) Patient with electrophysiology-proven carpal tunnel disease with no clear ultrasound evidence of median nerve thickening (*dashed line*). Asterisks, flexor tendons; arrowheads, retinaculum; curved arrow, ulnar neurovascular bundle. (*C*) A 23-gauge needle (*thick arrow*) is inserted from the ulnar side and some low-solubility steroid is injected (*circles*) around the median nerve (*arrows*). (*D*) The steroid surrounds the half circumference of the nerve.

rate of correct site injections for ultrasound-guided procedures compared with the blinded injection procedure (75% vs 50%).[58]

Technique

The probe is placed on a longitudinal plane over the joint to visualize the trapezium, the metacarpal base, and the joint space. Then, with an out-of-plane approach, the needle is inserted vertically into the joint. Joint space is very small, thus we advise not to inject more than 0.5 mL to avoid severe pain due to joint distension. In general, 0.5 mL of low-solubility steroid is enough to provide pain relief and can be followed by HA injection 2 weeks apart.

Trigger Finger

Trigger finger is chronic stenosing tenosynovitis of the flexor tendons of the hand, caused by inflammation and subsequent narrowing of the flexor pulleys (A1 in particular), with consequent pain, snapping, and reduced range of motion of the affected finger.[59,60] Treatment of trigger finger includes activity modification, nonsteroidal anti-inflammatory drugs, joint immobilization,[61] open and percutaneous release,[62] and also ultrasound-guided procedures.[63] Bodor and Flossman[64] reported results at 1-year follow-up, stating ultrasound-guided injection had good results in 90% of cases, with disappearance of symptoms after a single injection, versus 44% for blind injection, as reported by Rozental and colleagues.[65]

Technique

The patient is seated with the hand over the examination bed, with palm facing up. The probe is aligned along the major axis of flexor tendons to visualize the affected pulley. Short-axis approach also can be possible, especially for the thumb, where accessibility of the A1 pulley might be more difficult. Ethyl chloride spray might be used to numb hand skin, which is very sensitive. A thin needle (ideally 25 gauge) is inserted laterally to the probe with an in-plane approach and the tip is inserted into the tendon sheath. There, a small amount of anesthesia can be injected to confirm needle placement. Then, 1 mL of low-solubility steroid can be injected. This procedure can be repeated, injecting up to 2 mL of HA 2 weeks apart with the same technique. Lapègue and colleagues[66] described the ultrasound-guided release of A1 pulley. With a technique similar to that reported previously, after local anesthesia, a 21-gauge needle purposely curved at 140° was inserted into the affected pulley. There, several punctures were performed to achieve pulley release.

SUMMARY

Ultrasound-guided interventional procedures of the upper limb can be performed to treat several pathologic conditions. Almost all procedures are effective, safe, and well tolerated with very low rate of minor complications. They should be strongly considered as first-line approach because their minimal invasiveness and excellent patient tolerability.

REFERENCES

1. Pourcho AM, Colio SW, Hall MM. Ultrasound-guided interventional procedures about the shoulder. Phys Med Rehabil Clin N Am 2016;27(3):555–72.
2. Sconfienza LM, Albano D, Allen G, et al. Clinical indications for musculoskeletal ultrasound updated in 2017 by European Society of Musculoskeletal Radiology (ESSR) consensus. Eur Radiol 2018. https://doi.org/10.1007/s00330-018-5474-3.
3. Javed S, Sadozai Z, Javed A, et al. Should all acromioclavicular joint injections be performed under image guidance? J Orthop Surg 2017;25(3). 230949901773163.
4. Partington PF, Broome GH. Diagnostic injection around the shoulder: hit and miss? A cadaveric study of injection accuracy. J Shoulder Elbow Surg 1998;7(2):147–50.
5. Edelson G, Saffuri H, Obid E, et al. Successful injection of the acromioclavicular joint with use of ultrasound: anatomy, technique, and follow-up. J Shoulder Elbow Surg 2014;23(10):e243–50.
6. Messina C, Banfi G, Orlandi D, et al. Ultrasound-guided interventional procedures around the shoulder. Br J Radiol 2015;89(1057):20150372.
7. Messina C, Banfi G, Aliprandi A, et al. Ultrasound guidance to perform intra-articular injection of gadolinium-based contrast material for magnetic resonance arthrography as an alternative to fluoroscopy: the time is now. Eur Radiol 2016;26(5): 1221–5.
8. Uppal HS, Evans JP, Smith C. Frozen shoulder: a systematic review of therapeutic options. World J Orthop 2015;6(2):263.
9. Wu T, Song HX, Dong Y, et al. Ultrasound-guided versus blind subacromial—subdeltoid bursa injection in adults with shoulder pain: a systematic review and meta-analysis. Semin Arthritis Rheum 2015; 45(3):374–8.
10. Fawcett R, Grainger A, Robinson P, et al. Ultrasound-guided subacromial–subdeltoid bursa corticosteroid injections: a study of short- and long-term outcomes. Clin Radiol 2018;73(8):760.e7-12.
11. Lanza E, Banfi G, Serafini G, et al. Ultrasound-guided percutaneous irrigation in rotator cuff calcific tendinopathy : what is the evidence ? A systematic

review with proposals for future reporting. Eur Radiol 2015;25(7):2176–83.

12. Messina C, Sconfienza LM. Ultrasound-guided percutaneous irrigation of calcific tendinopathy. Semin Musculoskelet Radiol 2016;20(5):409–13.

13. Cacchio A, Rompe JD, Serafini G, et al. US-guided percutaneous treatment of shoulder calcific tendonitis: some clarifications are needed. Radiology 2010; 254(3):990.

14. de Witte PB, Selten JW, Navas A, et al. Calcific tendinitis of the rotator cuff: a randomized controlled trial of ultrasound-guided needling and lavage versus subacromial corticosteroids. Am J Sports Med 2013;41(7):1665–73.

15. Bazzocchi A, Pelotti P, Serraino S, et al. Ultrasound imaging-guided percutaneous treatment of rotator cuff calcific tendinitis: success in short-term outcome. Br J Radiol 2016;89(1057):20150407.

16. Chianca V, Albano D, Messina C, et al. Rotator cuff calcific tendinopathy: from diagnosis to treatment. Acta Biomed 2018;89(1–S):186–96.

17. Farin PU, Jaroma H, Soimakallio S. Rotator cuff calcifications: treatment with US-guided technique. Radiology 1995;195(3):841–3.

18. Orlandi D, Mauri G, Lacelli F, et al. Rotator cuff calcific tendinopathy: randomized comparison of US-guided percutaneous treatments by using one or two needles. Radiology 2017;285(2):518–27.

19. Serafini G, Sconfienza LM. Treament of calcific tendinitis of the rotator cuff. Ultrasound-guided musculoskeletal procedures. Milano (Italy): Springer Milan; 2012. p. 29–35.

20. Sconfienza LM, Serafini G, Sardanelli F. Treatment of calcific tendinitis of the rotator cuff by ultrasound-guided single-needle lavage technique. Am J Roentgenol 2011;197(2):W366.

21. Fabbro E, Ferrero G, Orlandi D, et al. Rotator cuff ultrasound-guided procedures: technical and outcome improvements. Imaging Med 2012;4(6):649–56.

22. Sconfienza LM, Bandirali M, Serafini G, et al. Rotator cuff calcific tendinitis: does warm saline solution improve the short-term outcome of double-needle US-guided treatment? Radiology 2012;262(2):560–6.

23. Aparisi Gómez MP, Aparisi F, Bazzocchi A. Osseous involvement in calcific tendinitis: unusual in the usual. Arthritis Rheumatol 2018. https://doi.org/10.1002/art.40755.

24. Barker SL, Bell SN, Connell D, et al. Ultrasound-guided platelet-rich plasma injection for distal biceps tendinopathy. Shoulder Elbow 2015;7(2):110–4.

25. Stone TJ, Adler RS. Ultrasound-guided biceps peritendinous injections in the absence of a distended tendon sheath. J Ultrasound Med 2015;34(12):2287–92.

26. Unverferth LJ, Olix ML. The effect of local steroid injections on tendon. J Sports Med 1973;1(4):31–7.

27. Hashiuchi T, Sakurai G, Morimoto M, et al. Accuracy of the biceps tendon sheath injection: ultrasound-guided or unguided injection? A randomized controlled trial. J Shoulder Elbow Surg 2011;20(7):1069–73.

28. Potter HG, Hannafin JA, Morwessel RM, et al. Lateral epicondylitis: correlation of MR imaging, surgical, and histopathologic findings. Radiology 1995;196(1):43–6.

29. Smidt N, Assendelft WJJ, Van der Windt DAWM, et al. Corticosteroid injections for lateral epicondylitis: a systematic review. Pain 2002;96(1–2):23–40.

30. Sorani A, Campbell R. Image-guided elbow interventions: a literature review of interventional treatment options. Br J Radiol 2016;89(1057):20150368.

31. Mishra AK, Skrepnik NV, Edwards SG, et al. Efficacy of platelet-rich plasma for chronic tennis elbow. Am J Sports Med 2014;42(2):463–71.

32. Del Buono A, Franceschi F, Palumbo A, et al. Diagnosis and management of olecranon bursitis. Surgery 2012;10(5):297–300.

33. Weinstein PS, Canoso JJ, Wohlgethan JR. Long-term follow-up of corticosteroid injection for traumatic olecranon bursitis. Ann Rheum Dis 1984;43(1):44–6.

34. Smith DL, McAfee JH, Lucas LM, et al. Treatment of nonseptic olecranon bursitis. A controlled, blinded prospective trial. Arch Intern Med 1989;149(11):2527–30.

35. Sconfienza LM. Intra-articular injections. Ultrasound-guided musculoskeletal procedures. Milano (Italy): Springer Milan; 2012. p. 83–5.

36. Cunnington J, Marshall N, Hide G, et al. A randomised, controlled, double blinded study of ultrasound guided corticosteroid joint injection in patients with inflammatory arthritis. Arthritis Rheum 2010;62(7):1862–9.

37. Kim TK, Lee JH, Park KD, et al. Ultrasound versus palpation guidance for intra-articular injections in patients with degenerative osteoarthritis of the elbow. J Clin Ultrasound 2013;41(8):479–85.

38. Colio SW, Smith J, Pourcho AM. Ultrasound-guided interventional procedures of the wrist and hand. Phys Med Rehabil Clin N Am 2016;27(3):589–605.

39. Dubreuil M, Greger S, LaValley M, et al. Improvement in wrist pain with ultrasound-guided glucocorticoid injections: a meta-analysis of individual patient data. Semin Arthritis Rheum 2013;42(5):492–7.

40. Moran SL, Duymaz A, Karabekmez FE. The efficacy of hyaluronic acid in the treatment of osteoarthritis of the trapeziometacarpal joint. J Hand Surg Am 2009;34(5):942–4.

41. Orlandi D, Corazza A, Fabbro E, et al. Ultrasound-guided percutaneous injection to treat de

Quervain's disease using three different techniques: a randomized controlled trial. Eur Radiol 2015;25(5):1512–9.

42. McDermott JD, Ilyas AM, Nazarian LN, et al. Ultrasound-guided injections for de Quervain's tenosynovitis. Clin Orthop Relat Res 2012;470(7):1925–31.

43. Jeyapalan K, Choudhary S. Ultrasound-guided injection of triamcinolone and bupivacaine in the management of de Quervain's disease. Skeletal Radiol 2009;38(11):1099–103.

44. Leslie BM, Ericson WB, Morehead JR. Incidence of a septum within the first dorsal compartment of the wrist. J Hand Surg Am 1990;15(1):88–91.

45. Teh J, Vlychou M. Ultrasound-guided interventional procedures of the wrist and hand. Eur Radiol 2009; 19(4):1002–10.

46. Katz JN, Simmons BP. Carpal tunnel syndrome. N Engl J Med 2002;346(23):1807–12.

47. Omar G, Ali F, Ragaee A, et al. Ultrasound-guided injection of carpal tunnel syndrome: a comparative study to blind injection. Egypt Rheumatol 2018; 40(2):131–5.

48. McDonagh C, Alexander M, Kane D. The role of ultrasound in the diagnosis and management of carpal tunnel syndrome: a new paradigm. Rheumatology 2015;54(1):9–19.

49. Smith J, Wisniewski SJ, Finnoff JT, et al. Sonographically guided carpal tunnel injections: the ulnar approach. J Ultrasound Med 2008;27(10):1485–90.

50. Thornburg LE. Ganglions of the hand and wrist. J Am Acad Orthop Surg 1999;7(4):231–8.

51. Callegari L. Articular ganglia drainage. Ultrasound-guided musculoskeletal procedures. Milano (Italy): Springer Milan; 2012. p. 97–100.

52. Richman JA, Gelberman RH, Engber WD, et al. Ganglions of the wrist and digits: results of treatment by aspiration and cyst wall puncture. J Hand Surg Am 1987;12(6):1041–3.

53. Paul AS, Sochart DH. Improving the results of ganglion aspiration by the use of hyaluronidase. J Hand Surg Br 1997;22(2):219–21.

54. Zeidenberg J, Aronowitz JG, Landy DC, et al. Ultrasound-guided aspiration of wrist ganglions: a follow-up survey of patient satisfaction and outcomes. Acta Radiol 2016;57(4):481–6.

55. Joshi R. Intraarticular corticosteroid injection for first carpometacarpal osteoarthritis. J Rheumatol 2005; 32(7):1305–6.

56. Swindells M, Logan A, Armstrong D, et al. The benefit of radiologically-guided steroid injections for trapeziometacarpal osteoarthritis. Ann R Coll Surg Engl 2010;92(8):680–4.

57. Ingegnoli F, Soldi A, Meroni PL. Power Doppler sonography and clinical monitoring for hyaluronic acid treatment of rhizarthrosis: a pilot study. J Hand Microsurg 2011;3(2):51–4.

58. To P, McClary KN, Sinclair MK, et al. The accuracy of common hand injections with and without ultrasound: an anatomical study. Hand (N Y) 2017; 12(6):591–6.

59. Newport ML, Lane LB, Stuchin SA. Treatment of trigger finger by steroid injection. J Hand Surg Am 1990;15(5):748–50.

60. Makkouk AH, Oetgen ME, Swigart CR, et al. Trigger finger: etiology, evaluation, and treatment. Curr Rev Musculoskelet Med 2008;1(2):92–6.

61. Ryzewicz M, Wolf JM. Trigger digits: principles, management, and complications. J Hand Surg Am 2006;31(1):135–46.

62. Benson LS, Ptaszek AJ. Injection versus surgery in the treatment of trigger finger. J Hand Surg Am 1997;22(1):138–44.

63. Callegari L, Spanò E, Bini A, et al. Ultrasound-guided injection of a corticosteroid and hyaluronic acid. Drugs R D 2011;11(2):137–45.

64. Bodor M, Flossman T. Ultrasound-guided first annular pulley injection for trigger finger. J Ultrasound Med 2009;28(6):737–43.

65. Rozental TD, Zurakowski D, Blazar PE. Trigger finger: prognostic indicators of recurrence following corticosteroid injection. J Bone Joint Surg Am 2008; 90(8):1665–72.

66. Lapègue F, André A, Meyrignac O, et al. US-guided Percutaneous Release of the Trigger Finger by Using a 21-gauge Needle: A Prospective Study of 60 Cases. Radiology 2016;280(2):493–9.

Moving?

Make sure your subscription moves with you!

To notify us of your new address, find your **Clinics Account Number** (located on your mailing label above your name), and contact customer service at:

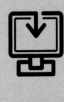

Email: journalscustomerservice-usa@elsevier.com

800-654-2452 (subscribers in the U.S. & Canada)
314-447-8871 (subscribers outside of the U.S. & Canada)

Fax number: 314-447-8029

Elsevier Health Sciences Division
Subscription Customer Service
3251 Riverport Lane
Maryland Heights, MO 63043

*To ensure uninterrupted delivery of your subscription, please notify us at least 4 weeks in advance of move.

ELSEVIER